taking **charge** of DIABETES

taking **charge** *of*

Australian
Diabetes
Council

DIABETES

A practical guide to managing your health and wellbeing

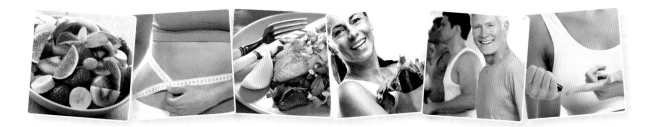

Reader's
Digest

About this book

Diabetes is a bit like an uninvited house guest: you didn't want it in the first place, and it won't go away. Worse still, it demands daily attention. But, while you can't send diabetes home, you can minimise the impact that it has on your health and quality of life.

Unlike most diseases, diabetes is patient-centred – meaning that you are the one in control. Your diabetes team will help you to formulate a game plan for keeping your blood glucose in line, but it's up to you to make sensible food choices, monitor your blood-glucose levels and figure out a physical activity program that you'll really stick with. That's the bad news (because yes, it will take a bit of effort on your part); it's also very good news because it means that you're in control. And *Taking Charge of Diabetes* will show you how to take the reins.

Australian Diabetes Council has been involved in the production of this book. It is a not-for-profit, non-government organisation offering information, support and advice for all people with diabetes. It is a leading diabetes consumer organisation in Australia, with the common purpose of helping those with the condition to live long and healthy lives.

Taking Charge of Diabetes has been designed to help you to learn as much as you can about diabetes and to serve as a useful, ongoing reference when you need specific information about your condition. It has not been designed to take the place of valuable advice you will receive from your diabetes team.

Each chapter is packed with information that will help you to manage your diabetes. If you're at risk for developing diabetes but aren't sure if you have it, you'll learn how to find out – a critical first step that millions of people throughout the world haven't taken. And if you do have diabetes, you'll discover a host of practical strategies for everything from meal planning to weight loss to finetuning your regimen for the best possible blood-glucose control.

The overall message is positive and one of hope. Health professionals have made huge strides in their ability to predict, diagnose and treat diabetes with a wide variety of therapeutic options. And now we know just how vital healthy eating and physical activity are in keeping the condition, and its potential complications, under control. By putting into action the lifestyle advice that will help you to manage your blood glucose, you'll feel better than you've ever felt before.

The Editors

Contents

CHAPTER 1
Take charge today 8

CHAPTER 2
Understanding diabetes 28

CHAPTER 3
Monitoring & measuring 56

CHAPTER 4
Eat to manage diabetes 82

CHAPTER 5
Exercise is medicine 108

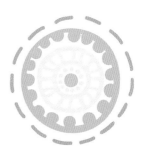

CHAPTER 6

Medications & surgery 142

CHAPTER 7

Preventing complications 166

CHAPTER 8

Complementary therapies 190

CHAPTER 9

Living well with diabetes 208

CHAPTER 10

Breakthroughs of the future 230

CHAPTER 11

Recipes 246

Resources directory 274

Index 276

CHAPTER 1
----

take *charge* today

Whether it be type 1 or type 2 diabetes, this is a serious disease, but it's well within the power of those who have it to control both high blood glucose and the complications it can cause. If you have type 1 diabetes, you have probably already been diagnosed, as symptoms are usually quite sudden. If you're at risk for type 2 diabetes or don't know if you have it, because it can be symptomless, then see your doctor and get the tests you need. Then take charge today! Taking steps such as eating right, losing weight and taking medication or insulin, if necessary, will make you feel better both physically and mentally – now and over the long haul.

Diabetes is a condition in which the amount of glucose in the blood is too high because the body is unable to use it properly. This is because the body's method of converting glucose into energy is not working as it should. There are two main types of diabetes: type 1 and type 2, which you will read about in the following pages.

You can look at diabetes in two ways. One is the big picture, which is not very pretty. Diabetes is the sixth-deadliest disease in Australia and New Zealand, and it's becoming increasingly more common. The other is the small-scale picture, the scale of one – you. Here, the news is much brighter. More than ever before, diabetes is a disease you can manage effectively. And the tools available to help you are getting better all the time.

On the large scale, you can't ignore the fact that if you have diabetes, you've got plenty of company. Across the country (and throughout the world), rates of diabetes have grown to epidemic proportions. Today, about 366 million people have diabetes worldwide and this number is increasing by more than 8 million each year. Just as alarming, rates among children, who in the past rarely developed the most prevalent form of diabetes (type 2), are climbing as well.

The silver lining in this cloud of gloom and doom is the fact that few serious diseases allow you to fight back as much as diabetes does. If you take the right steps to keep the condition under your control, you can live a full and active life. In fact, some people who are committed to managing their diabetes say that because of action they took, they now feel healthier overall than they have in years.

Your take-charge tool kit

If there's an upside to the diabetes epidemic, it's that chronic diseases that threaten growing numbers of people capture the interest of researchers (and the companies and federal health agencies that fund them). As a result, the past decade has seen significant advances in the way doctors understand, prevent and treat diabetes. New findings have improved three key components of diabetes treatment:

Blood-glucose management. Complications of diabetes, such as cardiovascular problems, poor vision, kidney disease and nerve damage, were once thought inevitable no matter how hard you tried to manage erratic swings in blood glucose. But that thinking has changed. Several major studies from around the world have shown that if you bring blood glucose into a normal range with medication(s), insulin, healthy eating, physical activity or some combination of these, you can significantly reduce your risk of complications. If you're diagnosed before you develop complications, you may sidestep diabetes-related health problems completely, sometimes with lifestyle changes alone. Meanwhile, technology to monitor blood glucose continues to improve and is now very convenient and relatively pain-free.

Lifestyle. Healthy eating and physical activity are powerful tools for helping to lower blood glucose. Recent research into how foods affect

> **? DID you KNOW...**
>
> Diabetes is often hiding in plain sight. Many people who have it but don't know it are already being treated for heart-disease risk factors, such as high blood pressure or high cholesterol – yet they haven't been given a simple blood-glucose test. By educating people about the risk factors, those at risk are more likely to ask for a test, to avoid the serious health problems untreated diabetes can bring.

blood glucose has shown that your eating plan need not be as restrictive as experts once believed. In fact, healthy eating guidelines are essentially the same for everyone, whether or not they have diabetes. And your work-outs don't have to be as vigorous as once thought. Even short bouts of activity throughout the day add up to significant benefits to your health.

Medication. Earlier generations of diabetes medications for type 2 diabetes have been bolstered by a growing roster of newer medications that tackle the disease in a variety of different ways. In many cases, you can combine these medications to take advantage of their different modes of operation. The fact that there are also many varieties of insulin (which regulates the body's use of blood glucose) offers more flexibility in finding a regimen that matches the lifestyle of people with type 1 diabetes as well as those with type 2 diabetes who require insulin.

Dealing with the diagnosis

Hearing that you have a chronic disease is never easy. One day it seems you have a clean bill of health (although you may have felt that something was wrong), and the next you have a condition for the rest of your life. But don't despair. Now that you've been diagnosed and are being treated, you are well on the way to a healthier, happier life.

Still, it can be tough to be optimistic initially. You might feel as if your body has betrayed you or that it's out of control. Some people assume that the worst they've heard about diabetes (accurate or not) lies just around the corner, and they jump to panicky conclusions like 'I'll go blind!' or 'I can never eat dessert again!' Others are nonchalant, figuring that they've managed to get by up to now with diabetes, so 'worrying about it won't get me anywhere'.

You're possibly somewhere in the middle of the spectrum between panic and denial. You may even be relieved to finally know why you've been feeling so bad. All of these emotions are completely normal. In fact, you can anticipate moving through several emotional stages after being diagnosed. Typically, an I-can't-believe-it phase gives way to feelings of anger and the realisation that there's a long road ahead, which can sometimes lead to depression. To deal with the dismay a diagnosis can produce, consider these points:

✅ **View your emotions as progress.** The next time you snap at a family member or find yourself in a fog and staring out the window, play the moment out as a mental movie – an emotional scene in an unfolding story that continues to move progressively towards something better. When you accept your feelings as a natural, important part of an ongoing process, it's an indication you're actually working through them and going ahead with the rest of your life.

✅ **Talk to someone.** Sharing emotions with a loved one, joining a support group or attending a session about diabetes in which you can meet others with the disease can help put your feelings in perspective and make you feel less alone.

✅ **Think short term.** You may feel overwhelmed by all the changes you have to make in your life, the new self-care skills you have to learn and the sheer volume of medical information you need to absorb. Rest assured that eventually it will all seem second nature. For now, focus on immediate goals ('Today I'll meet my dietitian') that will move you further down the road.

✅ **Forge ahead.** The key is not to let your diabetes diagnosis paralyse you. The sooner you take action, the sooner you'll feel that you have got your life back under control – and the sooner you'll start to feel better.

What you can expect

When you're diagnosed with either type 1 or type 2 diabetes, your doctor will need to cover a lot of ground in a short time. They will want to know virtually everything about you: eating patterns, weight history, blood pressure, medications you're taking, whether you smoke or drink, any family history of heart disease and any treatment you've received for other problems. If you're a mother, you may also be asked about the development of your children. Rest assured that your doctor isn't prying. All of this information has a bearing on your condition and the management program that you'll follow.

Do you have type 1 diabetes?

When you are first diagnosed with type 1 diabetes, you will be given a lot of new information as you learn to live with the condition. Once the initial adjustment is over, it is normal to feel overwhelmed, isolated or uncertain, however, these are feelings that will usually pass. Ask your doctor or diabetes specialist for a referral to a psychologist or counsellor to discuss any concerns you have and to help you through this period until you feel you are coping better.

There are four key things you need to learn about effectively managing your diabetes and your diabetes team will help you to do this:

1 **Insulin.** As you have type 1 diabetes, your body doesn't make any insulin. You will therefore need daily insulin injections and will be shown how to inject or how to use an insulin infusion pump.

2 **Testing.** Regularly monitoring your blood-glucose levels is the only way to know exactly what they are doing at any given time of day or night. A wide range of blood-glucose meters with varying features is available and your diabetes educator will help you to choose the one that is most suited to you and your lifestyle.

3 **Finding the balance.** To manage your blood-glucose levels, you need to aim for a balance between the amount of food you eat, the exercise you do and the insulin you take. You will need to consider the timing, amount and type of carbohydrate foods you eat, as well as the timing, amount and type of insulin you take. This may sound daunting at first but your diabetes team will provide you with support and

> **! CAUTION**
>
> People with type 1 diabetes are more likely to develop other autoimmune conditions, including thyroid and coeliac disease. Make sure your doctor checks your thyroid function and orders screening tests for coeliac disease.

Can a vaccine prevent type 1 diabetes?

The Intranasal Insulin Trial (INIT II) began in Australia in 2006 with the aim of developing a vaccine for type 1 diabetes. The study is testing whether intranasal insulin administration to children and young adults with a family history and positive antibodies for the disease will delay or even prevent the onset of type 1 diabetes. Based on previous research that suggested that intranasal insulin can induce protective immunity, thus acting as a vaccine against type 1 diabetes, the INIT II trial is designed to test the effectiveness of this potential vaccine and to assist in finding a suitable dose range in a larger population. The trial is taking place at several centres across Australia and New Zealand with first-degree and second-degree relatives of people with type 1 diabetes.

your accredited practising dietitian will help to develop an eating plan that suits you and your lifestyle.

4 **Recognising highs and lows.**
Understanding the signs when your blood-glucose levels get out of balance (such as low or high blood-glucose levels) and knowing what to do should this occur are essential to your ongoing health and wellbeing.

Who will help. Diabetes is best managed by a team in which you and your family are the key players. Other team members are your doctor, a diabetes educator, a dietitian, a diabetes specialist, a podiatrist and an eye specialist or optometrist. Your team may also include a social worker, psychologist and other healthcare professionals such as an exercise physiologist or physiotherapist. When you're first diagnosed with type 1 diabetes, you will be referred to these members of your team who will support you in managing your diabetes effectively.

Regular tests and why they're important. Following your diagnosis, your doctor will arrange a series of tests, which should be conducted on a regular basis. While having diabetes puts you at risk of developing certain complications over time, well-managed blood-glucose levels greatly reduce that risk. Other preventative measures include managing your blood pressure, blood cholesterol and not smoking. The good news is that regular checks can detect early signs of complications long before they actually affect your health, and, if found, a great deal can be done through prompt and appropriate treatment to delay and even prevent damage occurring.

Regular tests your doctor will arrange for you should include:

- an HbA1c blood test that measures your average blood-glucose control over the past 3 months
- an eye check by an ophthalmologist or optometrist who looks into your eyes to see

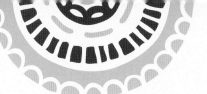

WHEN DIABETES STRIKES YOUR CHILD

Treating diabetes in a child can be more challenging than dealing with the disease yourself. Depending on their age and temperament, children vary in their ability – or desire – to understand what's happening to them, take care of themselves and follow your instructions. But you can put your child on the road to responsible self-care with either type 1 (the most common type in children) or type 2 diabetes if you bear these principles in mind:

Toddlers and pre-schoolers

Learn to recognise how hypoglycaemia (too little glucose in the bloodstream) and hyperglycaemia (too much glucose in the bloodstream) affect your child's behaviour, since they simply don't have the words to tell you how they feel themselves. Expect some battles over insulin injections and blood-glucose tests around toilet-training time, as your child starts to assert themselves more, but stick to your guns to get them done. Don't worry too much if blood glucose ranges between 8 mmol/L and 11 mmol/L (higher than what's recommended for adults). Children need a balanced food plan for normal development. Forget trying to control when your child eats. Instead, accept irregular eating patterns and discuss with your doctor using shorter-acting insulin or bolus from a pump when your child does have a bite.

Primary school kids

As your child develops physically and mentally, they'll be better able to understand why their treatment is necessary and become more willing to cooperate with its demands. Educate them about how caring for their condition now will protect their health in the future, but don't scare them with the details of complications. Tighter glucose control now becomes more important, especially at night, when the risk of hypoglycaemia is at its highest. Also make sure they have a bedtime snack and don't skip meals. Encourage them to participate in school and social activities to build friendships, promote self-esteem and make them feel less different from other kids. At about eight years old your child can probably start taking on some of the responsibility for injections and blood tests themselves – maybe even with the help of teachers or classmates, who may benefit from the opportunity to learn about diabetes.

Pre-teens and adolescents

Control – over a number of things – now starts falling into your child's hands. Studies find that tight blood-glucose control as early as 13 years of age can prevent complications in adulthood, so encourage them to take charge – but don't expect the thought of future consequences to motivate them too much. Now's not the time to completely let go of the reins: worries about what other kids think might cause them to skip steps in their care. Make an issue of it, expect an argument – but be confident that using you as an excuse ('My parents make me do it') can help them do the right thing. Gradually give your child more responsibility as they are able to handle it. By the time they're choosing which university to attend, responsibility should pass to them.

if any eye disease (diabetic retinopathy) is present

- a kidney test called a microalbuminuria test to check that your kidneys are working as they should
- cholesterol/triglyceride blood test to check for high levels – more common in people with diabetes, as well as
- regular checks by health professionals of your feet, blood pressure, weight and regular visits to the dentist.

Do you have type 2 diabetes?

If you don't know the answer to this question but feel you have cause to wonder, that's reason enough to see a doctor. In its early stages, when it's easiest to manage, diabetes can be sneaky and silent, slowly causing damage throughout your body without obvious symptoms. But if you're alert to subtle signs, it can be treated at the outset to avoid the development of further complications.

It's human nature not to look for problems if they haven't already found you – which explains why up to 50 per cent of people with type 2 diabetes don't even know they have it. According to statistics, half of all people who finally go to their doctor to be tested for type 2 diabetes have already developed some degree of complications.

How can you recognise when diabetes is at your door? There are three fundamental ways.

Figure your risk factors. The first thing to look at is whether any element of your background makes you more likely than the general population to develop diabetes. Among the most important factors to evaluate are:

Family history. If anyone in your immediate family – a parent, sibling or grandparent – has had type 2 diabetes, you have a higher chance of developing the disease yourself. The extent of the risk depends on the type of diabetes and how closely related you are to the person who has it (the risk is highest among identical twins).

Cultural group. The most common type of diabetes (called type 2) is most prevalent in people from the Pacific Islands, the Indian sub-continent, the Middle East or those of Chinese cultural background. Aborigines and Maori have four times more chance of developing type 2 diabetes than Caucasians.

Weight. Being overweight significantly raises your risk of developing type 2 diabetes. That makes it one of the most important risk factors because it's one you can manage.

Age. Type 1 usually occurs in children or teens but is sometimes diagnosed after the age of forty. Type 2 generally develops after the age of 40, although it's becoming increasingly common in younger people, even children.

Keep a sharp eye for symptoms. While the signs of diabetes can be subtle at first, they're not impossible to pick up on. The longer untreated diabetes progresses, the more likely is the development of complications. Common symptoms of diabetes are:

- excessive thirst and increased appetite
- frequent urination
- fatigue
- blurred vision
- weight loss
- frequent infections
- tingling in your hands and feet
- sexual dysfunction.

✅ **Get tested.** Although urine and finger-prick tests can reveal a higher than normal blood-glucose level, you need one or more of three laboratory blood tests to diagnose diabetes. These tests will be organised by your doctor.

Blood screenings at health fairs or shopping centres can provide inaccurate results and are best avoided. Your doctor will advise you about which tests you need and whether you'll need to be tested again and when.

Following your diagnosis, a full assessment for potential complications will need to be done as these may already be present.

Your doctor will also want to do a thorough physical examination, including a cardiac work-up and a careful look at your mouth, feet, eyes, abdomen, skin and thyroid gland. You'll have a range of tests, including a blood-lipid test for cholesterol (among other things), a blood pressure check and at least two different blood glucose–related tests – one test that shows what your blood glucose is right now and the

other, what it has averaged for the past 2 to 3 months (an HbA1c test).

Who will help. It may seem like a lot to begin with, but this initial assessment is the most important phase of your overall care. Other parts of this phase will include introducing you to the other members of your diabetes healthcare team. Eventually, you'll get to the point where you're in charge from one day to the next and your team is a valuable and reliable resource for follow-up assessments, support and advice.

Will you need insulin?

If you have type 2 diabetes, your requirement for insulin will depend on a number of factors, including:

- **How much insulin your body makes on its own.** In type 2 diabetes, your body's insulin-making ability is partially impaired, and the extent of the impairment is different from one person to the next.

- **How well your body uses the insulin it has.** If your cells have trouble using the insulin that's naturally available to them, you may need supplemental doses.

- **Your blood-glucose levels.** How high above normal your blood-glucose levels tend to be will help guide your doctor in deciding whether insulin is necessary.

- **How effective other forms of treatment have been.** As a rule with type 2 diabetes,

Two-hour oral glucose tolerance test results

The figures below show results for the 2-hour oral glucose tolerance test, and likely treatment.

< 7.8 mmol/L[1]
Pre-diabetes: impaired fasting glucose

Likely treatment: healthy eating, physical activity; weight loss[2]

> 7.8 mmol/L but < 11.0 mmol/L
Pre-diabetes: impaired glucose tolerance

Likely treatment: healthy eating, physical activity; weight loss[2]

11.1 mmol/L or above
Type 2 diabetes

Likely treatment: healthy eating, physical activity; possibly tablets and/or insulin; weight loss[2]

[1] after having a glucose drink   [2] if overweight

insulin will be introduced when lifestyle measures and oral medications fail to bring your blood glucose under control.

Where do you stand?

Any glucose test that is higher than normal but not high enough to diagnose diabetes needs further checking. Depending on your initial result, your doctor may order an oral glucose tolerance test (OGTT) to find out more. In New Zealand and parts of Australia, HbA1c is also used to diagnose type 2 diabetes. Currently, an OGTT is only performed if fasting blood glucose is 5.6 mmol/L to 6.9 mmol/L inclusive. As a general guideline this test will give the following results:

- If your fasting blood glucose is less than 7 mmol/L and your 2-hour blood glucose is between 7.8 mmol/L and 11 mmol/L, you have pre-diabetes, which is also known as impaired glucose tolerance (IGT) – a condition in which elevated blood-glucose levels significantly raise your risk of developing diabetes. You'll be advised to start eating a healthier diet and to undertake regular physical activity. Weight loss may be required and sometimes tablets are also prescribed.

- If your fasting blood glucose is 7 mmol/L or more and your 2-hour blood glucose is 11.1 mmol/L or more, type 2 diabetes is diagnosed. The initial treatment for this involves healthy eating and physical activity, perhaps taking medication in the form of tablets and possibly even insulin, depending on how high your blood-glucose level is. In addition to these measures, you will be guided by the advice of your doctor based on the regular blood-glucose testing you will do at home following your diagnosis (see pages 64–72).

- Another pre-diabetes condition is impaired fasting glucose (IFG), where your fasting blood glucose is between 6.1 mmol/L and 6.9 mmol/L and your 2-hour blood glucose is less than 7.8 mmol/L.

What's the plan?

Once you have diabetes, you've got it for life, until a cure is found. However, the good news is that by controlling and lowering your high blood-glucose levels you can significantly reduce your risk of developing the serious health problems that often go along with having diabetes.

Bringing diabetes under control is an important task and there's no one better qualified to do it than you. Taking charge of diabetes doesn't have to be a full-time job, but you have to be mindful of it throughout your entire day, whether you're eating, working or going to bed. You'll have a team of people to help you, including your doctor, diabetes educator, dietitian, exercise specialist, podiatrist and eye specialist. However, they are not the key players in this scenario – you are. And your success ultimately depends on managing a treatment plan that puts you in charge. These are the key steps you need to take to get your diabetes under control.

Start damage control immediately

Think about what happens when you spill honey: it gets on your fingers, sticks to everything you touch and generally makes a complete disaster area of the kitchen bench. Now try imagining a honey spill taking place inside your bloodstream – which is essentially what high blood glucose is. What happens? Cells, proteins and fats get stickier, slowing down your blood circulation, holding back

tissue repair and encouraging material to stick to your artery walls and cause clots. In short, excess blood glucose gums up your entire body.

You don't leave honey on your benchtop. Likewise, blood glucose needs to be cleaned up as quickly and thoroughly as possible because the 'stickiness' only gets worse. Doing so can make you feel better right away. And even if you have no symptoms of diabetes, taking this action will start to reduce your risk of such problems as these:

- damage to delicate blood vessels at the back of the eye (the retina), which can lead to vision problems
- damaged capillaries in the kidneys that filter waste from your body via the bloodstream
- impaired nerve function due to less nourishment from damaged blood vessels
- damage to artery walls that makes high blood pressure, heart attack and stroke more likely.

These complications wreak all kinds of havoc, including impaired healing, infections, lack of sensation that can lead to injury (especially in the feet), loss of vision, swollen ankles, fatigue, sexual dysfunction – the list can be long. Fortunately, the following steps will help you clean up the excess blood glucose and halt potential complications.

Know the problems and the solutions

That's the rule in business, sports and politics, and it's just as important when you're maintaining quality of life. The power to tame

Take-charge tips

While there may seem to be a lot of details to deal with in the first days of a diagnosis, the steps you need to take boil down to a handful of key objectives:

○ Learn how to test your own blood glucose using finger prickers, test strips and a blood-glucose meter.

○ Use the results to determine your average blood-glucose levels and how they tend to fluctuate throughout the day.

○ Learn more from your doctor, dietitian or diabetes educator about how to help stabilise your blood glucose with healthy eating and physical activity, and don't be shy about asking questions related to these measures.

○ Research everything you can about diabetes – a step you're already taking.

○ Schedule an eye examination following your diagnosis. While high blood glucose can temporarily cause blurry vision, an examination will screen for damage that may have already occurred in those who may have had undiagnosed type 2 diabetes for some time.

diabetes is within your grasp, but to use it you need some know-how. That means grappling with information about your particular type of diabetes, medications, insulin varieties, blood-glucose tests, meal planning and physical activity, to name a few. But the details are not insurmountable, and you've got plenty of people to give you a hand – including your diabetes team whose role is to impart knowledge and clear up your confusion.

Keep tabs on blood glucose

Diabetes can be a silent disease because you can't feel your blood glucose unless it becomes too high or low – two situations that are best avoided. How can you tell what's going on with the blood inside your body? Only one way: get a bit of blood outside of your body and analyse it. This isn't something you need to run to your doctor for (though certain tests need to be performed in a surgery). Handy, easy-to-use and relatively painless lancets, test strips and blood-glucose meters let you check your own blood glucose anywhere, any time. Some people take blood-glucose readings four or more times a day, depending on the type of diabetes treatment they are receiving.

The blood-glucose readings that you yourself – not your doctor – gather every day are a fulcrum by which you gain leverage over your disease. They provide data that will constitute a critical component of your care by allowing you to see how your blood glucose varies throughout the day and how much it swings in response to food, physical activity, stress or anything else that may affect it. They will help guide the way you manage your diabetes and when you administer insulin (if you need it).

Lose body baggage

Nothing signals more clearly that you're at risk for type 2 diabetes than being overweight (which accounts for 8–9 out of 10 cases of the disease). Excess baggage – especially around the middle – makes you more likely to develop insulin resistance, a condition in which cells don't use glucose (a form of sugar) as well as they should. The result is that glucose accumulates in the blood. Wearing a spare tyre also increases the body's demand for insulin, which the pancreas (the maker of insulin) may have trouble meeting – again resulting in high blood glucose. Of course, there are other dangers in being overweight – high blood pressure, high cholesterol and heart disease among them. Studies show that 60 to 80 per cent of people with type 2 diabetes will develop and die of cardiovascular disease including heart attack and stroke.

Losing weight may be the single most important thing you can do to manage type 2 diabetes. And there's no need for anything extreme; a slow and steady drop in weight keeps the kilograms off more efficiently than all of those crash diets you're unlikely to stick to. And rest assured that you don't have to slim down to supermodel size. Even losing small amounts of weight can make a significant difference to your health and wellbeing. Your dietitian is there to help and guide you with this.

Deconstruct your diet

In terms of what you eat as part of your eating plan, it may surprise you to learn that the principles of healthy eating for people with diabetes are essentially the same as for everyone. A dietitian can show you how to include ample amounts of appetising edibles in your eating plan (including some of your favourites, within limits of course), yet still keep kilojoules down so you lose weight. If you have type 1 diabetes, you'll need to carefully balance your daily carbohydrate intake with your insulin to keep your blood glucose from soaring too high or dropping too low. Whatever type of diabetes you have, there are nine food strategies that you can put into action straight away:

1 Keep physically active and eat according to your energy needs.

2 Eat high-fibre foods, such as wholegrain bread and cereal and plenty of fruit and colourful vegetables (at least five portions a day).

3 Choose low-glycaemic index wholegrain foods whenever possible.

4 Cut down on fat, especially saturated fats found in high-fat snacks and fried fast foods. Replace saturated fats with the healthier fats found in nuts, fish, avocado and olive oil.

5 Eat lean red meat in moderation. Include grilled fish, skinless chicken, legumes and soy products in your eating plan.

6 Limit added sugar and foods and drinks high in added sugar.

7 Reduce your salt intake: avoid processed foods that are high in salt and don't add salt to cooked foods.

8 Keep your alcohol consumption to the recommended limits (see also pages 100–2).

9 Eat some – but not too much – starchy foods (carbohydrate) at every meal.

Get physical

Physical activity gobbles up glucose, and this usually lowers your blood glucose. If you exercise regularly, it also enables your cells to better use glucose, even when you're not active. That can make you require less insulin or medication. Physical activity also helps you lose weight, lower your cholesterol and blood pressure, and makes your heart and lungs more powerful, all of which contribute to cutting your risk of complications from diabetes.

Hate to exercise? Don't worry. Your activity plan doesn't have to be any more involved than making sure you pump up your heart rate and breathe a little harder most, if not all, days of the week, preferably for 30 minutes at a time (or 1 hour if you want to lose weight). Classic aerobic activities such as walking, running and cycling are ideal, but ordinary jobs, such as washing your car, mowing the lawn and cleaning your house, all help.

Beat back related risks

Eating healthily, getting regular physical activity and losing weight (if you need to) are among the most important things you can do to prevent complications from diabetes – but they're not the only steps you can take.

✅ **Quit smoking.** Besides making a mess of your lungs and increasing your risk of cancer, smoking narrows arteries, which raises your risk of heart attack and stroke and cuts circulation to your legs, making it harder for wounds to heal (especially on the feet). It also raises blood pressure and increases the risk of kidney and nerve damage.

✅ **Take the pressure off.** High blood pressure contributes to cardiovascular disease, stroke, eye disease, kidney disease and nerve damage. Eating plenty of fruit, whole grains and coloured vegetables will help bring your blood pressure down, as will eating less salt and limiting processed and takeaway foods. Choose lean meat, chicken, fish and low-fat dairy foods, and limit alcohol to recommended limits (see pages 100–2). If you are overweight, losing weight will help to drop your blood pressure.

✅ **Lower your lipids.** Keeping your cholesterol and triglycerides under control will significantly reduce your risk of cardiovascular disease.

Get on a schedule

Once you become accustomed to changes in your healthy eating and physical activity habits and learn to handle medications, day-to-day life will start to seem routine again. But check in with your doctor regularly to make sure that everything is going according to plan. Your doctor will organise a range of tests including an eye examination, a cholesterol test and blood and urine tests to check kidney, liver and thyroid function. A blood test called an HbA1c will also be done to measure your average blood-glucose level over the previous 10 to 12 weeks.

Where to get support

You're in charge of managing your game plan from day to day (and hour to hour) because you're the one who's always there – but you're certainly not alone. In fact, one of your most important jobs as the manager – and boss – of your care is to line up a team of professionals to help you.

Your first stop is your doctor, who probably diagnosed your diabetes. Your family doctor is a general practitioner (GP), not a diabetes specialist, but just because you have a specific disease doesn't mean you must bid your regular doctor goodbye. Your doctor may wish to refer you to a diabetes specialist for expert advice if you have type 2. However, you should be referred to a diabetes specialist if you have type 1. Your GP will arrange essential check-ups on a regular basis and readily refer you to a range of specialists if you should need them. These tests and check-ups may include:

- the initial diagnosis of your diabetes
- initial and ongoing treatment
- coordination of care and referral to other members of your diabetes team, including your diabetes educator, dietitian, podiatrist, eye specialist, exercise specialist and possibly a diabetes specialist
- annual medical check-ups
- regular review of your medication and/or insulin routines.

You can also expect to draw on the talents and experience of the other specialised members of your diabetes team.

Your diabetes specialist

A diabetes specialist is a doctor who concentrates specifically on the management of diabetes, and is often called an endocrinologist. (An

endocrinologist specialises in the study of hormones.) An endocrinologist will know more than most general practitioners about how to match your diabetes treatment to your fluctuating blood-glucose levels, eating and physical activity patterns, and this specialist doctor will be up on the latest diabetes medications and research.

While some general practitioners have expertise and skills in special interest areas such as diabetes, other GPs have more limited skills in that area. Larger practices will often cross-refer people with diabetes to other general practitioners within the practice who have an interest and special skills in diabetes. This means that there is some flexibility as to which professional to see for specific concerns.

Arrangements can be different in country areas where there may be a lack of specialist care. In these circumstances, GPs often develop extra skills to fill gaps where specialists are not available.

Because of the importance of self-management of diabetes, good communication between people with the condition and their health professionals is critical. The more candid the communication, the better the care will be, so talk openly with your general practitioner about whether you need an endocrinologist. If you have type 1 diabetes, it is best to have an endocrinologist involved in your diabetes care.

Your diabetes educator

The time you get with your family doctor is rarely enough to learn all the ins and outs of dealing with diabetes. That's where a diabetes educator, usually a nurse or dietitian with a

Where to get more information

State & Territory Diabetes Organisations in Australia

Not-for-profit, non-government consumer organisations offering information, support and advice for all people with diabetes:

ACT: www.diabetes-act.com.au

NSW: www.australiandiabetescouncil.com

NT: www.healthylivingnt.org.au

QLD: www.diabetesqld.org.au

SA: www.diabetessa.com.au

TAS: www.diabetestas.com.au

VIC: www.diabetesvic.org.au

WA: www.diabeteswa.com.au
   or phone 1300 136 588

National Diabetes Services Scheme (NDSS)

Ask about registering with NDSS for subsidised products.
www.ndss.com.au

Juvenile Diabetes Research Foundation

A not-for-profit organisation dedicated to funding the search for a cure for type 1 diabetes.
www.jdrf.org.au

Diabetes New Zealand

A not-for-profit, non-government consumer organisation offering information, support and advice for all people with diabetes.
www.diabetes.org.nz

Diabetes Youth New Zealand

A voluntary incorporated society dedicated to providing support for children and young people with diabetes and their families.
www.diabetesyouth.org.nz

(For a full listing of organisations, including the Aboriginal Medical Service, look in the Resources Directory at the back of this book.)

special interest in diabetes care, comes in. You will learn how to prepare and administer insulin and perform blood and urine tests, how to balance your eating and physical activity with your blood-glucose readings and hear more about how diabetes affects your body.

A diabetes educator is usually a walking diabetes library who may run classes on diabetes, at which you can get more background information and meet other people with diabetes. As such, your diabetes educator/specialist should be a registered health professional who specialises or is training in the area of

diabetes education and care. In Australia, a Credentialled Diabetes Educator (CDE) has met the criteria set down by the Australian Diabetes Educators Association (ADEA).

Your dietitian

Making positive changes in the types of foods you eat, learning how to modify recipes and losing weight – your dietitian can help you with all of this. Meal planning is key to your care whether you are trying to lose weight or improve your blood-glucose levels. A Registered/Accredited Practising Dietitian

(APD) will help you find health and pleasure in what you eat by matching your food to your medication or insulin dose, your physical activity habits and your daily schedule. If your treatment changes, your dietitian can help you adjust. Most of your contact with a dietitian will be at the beginning of your care, but checking in once or twice a year or whenever your diabetes treatment changes is a good idea.

Your eye doctor

Because diabetes is a leading cause of eye disorders and even blindness, you constantly need to guard against vision problems. The medical doctor qualified to diagnose and treat eye damage from diabetes is an ophthalmologist – an eye specialist. Your eyes need to be checked by an eye specialist or an optometrist every 1 to 2 years. They will check the blood vessels at the back of your eyes (retina) for any damage. Plan to visit your eye specialist as recommended, but don't wait for your next check-up if you notice changes in your vision or feel pain or pressure in your eyes – possible signs of damage that require immediate attention. Proper examination involves pupil dilation with drops so someone will need to drive you home. Retinal photography is another accurate method. Reading a wall chart is not sufficient.

Your podiatrist

High blood glucose makes you prone to foot problems partly because it hinders circulation, as blood has trouble getting all the way from the heart to the feet and back. Small sores and calluses, which are common with diabetes, can quickly become worse if you don't keep on top of them with the help of a podiatrist, a practitioner who specialises in foot care, or your GP. While your doctor or nurse will check your feet every 6 months, you need to check your feet, too – every day. But your podiatrist is the best person to treat sores, calluses, corns, bunions, infections or any other problem that may develop. A podiatrist can also give you guidance on keeping your feet healthy, including cutting your toenails and choosing the right shoes. Ask your doctor or endocrinologist to refer you to a podiatrist if you have concerns about your feet.

Your dentist

As every cavity-prone eight-year-old knows (or will eventually find out), bacteria thrive on sugar. Unfortunately, if you have diabetes, high blood glucose makes you prone to the destructive effects of gingivitis – infection of the gums – even if you faithfully brush your teeth every day. There's no reason to change your dentist if you have diabetes; you just need to make sure you actually go for a check-up and a cleaning every 6 months, as we all should (but often don't). Make sure that you tell your dentist you have diabetes, however, and ask how you can improve your brushing and flossing techniques in order to keep problems to a minimum.

Your pharmacist

The special training that pharmacists receive about how medicines affect the body (in both good ways and bad) and how medicines interact with each other can make them an invaluable source of information. Try to find a pharmacist who works well with you; you may end up seeing them more often than anybody else on your team. Then keep going back to the same pharmacy so the pharmacist can keep an up-to-date record of all your medications. Whenever you start a new medication, including over-the-counter remedies, or make a change in your prescriptions, your pharmacist can explain how your body may react. They can also give you a printout of all your medications (with their doses and side effects) to take with you when you see other members of your medical team.

Exercise specialist

Accredited Exercise Physiologists (AEPs) are university-trained exercise specialists who can assess your exercise capacity and prescribe a safe and effective program, taking into account your lifestyle and general health plus any barriers to exercise such as joint, muscle or mobility problems. Some physiotherapists can also design you a tailored exercise program.

The team approach

Now that you understand the specific roles of each member of your diabetes team, you will know that you are definitely not alone. Each member of your diabetes team brings special skills and knowledge to your total healthcare plan to ensure you have all the professional care and support you need to manage your condition in the very best way. For optimum diabetes care, see your doctor regularly and have an extended consultation every 6 to 12 months.

Ready to fight back

You know exactly what kind of opponent you're up against, you understand the tools at your disposal, you've formulated a battle plan and lined up a team to help you put it into action. So what will it take to win the fight? The same things it takes to succeed in just about any other worthy struggle: patience, strength, determination, good communication skills, the ability to cooperate with your team and confidence that you will prevail. Last but not least, a positive attitude!

An attitude of confidence may be the most important quality of all. It's easy to feel (especially right after your diagnosis) that diabetes has already won the battle. It's stolen your health and made you feel like a 'diseased' or 'damaged' person – a statistic. So what's the use of fighting when you know your essential condition won't change? Such bleak thoughts are the seductions of pessimism and defeatism. If you buy into them (and most people do – at least a little bit some of the time), then diabetes really has won after all. Acknowledge these feelings when you have them, but don't let them linger. Just keep moving forward.

The truth is that diabetes is much like the classic playground bully who pushes you down and then turns his back because he doesn't expect you to get up and fight back. Standing up for yourself when diabetes lets down its guard means that you have refused to become

Rights and responsibilities

As a general rule, the best that your life can offer will mostly be up to you. Therefore, if you have diabetes it is vitally important to be aware of your rights and responsibilities, and to act on them.

Rights:

- Free registration with the National Diabetes Services Scheme (NDSS). Contact your diabetes association.

- Ongoing care from your diabetes team – regardless of financial, religious or cultural status – whose qualifications you have the right to know.

- Diabetes education that's appropriate to you and your culture and, if required, access to qualified health interpreters.

- Test results explained and copies provided.

- A complete care plan with agreed management goals.

- Regular checks for complications and education updates.

- Referral to specialists for prevention or treatment of complications.

Responsibilities:

- Live life to the fullest, keeping diabetes as important but not the sole focus in your life.

- Know your diabetes team and stay closely connected.

- Ask questions and be sure that you understand the answers.

- If you are taking insulin or tablets that can cause hypos, test before you drive and don't drive if 5 mmol/L or less.

- Have management goals that suit you and are achievable.

- Do your best to follow your care plan and meet goals.

- Seek a second opinion if you're unable to manage your planned routine as expected.

- Wear medical identification.

- Get extra support from family, carers, friends and colleagues.

- Be sure family, friends and workmates know what to do or who to contact in an emergency.

- Dispose of lancets, needles and contaminated waste properly.

a victim of the disease. And you'll find that diabetes often backs down in the face of sound treatment options – though you don't ever want to turn your back on it.

If you're willing to fight, you'll find plenty of weaknesses in diabetes to exploit. Don't forget that you've got support to back you up and help you overcome the meanest tricks diabetes can pull. But it's still your battle. Roll up your sleeves, make a fist and prepare to knock diabetes off its feet.

understanding diabetes

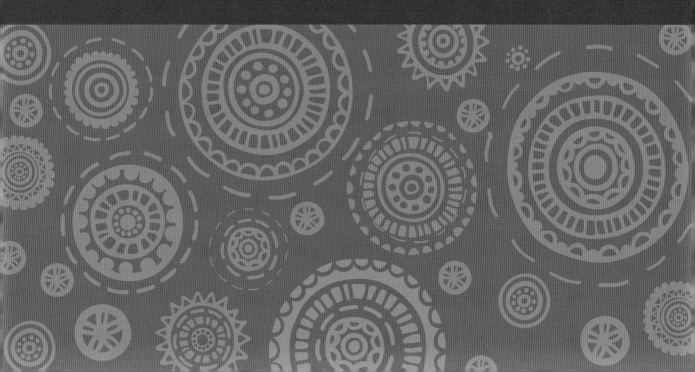

You can't see it, you usually can't feel it – so what exactly is diabetes? It's a complex disease, to be sure, which can affect your entire body, and it can seem difficult to get your mind around. But understanding diabetes braces you for battle with your condition. In fact, education is a cornerstone of care. The more you know about diabetes, the better you'll be able to use all the tools at your disposal to keep blood glucose in check and avoid complications that can compromise your enjoyment of life.

What exactly is diabetes? Unlike, say, high blood pressure, the term doesn't exactly paint a clear picture. Even doctors sometimes have a hard time describing it. Is it an endocrine disorder, a blood-related disease, a metabolic problem? Actually, it's all three – and then much more.

If you don't understand what diabetes is all about, you're not alone. But it's worth finding out, because whenever you're faced with an important mission (and managing diabetes certainly qualifies), taking effective action means gathering good intelligence first.

Aside from being complex, diabetes is often the subject of misconceptions. For example, many people think it comes from eating too much sugar, but that's not the case. It's also often assumed that having diabetes means constantly jabbing syringes full of insulin into your body, but – while people with type 1 diabetes need insulin to survive – millions of others can control their disease by making relatively simple lifestyle changes.

And then there's the idea that people with diabetes are defined by the term diabetic. This may seem like a small point, but it's worth making. You are not your disease, and your life isn't about diabetes, even if managing it demands a lot of your attention. Rather, you have diabetes and diabetes is a condition that you can control day by day, so that you can take part in and enjoy the truly important aspects of your life that really define who you are.

A hidden fuel spill

Imagine that the nation's intricate system of roads, streets and highways is your body and that the millions of cars humming along this system are your cells. Every car needs regular replenishment with fuel, and, fortunately, petrol is abundant. When everything is working normally, cars and petrol come together, fuel tanks open, petrol is dispensed and the cars go about their business, brimming with the energy they need to run.

Now suppose something goes fundamentally wrong. The petrol flows out of the pump, but there's nobody around to open the cars' fuel tanks. The petrol spills all over, floods the roads, rushes down the gutters and pollutes the entire system. That's the nature of diabetes.

In the real-life disease, the source of energy (that is, the 'petrol') is a substance called glucose, and the petrol-station attendant who opens the tank is equivalent to a hormone called insulin.

Why glucose matters

Glucose, also known as blood glucose, is the major source of energy powering your brain, organs, muscles and tissues – all your body's functions. In fact, glucose is one of nature's great dynamos, providing an almost universal energy source for living things. Scientists know down to the molecule how it's made and what it does, but, interestingly, they have never been able to create it in a lab. Only plants can make

glucose through the magic mix of sunlight, water and other elements, and pass this energy along to other creatures through the food chain.

When you eat, your body breaks down the food into smaller, simpler components that move through the small intestine and into the bloodstream. Once in the blood, these nutrients are carried to cells throughout the body.

Different foods break down into different types of nutrients. Protein breaks down into amino acids, which are often used to build or repair tissue. Fat breaks down into fatty acids, which are mostly stored as energy reserves. Carbohydrates (including everything from bread and pasta to some fruits and vegetables) mainly break down into glucose, which is used almost immediately for energy. In order to feel your best, you need enough glucose powering your cells at all times.

With diabetes, however, glucose in the blood doesn't make it into cells. Because of this, the cells are deprived of energy, which explains why fatigue is one of the hallmarks of diabetes. And since the glucose can't enter cells, it builds up in the blood. High blood glucose wreaks havoc with the body. In the short term, for example, the excess glucose essentially soaks up water from the bloodstream, creating a paradoxical condition in which you need to urinate more often while feeling parched with thirst. Too much glucose can also hinder the immune system's infection-fighting white blood cells, making you more vulnerable to illness. Over the long haul, persistently high blood glucose can lead to serious complications, such as damaged nerves, kidneys, eyes, blood vessels, liver and heart.

The blood-glucose problem

In uncontrolled diabetes, blood-glucose levels tend to spike after meals and remain high throughout the day. In people without diabetes, levels stay within the normal range, despite small fluctuations.

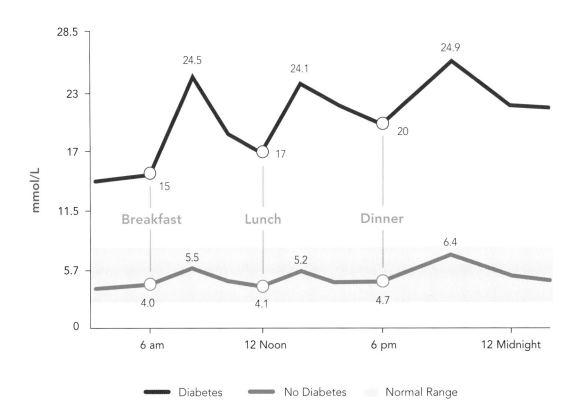

A wild blood-glucose ride

Blood glucose fluctuates normally throughout the day, rising after you eat a meal. In people who don't have diabetes, these fluctuations in glucose levels stay within a span (measured in units of millimoles of glucose per litre of blood) that ranges from about 4 to 7 mmol/L. When you have diabetes, though, the patterns become more erratic:

- ✳ Blood-glucose levels spike to mountainous heights (rather than gentle hills) after meals.
- ✳ Blood-glucose levels drop more slowly as the body metabolises the food you've eaten.
- ✳ Blood-glucose levels are, on average, higher than what is considered to be normal and healthy.
- ✳ The less you control your diabetes, the more likely your blood glucose is to swing wildly between highs and lows or simply stay high all the time.

Insulin's inside job

Glucose may inflict the damage done by diabetes, but it isn't really to blame. Instead, the real troublemaker is the hormone insulin, manufactured by the pancreas. Insulin's job is to 'unlock' cells so that glucose can enter. As glucose leaves the bloodstream and enters cells, blood glucose levels fall. When that happens, insulin levels also plummet so that blood-glucose doesn't get too low – a condition called hypoglycaemia.

When you have diabetes, the delicate dance of glucose and insulin is thrown out of step, either because the pancreas has trouble manufacturing

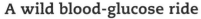

Insulin opposites

Insulin isn't the only hormone that can affect blood-glucose levels. A number of others, sometimes called insulin antagonists, or counterregulatory hormones, have the opposite effect of insulin. These include:

- Glucagon. Produced in the pancreas along with insulin, glucagon blocks insulin's ability to lower blood glucose by causing the liver to release stored glucose when the body requires it.

- Adrenaline. This so-called stress hormone is released when the body perceives danger. Adrenaline raises blood glucose in order to make more energy available to muscles.

- Cortisol. Another stress hormone, it can also raise blood-glucose levels.

- Growth hormone. Produced by the pituitary gland in the brain, it makes cells less sensitive to insulin.

insulin in the first place or because the body's cells have difficulty letting insulin do its job. The term that describes this latter condition is insulin resistance – a critical breakdown in the body's ability to utilise insulin properly. Insulin resistance is the underlying cause of the vast majority of type 2 diabetes cases.

Scientists are still struggling to understand exactly what goes physiologically wrong with a person's body in order to cause insulin resistance. (In one fairly recent medical textbook containing a diagram of how insulin may work at the cellular level, many steps in the process are simply illustrated with question marks.) But the sheer complexity of normal insulin function allows plenty of opportunity for things to go awry. It's possible, for example, that insulin resistance occurs when problems develop in the normal chain of chemical reactions that must occur to permit glucose to be transported through cell membranes. Or perhaps an intricate system of proteins in cells, sometimes called the metabolic switch, loses its ability to sense the presence of insulin and react accordingly.

Even if the biology is still a bit mysterious, however, it's important to remember that the factors known to raise the risk of type 2 diabetes are already fairly well understood.

Typecasting: a key to understanding

Diabetes was long assumed to be one disease. But researchers have come to realise that it actually takes several forms, which, while fundamentally similar, differ in many important ways. The two main forms are known as type 1 and type 2. (Other types are far less common.) Both occur when glucose can't enter cells. As a result, they share many symptoms. These include:

Feeling exhausted. When cells can't get glucose and are deprived of energy, you can suffer from both physical and mental fatigue. The brain, in fact, is a glutton for glucose, using far more glucose for its weight than do other types of tissue. Mental fatigue can make you fuzzy-headed and emotionally brittle, while physical fatigue can make your muscles feel weak.

Frequent toilet breaks. When the body is awash in blood glucose, the kidneys, which recirculate nutrients and filter out waste products, are among the first to know. When overwhelmed by glucose, they try to flush the excess out of your system by boosting production of urine, especially after blood-glucose levels reach or exceed about 10 mmol/L.

Unquenchable thirst. As urine is excreted, you lose fluid. To urge you to replace it, the body triggers a persistent thirst.

Snack attacks. The irony of diabetes is that although your body is overflowing with nutritional energy, your cells are starving. Deprived of sustenance, they tell the body's appetite system to send a call for more food – which only creates more glucose that can't be properly used.

Blurry vision. Diabetes can degrade your eyesight in two seemingly contradictory ways. In one, lack of body fluid due to loss of urine can dry out the eyes, constricting the lens and distorting vision. In the other, excess blood glucose can cause the lens to swell, also creating distortion. Both of these effects are temporary, although diabetes can cause other complications that may eventually result in serious visual impairment and even blindness.

A pancreas primer

The pancreas is a fist-sized organ that resembles an overgrown tadpole. It lies just behind and below the stomach. In its 'tail', cells known as beta cells (which are clustered in clumps called the islets of Langerhans) produce insulin and release it when needed. Other cells called acinar cells secrete enzymes that help break down proteins, carbohydrates and fats. Normally, the pancreas acts as a kind of glucose meter, closely monitoring levels in the blood and releasing insulin in spurts to mirror glucose levels. It also helps regulate a process in which the liver stores glucose as glycogen and then releases it back into the bloodstream to raise glucose levels when they fall too low. Certain diabetes drugs work to improve the function of the pancreas.

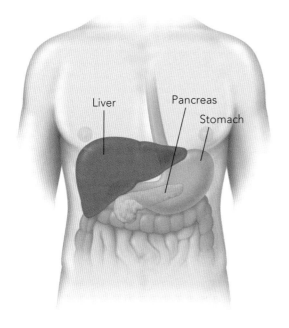

Liver

Pancreas

Stomach

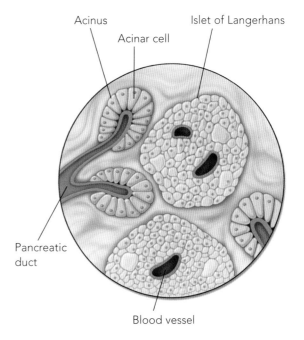

Acinus

Acinar cell

Islet of Langerhans

Pancreatic duct

Blood vessel

More infections. Having too much glucose in your blood makes immune-system cells less effective at attacking viruses and bacteria that cause infection. To make matters worse, some of these invaders actually feed on glucose, making it easier for them to multiply and become an even bigger threat. This can result in frequent upper respiratory illnesses like colds and flu, as well as urinary tract infections, gum disease and, in women, vaginal yeast infections.

Tingling hands and feet. High blood glucose can damage nerves, a condition that may first become noticeable in the touch-sensitive extremities as a tingling or burning sensation. Damage caused by excess blood glucose can also affect nerves in the digestive tract, provoking nausea, diarrhoea or constipation.

Type 1: an insulin no-show

So what makes the two types different? Firstly, type 1 is less common, accounting for only 10 to 15 per cent of all diagnosed cases of diabetes in Australia, 5 per cent of Maori and Pacific Islanders, and 11 per cent of Caucasians in New Zealand. With type 1 diabetes, the body's immune system destroys special cells in the pancreas that manu-facture insulin. These cells, called beta cells, are the only places in the body where insulin is produced. Without them, the body lacks the insulin it needs to move glucose out of circulation and control high blood glucose. Other major characteristics of type 1:

Injections are necessary. Because the body can't produce insulin, people with type 1 need an outside supply of the hormone, self-administered by daily injections. That's why type 1 used to be called insulin-dependent diabetes mellitus, or IDDM. This term is no longer used because people with type 2 diabetes sometimes need to take insulin as well. But the fact that injections are essential for people with type 1 diabetes to survive remains one of the key characteristics of this form of the disease.

It strikes early. Type 1 diabetes is usually diagnosed during childhood, or early adulthood, but can occur at any age. Because it's widely seen as a disease of the young (although you continue to have it your entire life), type 1 is sometimes called juvenile-onset diabetes. This term, too, has fallen out of favour, both because adults can get type 1 diabetes and because rates of type 2 diabetes in children are exploding.

It strikes fast. The onset of type 1 diabetes is rapid compared with the onset of type 2 diabetes, which can take years to develop. If you (or your child) have type 1 diabetes, such classic symptoms as fatigue, excessive thirst and frequent urination will probably become worse over a period of just days or weeks.

There is a 'honeymoon' period. In the first several months after type 1 diabetes is diagnosed and treatment begins, many people seem to improve as the pancreas temporarily begins to increase insulin production once again. This period of remission may last for as long as a year and sometimes even longer, during which blood-glucose levels become more stable and insulin doses are reduced or may not even be necessary for a period of time. While all honeymoons must come to an end, researchers see this period as a potential window of opportunity. One day in the future it may allow yet-to-be-perfected therapies to preserve beta cell function before it becomes too late.

Blood glucose swings wildly. With type 1, the pancreas loses its ability to monitor and control blood glucose. Blood-glucose levels tend to spike and crash with greater volatility than in people who have type 2 diabetes, who usually still produce some insulin of their own. With type 1, the job of the pancreas essentially falls to you. You control your blood-glucose level with the timing and dosage of your insulin injections. This makes monitoring your blood glucose critically important (see Chapter 3).

Diabetes at a glance

	TYPE 1	TYPE 2	GESTATIONAL
Common symptoms	Sudden onset; marked thirst and hunger; frequent urination; fatigue; nausea and vomiting; weight loss	Slow, difficult-to-detect onset; marked thirst; frequent urination; fatigue; slow wound healing; tingling hands or feet; frequent infections; weight loss/gain	Most women have no symptoms
Age at onset	Usually children and young adults	Usually 40 or older, although rates are escalating among younger people, even children	Child-bearing years
Physical condition	Usually lean or normal weight	Usually overweight	Pregnant
Cause	The immune system destroys the pancreas cells that produce insulin	Lack of exercise, poor diet, and resulting obesity; family history	Hormones produced by the placenta hinder the function of insulin. Being overweight, poor diet and a family history of type 2 diabetes increase the risk.
Mainstay of treatment	Insulin injections plus healthy eating and physical activity	Lifestyle changes, possibly augmented by insulin and oral medications	Lifestyle changes, possibly augmented by insulin injections. Also self blood-glucose monitoring.

What causes type 1?

Type 1 diabetes seems to appear out of nowhere and, as yet, is not preventable – something that is definitely not true of type 2. So why does type 1 occur?

The bottom line is that researchers don't know yet. But clues can be found in the nature of the disease. Type 1 diabetes is thought to involve a misguided attack by the immune system on the body's own tissue – specifically, the beta cells of the pancreas. This type of attack is known as an autoimmune response. Other autoimmune diseases include lupus, multiple sclerosis, rheumatoid arthritis, Grave's disease and coeliac disease. Scientists are studying the different players involved with helping the body distinguish its own cells from foreign cells. Eventually they may be able to develop new therapies to prevent and treat type 1 diabetes. Meanwhile, the question still lingers as to why an autoimmune attack occurs in the first place. There appear to be a number of factors at work in type 1:

Genetics. Having a family history of type 1 diabetes may be the single most important risk factor in determining who will get the disease. Even so, the genetic connection is weak. If you already have the disease, your children or siblings have only about a 5 per cent chance of developing it. (For reasons that aren't well understood, men with type 1 diabetes have a slightly higher chance of transmitting it to their children than women with type 1 do.) Among identical twins, there's only a 30 to 40 per cent chance that the second twin will develop the disease if the first one has it.

Family history does make certain cultural groups more susceptible than others to type 1 diabetes. Caucasians are at the highest risk, as evidenced by studies showing that Caucasians living in New Zealand get type 1 diabetes more than non-white New Zealanders (Maori and Pacific Islanders), who share the same island environment.

Even though genetics doesn't completely predict the disease, scientists are currently working to gain a better understanding of the genes involved with type 1 diabetes, and they may someday be able to develop genetic therapies specifically for those people who are most at risk of developing that form of the disease.

> **? DID you KNOW...**
>
> The discovery of insulin, a major breakthrough in understanding and treating diabetes, came in the 1920s, following the earlier discovery that when beta cells of the pancreas were missing, people developed diabetes. Building on this observation, a team of doctors led by researchers Frederick Banting, Charles Best and John MacLeod extracted insulin from beta cells and injected it into diabetes patients. When the patients improved, the researchers knew they had made a major discovery – one that brought Banting and MacLeod the Nobel Prize for medicine. Another 50 years passed, however, before researchers fully understood the distinction between type 1 and type 2 diabetes.

Viruses. Could type 1 be caused by an infection? It's possible. One reason researchers think so is that the onset of the disease appears to follow a seasonal pattern, with the fewest new cases in summer and the most in winter – when many viral illnesses are more common. A number of viruses have been implicated as suspects, in particular mumps and rubella. Some studies have found that a high percentage of people newly diagnosed with type 1 have coxsackievirus (hand, foot and mouth disease) antibodies in their blood, suggesting that the body has been fighting this viral infection. In the lab, a cousin of the coxsackievirus has been shown to produce type 1–like symptoms in animals.

Some researchers question the merit of the virus idea, but a number of theories explain how it might work. One hypothesis is that the immune system may have trouble distinguishing between certain viruses and the insulin-producing beta cells in the pancreas. After fighting off the virus, the immune system continues the battle by attacking the pancreas. Other theories suggest that viruses may change the beta cells in ways that make them appear foreign to the immune system. Or they may destroy proteins in the pancreas that manufacture insulin.

Cow's milk. Some research has suggested a link between feeding children cow's milk before 3 or 4 months of age and the risk of developing type 1 diabetes. People with type 1 sometimes have higher levels of antibodies that bind to both a protein found in milk and a protein sometimes found on beta cells, but the

WHAT the STUDIES show

Harvard scientists using an imaging technique called X-ray crystallography recently obtained the first detailed, three-dimensional pictures of immune cells called T-cells attacking a foreign substance. The pictures revealed a previously unknown docking mechanism between cells that will help researchers better understand the rules of engagement in immune-system battles. Eventually, such knowledge may lead to therapies to help the body protect itself against specific kinds of attack. Meanwhile, US researchers at the University of Illinois have discovered a way to improve the properties of T-cell receptors. This may open the door to manipulating the immune system in new ways to fight a variety of auto-immune diseases.

significance of this isn't clear. A large ongoing study called TEDDY (The Environmental Determinants of Diabetes in the Young) is investigating the effect of early childhood diet, including cow's milk. Breastfeeding is recommended as the ideal milk for babies.

Free radicals. These unstable molecules are formed as a by-product of natural bodily functions (such as breathing) that involve the use of oxygen. Free radicals have a single, unpaired electron instead of the usual pair, making them unstable. As they circulate around the body, they try to latch onto other molecules, inflicting damage on healthy cells in the process. Normally, enzymes in the body neutralise free radicals and keep this damage to a minimum. But toxins, such as air pollution and tobacco smoke, can boost their numbers to levels the body can't adequately handle. Studies suggest that the insulin-producing cells of the pancreas may be particularly vulnerable to free-radical damage because they are less well guarded by protective enzymes than other parts of the body.

Type 2: a system breakdown

Compared with type 1, type 2 is far more common, accounting for 85 to 90 per cent of all cases of diabetes. It's also far more complex. High blood glucose is still the basic problem. But with type 2, the pancreas doesn't completely shut off insulin production. Instead, the body's use of insulin becomes impaired in any number of different ways.

- ❋ The beta cells of the pancreas are able to produce plenty of insulin, but they take their sweet time releasing it in response to the surge of glucose that follows a meal. The result is that by the time the pancreas puts out the large amounts of insulin the body is waiting for, glucose levels have already built up in the blood.
- ❋ The number of beta cells is lower than normal, so the pancreas has trouble keeping up with insulin demand.
- ❋ There's plenty of glucose and insulin, but cells don't allow insulin to do its job – a condition known as insulin resistance. The problem can be caused by any number of things – a lack of proteins called insulin receptors on cells (think of insulin as a key and the receptor as a lock), a mismatch of insulin and receptors (the keys don't fit the locks), or flaws in the chemistry that lets insulin pass into cells. Carrying extra weight also makes it harder for insulin to work. No matter what the problem, the result is the same – glucose can't get where it needs to go and stays in the bloodstream instead.

As insulin resistance occurs well before the development of diabetes, initially the pancreas produces extra insulin to overcome the resistance so blood-glucose levels remain well controlled. However, over time insulin resistance can worsen and the pancreas can't keep up with the additional demand, so blood-glucose levels rise, leading to type 2 diabetes.

The major symptoms of type 2 mirror those of type 1, but type 2 is different in other ways:

It takes time. Unlike type 1, type 2 develops slowly over time. Symptoms don't show up right away and in many cases, there are no symptoms at all. When you finally notice that something's wrong, you may already have had diabetes for many years. That can make type 2 diabetes seem a bit vague – if it appears so gradually, when does it actually begin? Doctors admit that it's sometimes tough to say exactly when any given case of diabetes got started – especially after the fact. But exact criteria based on blood-glucose levels clearly define when you have diabetes and when you don't. Once you have it, you can control it to a remarkable degree, but it never goes away. There is no such thing as 'mild' diabetes.

Adults suffer most. Type 2 diabetes is sometimes called adult-onset diabetes because it usually strikes after age 40 and is more likely to develop as you get older. One reason is that insulin resistance increases with age. In fact, more than 10 per cent of people over 60 years of age have type 2 diabetes. But, as with other terms for diabetes, 'adult onset' is becoming a misnomer because of the increasing prevalence of type 2 in children.

Blood glucose is more stable. Because the pancreas still produces and releases at least some insulin when it's needed, glucose levels in the blood don't tend to swing as wildly as they do with type 1 – even though, on average, unmanaged blood-glucose levels with type 2 are still too high.

What causes type 2?

The causes of type 2 diabetes have much more to do with lifestyle issues, particularly obesity. But weight doesn't tell the whole story. In fact, it's unlikely that type 2 develops because of any one thing. Instead, a number of factors appear to come together, potentially even magnifying each other, with unhealthy results. Among the factors that may come into play are the following:

? DID you KNOW…
Although the reasons are not understood, the incidence of type 1 diabetes is rising steadily, despite the fact that, unlike type 2 diabetes, the disease isn't clearly related to lifestyle. Researchers point to a virtual epidemic of type 1 diabetes, with rates as much as five times higher today in the Western world than 40 years ago. Still, rates of type 2 diabetes are rising faster than rates of type 1. In Australia the rate of new cases of type 1 diabetes is increasing at almost 3 per cent per year and is high compared to other countries.

Genetics. Again, patterns in twins indicate how strong the genetic link is – and it's much stronger with type 2 than with type 1. In the case of type 2, if one identical twin has diabetes, the chances of the other getting it are as high as 90 per cent. If one parent has type 2, there's a 20 to 30 per cent chance their children will develop it, too. (If both parents have type 2, the risk to children is about the same as that shared by identical twins.) This makes type 2 a serious concern for cultural groups that seem predisposed to it – and those groups are not the same ones that are most susceptible to type 1. Caucasians are more likely to get type 1, but type 2 is more prevalent among people from the Pacific Islands, Indian sub-continent, Middle East or of Chinese cultural background, along with Aborigines and Maori.

Metabolic syndrome or syndrome X

Insulin resistance is the earliest abnormality in type 2 diabetes. Several features associated with increased incidence of coronary artery disease combined with insulin resistance are:

- Hypertension
- Increased blood fats – high LDL ('bad' cholesterol) and low HDL ('good' cholesterol)
- Increased waist measurement (abdominal visceral fat)
- Obesity
- Sedentary lifestyle

Inactivity. Physical activity improves the body's use of insulin. This happens for a variety of reasons. Muscle, for example, uses glucose more efficiently than other types of tissue, and exercise builds muscle. Unfortunately, the opposite is also true. Lack of physical activity makes cells more prone to insulin resistance. It also contributes to weight gain.

Poor diet. How much you eat matters. But what you eat is also important. And the high-kilojoule foods so common today are more likely to add kilos.

Age. Type 2 diabetes becomes more common with age, in part because cells in older bodies tend to be more insulin resistant. But it's also true that people tend to become more sedentary with age. Their metabolism slows down, yet most eat just as much – or more. All of those elements are a prescription for an increased risk of diabetes.

Obesity: the big difference

Type 1 diabetes doesn't 'look' like anything – there's nothing to distinguish a person who has it from anybody else. That's usually not true of people with type 2 diabetes, who are overweight or obese in 80 to 90 per cent of cases. Being overweight is the single most important contributor to type 2 diabetes. It's no coincidence that the skyrocketing incidence of diabetes in recent years has been matched by obesity rates, which have doubled in the past 30 years.

The potbelly peril. Not all flab is created equal, though. Research studies have made it clear that fat around the midsection – what scientists call visceral adipose tissue and the rest of us call a spare tyre – contributes to type 2 diabetes more than fat located on the hips, thighs or other parts of the body. To get an idea of your risk, just take a look in a mirror: if your shape resembles an apple (thickest around the middle) more than a pear (thickest below the waist), your disease risks are higher. It's not clear why this is true, but excess belly fat seems linked with high levels of fatty acids that contribute to insulin resistance, perhaps through processes involving the nearby liver, which stores glucose.

Size really does matter

- Healthy eating, ideal body weight and regular physical activity are important objectives in managing type 2 diabetes.

- Body Mass Index (BMI) = weight (kilograms)/ height^2 (metres)

- The healthy BMI is 20–25, overweight 25–30, obese over 30.

- As a guide, a person's healthy weight is approximately: height (centimetres) – 100.

Abdominal circumference (cm) chart

	HEALTHY	OVERWEIGHT	OBESE
Men	<94	94–102	>102
Women	<80	80–88	>88

Weight for height chart for men and women
(from 18 years onwards)

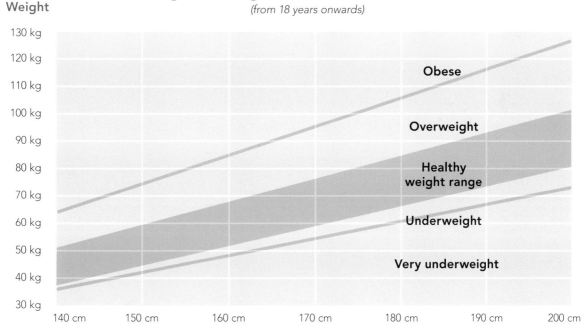

Other 'diabesity' dangers. Diabetes isn't the only chronic disease linked to abdominal fat. A spare tyre is also a critical risk factor for heart disease and a raft of conditions that go along with it, such as high blood pressure and elevated levels of such blood fats as cholesterol and triglycerides. In fact, obesity, insulin resistance and risk factors for heart disease appear together so often that researchers are beginning to think of them as different expressions of a single disorder sometimes called metabolic syndrome, or syndrome X.

It isn't clear how the different components of metabolic syndrome affect one another, but in 2001 a US study defined for the first time what to look for in diagnosing the condition. Some researchers now believe that about a quarter of the population has metabolic syndrome. What does this mean to you? If diabetes goes hand in hand with heart disease, taking charge of your blood glucose can help protect you against both.

Do your genes make you look fat? Like diabetes itself, obesity seems to run in families. Scientists believe that genes play a role in how well hormones, enzymes and other chemicals are able to control appetite by, for example, signalling the brain to stop eating or establishing how heavy the body thinks it ought to be. Does that mean you're a victim of genetic fate and can't do anything about your weight? Absolutely not. Genes may contribute to weight, but they don't tell the whole story. Some of the cultural groups in which obesity and diabetes rates are highest, for example indigenous Australians and New Zealanders, are not historically heavy people. Only when they took up a highly refined, high-kilojoule diet and became more sedentary after European colonisation did they 'adopt' obesity and diabetes, too.

You hold the key. If weight is such an important contributor to diabetes risk, that's actually good news because it's almost entirely within your control. You can manage your weight through healthy eating and physical activity – and you can control type 2 diabetes the same way. That may sound like a tough challenge, but it's an opportunity that people with type 1 don't have: to change the course of their disease just by making changes in the way they live.

Gestational diabetes: a disappearing act

At first, gestational diabetes sounds innocuous. It occurs in about 3 to 8 per cent of pregnant women during the second half of gestation (usually in the third trimester) as hormones guiding foetal development in the placenta interfere with normal insulin function. Gestational diabetes (GDM) doesn't usually have symptoms, and when the baby arrives, it usually goes away.

But don't imagine that gestational diabetes is strictly temporary or isn't worth taking seriously. GDM increases the risk of miscarriage (although a baby born of a mother with gestational diabetes is no more likely to have birth defects) and, because GDM often causes babies to grow large before birth, it can contribute to complications at delivery. (Having previously given birth to a child weighing 4 kg or more suggests you're at risk for GDM.) And most women who develop GDM do so because their pancreas is already weak (often due to obesity), making them vulnerable to getting type 2 diabetes later on – which occurs in a third to a half of cases.

Protecting your pregnancy

For many women, being diagnosed with gestational diabetes can be upsetting. However, working closely with your doctor can help you to keep within the blood-glucose levels found in a healthy woman who isn't pregnant. Fortunately, your pancreas still makes insulin,

WHAT the STUDIES show

A recent analysis found that women with menstrual cycles that are very irregular or long (more than 40 days) were about twice as likely to develop type 2 diabetes as women with normal periods. Obese women with irregular periods faced a nearly four-fold increase in diabetes risk. One possible reason is that women with menstrual irregularities are prone to polycystic ovary syndrome, a hormone disorder characterised by insulin resistance and thus linked to diabetes. The researchers advise women who have irregular periods to reduce their risk with weight control and physical activity.

so by being committed to your healthy eating plan and regular physical activity program, you will most likely be able to achieve your diabetes management goals and enjoy your pregnancy to the full. Your doctor may recommend that you:

- Ease insulin demand on the pancreas by spreading carbohydrate intake out in smaller, more frequent meals. Of course, you still need enough kilojoules to maintain a healthy pregnancy weight.
- Lower blood-glucose levels with regular activity such as walking or swimming.
- Make use of insulin injections if you have trouble managing blood glucose through healthy eating and physical activity.

Children are at risk, too

Type 2 diabetes is also known as adult-onset diabetes because it's a disease that starts in adulthood – that is, until recently. The past couple of decades have seen a marked increase in type 2 cases in children. Before the 1990s, type 2 accounted for less than 4 per cent of diabetes cases in children. Today, this figure is far higher and is constantly increasing at an alarming rate.

Why is this happening? Researchers point to a dramatic jump in juvenile obesity. Today many more Australian and New Zealand children are overweight. In an attempt to clarify the diabetes risk to heavy children, US researchers at Yale University, writing in *The New England Journal of Medicine* in March 2002, reported that, of 167 obese children and adolescents they studied, about a quarter were already glucose intolerant – one step down the path to having diabetes.

The director of Yale University's Pediatric Obesity/Type 2 Diabetes Clinic says that this is all very new, and we're still not exactly sure how to treat type 2 diabetes in children.

Insulin is the only drug currently approved for the treatment of diabetes in children. Oral diabetes medicines are not currently approved due to a lack of research on their effectiveness and safety in children. However, since type 2 in children appears to be similar to that of adults, it is assumed that these medications will be effective for use in both children and adolescents as well.

Less controversial are the benefits of addressing the various lifestyle issues that contribute to the growing obesity epidemic. More food is available to children at any time of the day than ever before. Generally, we heavily promote food consumption in children, especially high-kilojoule snacks and soft drinks, which are readily available from vending machines in schools and train stations. Super-sized portions are another problem. Children are used to enormous servings in restaurants. They don't even think about it.

On top of that, children are far less physically active now than they were in days gone by. Because of distance and safety issues, children seldom walk to school, and physical education is fast losing ground to more academic pursuits. Back at home, many children spend increasing amounts of time on sedentary activities, such as watching television, using computers or playing video games, instead of kicking a ball around the backyard or going for a swim. More families than ever before live in apartments, which could also lead to more sedentary habits.

If radical changes are to be made, then parents are the real focus of change. Parents need to learn more about proper nutrition and go outside to play more themselves, like most of our parents did 30 years ago. And if school lunch boxes even vaguely resembled the standard lunch-box fare of yesteryear, young people would be in a better position to gain perspective on everyday nutrition. It is, after all, about the everyday, not the exceptional.

Testing one, two, three

The most important thing to know about diabetes is whether or not you have it. Sounds pretty obvious, doesn't it? But diabetes can take even the smartest of us by surprise. And people with early signs of the disease need to monitor their condition closely, because relying on symptoms alone won't tell you if you've developed diabetes.

An estimated 50 per cent of the people in Australia and New Zealand who have type 2 diabetes are yet to be diagnosed. Millions more who are at risk for the disease and could stop it before it starts aren't taking preventive measures because they don't know they're in danger (see page 50).

Fortunately for people who have diabetes, the methods of testing are relatively easy and painless. There are three tests that measure blood glucose in slightly different ways: the fasting plasma glucose test (FPG), the random plasma glucose test and the oral glucose tolerance test (OGTT).

Two conditions known as Impaired Fasting Glucose (IFG) and Impaired Glucose Tolerance (IGT) are both characterised by higher than normal blood-glucose levels but not high enough to be diagnosed as type 2 diabetes. There is, however, a difference.

IFG is an early sign that a person's insulin is not working properly (insulin resistance). It's diagnosed when the fasting blood-glucose level is higher than the normal range, but does not rise abnormally after having a sweet glucose drink, whereas in IGT, it does. Without treatment, not everyone with IFG will progress to IGT or type 2 diabetes. Likewise, not everyone with IGT will progress to type 2 diabetes.

HbA1c measurement

In New Zealand, HbA1c measurement is the recommended diagnostic screening test for diabetes and should be measured by an accredited laboratory. If it is not possible to measure HbA1c or if there are concerns about its validity, then a plasma glucose test is recommended. HbA1c measurement is also used in parts of Australia.

Fasting plasma glucose test (FPG)

If your doctor recommends this test, an advance booking is definitely necessary, because accurate results depend on your preparing for the test in advance.

How it works. First, you must fast for at least 8 hours before taking the test, consuming nothing but water. That way, when blood is drawn, your gastrointestinal system has long since digested all food. As a result, your blood-glucose levels will be at their lowest ebb, providing the bottom measure of what's typical for you. If you're healthy, your reading will be 5.5 mmol/L or lower. If your reading is higher than normal levels, your doctor may want to repeat the test on a different day, just to be sure – though if your numbers are through the roof, this may not be necessary.

Random plasma glucose test

This test is also referred to as a casual plasma glucose test. Both 'casual' and 'random' refer to the fact that you can take the test at any time. No fasting is necessary.

How it works. The procedure is not very different from the fasting glucose test. Blood is drawn and sent to a lab. But when the results come back, the bar for diagnosis is higher because it's assumed you may have had glucose from food in your blood. In healthy people, normal insulin response usually keeps blood glucose under 8 mmol/L even after eating. If a random plasma glucose test shows a blood-glucose level of 11.1 mmol/L or higher and you have such symptoms as fatigue, excessive thirst or frequent urination, it's quite likely that you have diabetes.

Why it's used. Because it requires no preparation, the random plasma glucose test is often done as part of routine examination of blood samples. Your first hint at a diabetes diagnosis may emerge as the result of an annual physical and not from any special effort on your part.

✅ **Get confirmation.** If you don't have any obvious symptoms, don't rely on a single positive result from a random plasma glucose test as the final word. Doctors will almost always insist on confirming such results using a more exact test designed specifically to detect diabetes.

Oral glucose tolerance test (OGTT)

Raised blood-glucose levels means that a person's insulin is not working as it should be, placing them at risk of health problems. Therefore, such results must be checked further.

The oral glucose tolerance test is regarded as the gold standard for making a clear-cut diagnosis of type 2 diabetes but is only required when other blood test results are unclear.

How it works. Again, you first fast for at least 8 hours. But this time, that's only the start. When you get to your doctor's surgery, blood is taken to provide a point of comparison for additional blood samples that will be taken at 1-hour intervals for the next 3 hours. After the first blood draw, you drink a super-sweet solution containing about 75 g of sugar (about three times sweeter than an average soft drink). Each subsequent blood sample helps plot out a picture of how your body handles glucose over time. Results are compared to a normal range at each measure, but the 2-hour mark is especially critical. If your blood-glucose levels at that point are 11.1 mmol/L or higher, you have diabetes, final answer.

Why it's used. A more exact test is sometimes needed when results from other tests are less conclusive than your doctor would like. Let's say you have a strong family history of diabetes and are experiencing obvious symptoms but neither form of plasma glucose test has confirmed a diagnosis. Or one test indicates diabetes and a second test doesn't confirm it. In cases like these, you will require the gold standard (OGTT) for an unequivocal result. A version of the oral glucose tolerance test is also the preferred tool for detecting gestational diabetes, although the diagnostic criteria are different for pregnant women.

✅ **Watch what you ingest before the test.** Because of the test's sensitivity, OGTT needs to be done with proper preparation. It is important to let your doctor know if you're taking any kind of medication – including birth-control pills – or herbal or nutritional supplements, since they may boost blood-glucose levels and require the test to be delayed or repeated. For ideal results, some doctors recommend that you consume a lot of high-carbohydrate foods for 3 days before the test in order to mimic a standard diet.

Talk of other tests

The tests summarised above (and in the box at right) – the HbA1c measurement test, the fasting plasma glucose test, the random plasma glucose test and the oral glucose tolerance test – are the tests doctors commonly depend upon to make a definitive diagnosis. But you may have heard about other tests for measuring blood glucose. Some of these you'll read about in Chapter 3, but most are not – and in some cases, shouldn't be – relied upon to arrive at a diagnosis.

Glycated haemoglobin. Also called the HbA1c test, this is also used after a diagnosis to get a better idea of your blood-glucose patterns, as well as to monitor your condition as you continue living with the disease. Its

Diabetes by the numbers

Doctors make the determination of whether or not you have diabetes based on any one of the following measures:

Test: HbA1c
What it does: measures your average blood glucose over the past 4 to 6 weeks

You have diabetes if: you have symptoms of diabetes and your result is greater than or equal to 50 mmol/mol. If your result is 50 mmol/mol but you have no symptoms, the HbA1c will be repeated or a fasting plasma glucose test will be taken to confirm diabetes

Test: Fasting plasma glucose
What it does: measures glucose in blood after an 8- to 10-hour fast

You have diabetes if: your reading is 7 mmol/L or higher in two different tests taken on two different days

Test: Random plasma glucose
What it does: measures glucose in blood at any time, including after eating

You have diabetes if: your reading is 11.1 mmol/L or higher and you have symptoms of diabetes

Test: Oral glucose tolerance
What it does: following an 8-hour fast, measures blood glucose before and after you swallow a high-glucose solution

You have diabetes if: your 2-hour level is 11.1 mmol/L or higher

When to get tested

Anyone who ticks one or more of the boxes below is at risk of having type 2 diabetes. If you fit into that category, visit your doctor and ask to be tested.

○ I have/had a family member with diabetes and am 45 years of age or older

○ I have heart disease or have had a heart attack

○ I have/had a borderline high blood-glucose test or have been told that I have impaired glucose tolerance (IGT)

○ I am overweight and 45 years of age or older

○ I have high blood pressure and am 45 years of age or older

○ I am over 55 years of age

○ I had diabetes during pregnancy (gestational diabetes)

○ I am overweight and have polycystic ovarian syndrome

○ I am of Aboriginal, Torres Strait, Maori, Chinese, Indian, Middle Eastern or Pacific Islander heritage and am over 35 years of age.

(Many other cultural groups are also at an increased risk of developing type 2 diabetes.)

main benefit is that rather than assess your blood glucose at a specific moment in time, it surveys what happened with your blood-glucose patterns over 2 or 3 months by looking at glucose deposits on a specific type of cell. (See page 77 for more information.)

Urine test. Do doctors always have to use a needle? It's tempting to wonder why, if glucose appears in urine, they can't just measure that. High glucose levels in urine can indeed be an indication of diabetes. But the amount of glucose in the blood needed to raise glucose levels in urine varies from one person to the next, and sugary urine doesn't always correlate with high blood glucose. The bottom line is that a urine test is not accurate enough.

Finger prick. Tests in which a small drop of blood is squeezed from a fingertip onto a special test strip that's read by a glucose meter are a mainstay of home monitoring that many people with diabetes know intimately. While these tests give reasonably accurate results for daily tracking, they don't offer the kind of precision needed to make a diagnosis that will affect the rest of your life. While home testing has revolutionised people's control over their own blood-glucose levels, it is equally important that the person operating the machine is proficient in using the blood-glucose meter, as human error can result in inaccurate results. Older, non-digital devices in which the test strip is compared visually to a colour chart are even less reliable. A further method of testing that is no longer recommended is public screening in shopping centres and community fairs, as several factors can contribute to misleading results in these situations.

Pre-diabetes, or impaired glucose tolerance (IGT)

The diagnostic cut-offs for diabetes are very clear. However, there's a grey area in which blood-glucose readings don't add up to diabetes but don't indicate normal glucose levels, either. This used to be called border-line diabetes, but because that doesn't confirm whether or not you really have diabetes, in-between numbers are now known as impaired glucose metabolism. Two conditions fall into this category – impaired fasting glucose (IFG) and impaired glucose tolerance (IGT) – meaning that your cells are becoming insulin resistant. See the table below for the difference between IFG and IGT:

Having IFG or IGT doesn't necessarily mean type 2 diabetes is around the corner but does indicate a higher risk, with between 1 per cent and 10 per cent of people with IGT developing diabetes each year. A strong family history or being part of an at-risk cultural group raises your risk. But just as important, the more overweight and sedentary you are, the more likely that type 2 diabetes may develop.

A chance for change. A diagnosis of IGT is really a window of opportunity; think of it as an early warning that not every person gets. The potential power of this opportunity was brought home with the publication of results from a major US clinical trial, called the Diabetes Prevention Program, in early 2002. This study tried two main approaches to prevent diabetes in people with IGT: lifestyle modifications – healthy eating and physical activity – and an oral medication (metformin) used to treat type 2 diabetes. A third group took placebos instead of the real medication and made no lifestyle changes.

The result was that over the course of 3 years, people in the lifestyle group reduced their incidence of diabetes by an incredible 58 per cent – about twice as much as those who made no changes, and far more than

IFG or IGT?		
	IFG	**IGT**
Fasting blood-glucose level	More than 6.1 mmol/L but less than 7 mmol/L	Less than 7 mmol/L
Oral glucose tolerance results at 1 and 2 hours after having a sweet glucose drink	Less than 7.8 mmol/L	More than 7.8 mmol/L but less than 11 mmol/L

those who just took the medication. (Their incidence dropped by 31 per cent.) Another study called the Finnish Diabetes Prevention Study showed similar results. These stunning findings show that taking action can reverse IGT and may allow you to avoid type 2 diabetes if you're at risk.

When diabetes becomes an emergency

What if you simply decided to ignore your diabetes? While many complications of diabetes develop slowly over many years, blood glucose that's either too high or too low (due to treatment with insulin) can have immediate effects that quickly prove dangerous and even fatal. Fortunately, these complications can usually be treated easily by either you or your doctor. And close monitoring of your blood-glucose levels can prevent them from sneaking up on you. Later chapters will discuss some of these subjects in more detail, but you'll better understand diabetes if you have a working knowledge of these three conditions.

Diabetic ketoacidosis. This is mostly a problem for people with type 1, whose insulin deficit – barring treatment with supplemental insulin – allows no glucose at all into cells. In order to get energy, glucose-deprived cells instead start burning fat. The fat-burning process, however, produces highly acidic by-products known as ketones. When ketones build up in the blood (a condition known as ketoacidosis), they can cause shortness of breath, mental confusion and vomiting. Eventually, diabetic ketoacidosis, or DKA, can put you into a coma and even result in death.

DKA is less common these days, thanks to insulin treatment and easy-to-use self-monitoring devices, but it's still a medical emergency when it occurs. To treat it, doctors immediately replace fluids to flush out acid and make sure you receive adequate insulin, which can quickly get you out of danger.

Hyperosmolar syndrome. This condition is somewhat similar to diabetic ketoacidosis in that it's caused by extremely high blood glucose. But it affects primarily people with type 2 diabetes who don't know they have the disease or aren't monitoring it effectively. With hyperosmolar hyperglycaemic syndrome (HHS), blood glucose becomes so concentrated it makes the blood thick and syrupy. As the body reacts by forcing sugar out of the body in the urine, you can become severely dehydrated and experience such symptoms as cramps, rapid pulse, confusion and even convulsions and coma. Treatment involves fluid replenishment and insulin.

Hypoglycaemia. The most common acute complication of diabetes in people taking insulin or certain diabetes tablets is blood glucose that falls too low: hypoglycaemia. It's most common in people with type 1 since blood glucose is most likely to drop from having too much insulin or too little food. But

Can diabetes be cured?

Doctors often say you either have diabetes or you don't, based on your blood-glucose levels. But let's say you have type 2 and you do everything right. You change your eating habits, start an activity plan, lose a significant amount of weight and bring your blood-glucose numbers back to normal. Do you still have diabetes?

In one sense, type 2 diabetes can be seen as cured if all the measures that define it indicate that the condition at issue – high blood glucose – is no longer present. But this suggests that you can carry on with your life as if you never had diabetes – or that you won't have to worry about developing it in the future. And that would be a mistake.

Diabetes is a disease you have for life because, while you can keep it under control and live a normal life, the fact that you are controlling it is significant. Diabetes never goes away. If you were to stop controlling it – went back to a sedentary lifestyle and a

poor diet – your blood-glucose levels would rise again. Even if you continue practising your healthy eating and lifestyle habits, it's possible that your condition will change as you get older.

Think of it like parenting. Even when your children grow up and move out of the house, you still have children. Likewise, even after you've managed to get your diabetes under control, you still have the disease.

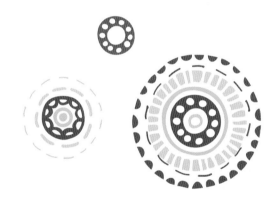

hypoglycaemia occurs in some people with type 2 as well, when glucose levels ebb because of insulin or drug treatments, perhaps made worse by other factors, such as going too long without eating.

Hypoglycaemia is both very unpleasant and potentially dangerous, so it must be dealt with immediately. The symptoms of hypoglycaemia – including feeling weak and shaky, mental confusion, rapid heartbeat, sweating and

double vision – can severely impair your ability to drive a car, operate machinery or do your job. Most cases can easily be treated by ingesting some fast-acting carbohydrate such as glucose tablets, jellybeans or sweet drinks. Although rarely the case, hypoglycaemia can be life threatening.

The agenda for action

By now, two points should be clear. First, diabetes is a serious, complex disease that has the potential to affect your overall health in a wide variety of ways. But second, it's well within your power to treat the underlying problem, prevent many – if not all – of the major complications and live a stimulating, productive and enjoyable life. In order to do this, you'll need to implement a big-picture plan in which you:

✔ **Be committed.** No, you don't need to obsess about your blood glucose. But studies have clearly demonstrated that closely monitoring your blood-glucose levels, to

Shooting down diabetes myths

Considering all the factors involved with diabetes, there's plenty of room for misinformation. Some of the more persistent misconceptions include:

Myth: If you develop diabetes, you can never eat sugar again.

Truth: People with diabetes can have a small amount of added sugar in the food they eat as part of their healthy eating plan.

Myth: I have just a touch of diabetes.

Truth: There is no such thing as a 'touch of diabetes', just as there is no such thing as a 'touch of pregnancy'. Once you have diabetes you will always have diabetes, until a cure is found.

Myth: I feel fine, so my blood glucose is fine.

Truth: High or low blood glucose doesn't always produce symptoms. Regular monitoring is the only way to know for sure where you stand.

Myth: I'm a pro at self-management; check-ups are just a waste of my time.

Truth: Your treatment program is never a done deal. Thanks to ongoing research, the medical community is constantly learning more about this complex condition and how best to deal with it. Regular check-ups are essential to help prevent complications from arising.

Myth: If I don't need insulin or medications, my diabetes isn't serious.

Truth: Diabetes is always serious. Healthy eating and physical activity can keep your blood glucose in check, but your cells are still insulin resistant and your condition could worsen if you don't control it.

help you keep as near to a normal range as possible, can dramatically reduce your risk of complications from diabetes.

✅ **Lose weight.** Just as being overweight is the biggest contributor to the vast majority of type 2 diabetes cases, dropping excess kilos is the single most important move you can make to assert control over your disease.

✅ **Eat smarter.** A healthy eating plan is the first step in controlling your weight. It's also a tool for managing your blood-glucose levels, blood fats and blood pressure. This doesn't mean you have to stop eating your favourite foods or subscribe to an eccentric diet. Instead, you'll want to follow a balanced eating plan that provides a variety of foods in moderate proportions.

✅ **Get moving.** Equally important to your weight and blood glucose is physical activity. The philosophy here is similar to that of your eating – nothing extreme is necessary. You just need to get your heart and muscles into action with moderate activities that are easy to do – and keep doing. Walking is a good example of a low-impact physical activity that is easy and pleasurable. Finding a routine you enjoy and can stick with is the key.

✅ **Take advantage of treatment.** While healthy eating and regular physical activity can go a long way, medication can make the difference between struggling with too high blood-glucose levels and taking charge of your condition.

In the following chapters, you'll find out how you can use all five of these strategies to bring down your blood glucose and help you lead a full and active life.

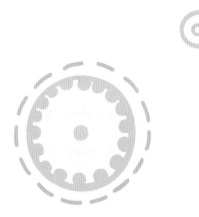

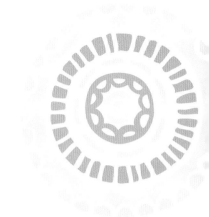

monitoring & measuring

Managing diabetes is all about vigilance. You can't know if your blood-glucose levels are where they should be unless you check them regularly. The idea of testing several times a day may seem dreary, but sophisticated tools make the task easier than you'd think, and they're getting better all the time. Along with results from other tests, your blood-glucose numbers are an all-important window on your disease and a key to managing it, and living with it, successfully.

Everything you do to treat your diabetes – whether it's physical activity, eating healthily, using insulin or taking medications – all serves one primary objective: controlling your blood-glucose levels. But how can you tell if your blood glucose is well controlled? Some people rely exclusively on their symptoms to determine how they're doing. For example, they watch for thirst and fatigue to tell them when their glucose levels are high, or trembling and dizziness to tell them when they're low. But gauging your blood glucose by symptoms alone is highly unreliable – and potentially dangerous. Blood glucose can easily soar too high or dip too low without sounding any obvious alarms, potentially leading to both short-term and long-term complications.

Fortunately, advances in blood-testing technology allow you to track your blood glucose in ways that weren't fully available to people with diabetes as recently as a generation ago. There are two basic methods for testing blood glucose, and both may need to be part of your management plan:

- Test your own blood at home (or anywhere else for that matter) using a small, portable blood-glucose meter – a method that is known as self-monitoring of blood glucose.
- See your doctor regularly to arrange regular tests, especially a haemoglobin test (HbA1c) that reveals average blood-glucose levels over the previous 10 to 12 weeks.

What you're after is crucial information, and the more precise that information is, the better. The more you know about the way your blood glucose behaves under specific circumstances, and the impact it has on your health, the more power you wield – power to control your glucose levels and, in turn, your life as a whole. Working without this information is like walking in pitch darkness without a torch – it's tough to know when you're veering off course or heading for a fall. Conscientiously monitoring your own blood glucose – and following up with regular check-ups – shines light on your diabetes, providing you with a clear perspective and allowing you to stride ahead with more freedom and confidence.

Worth the effort

Without a doubt, regular monitoring and measuring take a certain amount of dedication and discipline. Some people find it difficult. A study of over 3500 type 2 patients showed that more than a third never self-monitored their blood glucose. Yet numerous studies have shown that the people who fare best with diabetes are those who do the most to control their blood glucose with the help of careful monitoring.

One of the most important studies is the US Diabetes Control and Complications Trial (DCCT), which ended in 1993. For 10 years, it followed more than 1400 people with type 1 diabetes, comparing complications in those who closely monitored and controlled their blood glucose with those who were less vigilant. The results were that close monitoring and control reduced the risk of developing eye disease by 76 per cent, nerve disease by 60 per cent, kidney disease by 50 per cent and cardiovascular disease by 35 per cent. A more recent study called the United Kingdom Prospective Diabetes Study (UKPDS) produced similar results in people with type 2 diabetes.

Inspired by these findings, doctors have developed a form of treatment known as intensive therapy, in which patients, particularly those taking insulin or other medication, tightly control their blood glucose by carefully adjusting injections, food intake, physical activity and medications according to results from frequent self-monitoring. It's a disciplined approach that may not be right for everyone. But the idea that everyone with diabetes needs to monitor and control their blood glucose as best they can has gained wide acceptance. In fact, the DCCT and UKPDS show that any consistent reduction in blood glucose reduces the risk of complications.

No matter how much or how little blood-glucose testing you do, every bit of information you gather is valuable. You can then use this data to:

- See how different foods affect your blood glucose, so you can adjust your food intake as needed to keep glucose in check.
- Detect (or rule out) hypoglycaemia – that is, low blood glucose, the most common treatment complication in those taking insulin or some types of diabetes tablets – so you can deal with it quickly.

✸ Track the effect of medications so that you and your doctor can finetune dosages.

✸ Understand how blood-glucose levels swing when you're taking insulin or when you're sick, engaging in physical activity or drinking alcohol, so you can take steps to bring them back into line.

✸ Provide your doctor with a history of day-to-day blood-glucose changes, so you get better-informed treatment advice.

Setting blood-glucose goals

What blood-glucose readings should you aim for? First you need to know what's normal. In people without diabetes, the pancreas releases just the right amount of insulin when it's needed, allowing the body's cells to mop up glucose from the bloodstream and keep blood glucose steady at levels that rarely fall below 4 mmol/L or go above 8 mmol/L, even after eating. When you have diabetes, blood-glucose levels can vary much more widely, dropping much lower or spiking much higher than in people without diabetes. Swings will depend on the type of diabetes you have, how well your pancreas functions and other factors. Your goal is to bring these wild swings under control and attempt to keep your blood glucose as close to recommended ranges as possible.

Targets for glycaemic control

Recommended target ranges for people with diabetes may differ depending on your age, how long you have had diabetes, the type of diabetes medication and any other medication you are taking and if you have any other medical problems. It is strongly recommended that target ranges are developed for each individual in accordance with their needs and risks. Speak with your doctor and diabetes healthcare team about your individual target ranges.

For example, glucose targets for children are sometimes less stringent, while those for pregnant women may be tighter. Your goals may also depend on whether you're suffering from any complications. The bottom line is that you need to work out your own blood-glucose targets with your doctor.

If your blood-glucose levels are consistently outside your target range, you will need to work with your doctor to decide what steps to take. You may have to work more closely with your diabetes team, start taking or adjust medication or do more testing to get a better handle on your blood-glucose patterns.

What's the frequency?

How often you need to test depends mostly on what type of diabetes you have and how you're treating it.

Type 1. If you have type 1 diabetes, you're particularly sensitive to blood-glucose swings because, with the B cells in the pancreas out of commission, you rely on your insulin injections or pump to keep blood glucose in line. Balancing insulin with food, activity and other factors isn't easy, so it helps to test your blood-glucose levels several times a day (preferably at least four times), usually before and sometimes after each meal, at bedtime and occasionally overnight.

Why test before meals and not after? You already know food will make your blood glucose rise and that your insulin injection will handle it. By testing before the meal (and at bedtime), you can see how well your background insulin is maintaining blood-glucose levels between meals. This doesn't mean you should completely ignore what happens after eating. Your doctor may also advise you to take readings after meals and,

Targets for glycaemic control

Recommended target ranges for people with diabetes may differ depending on your age, how long you have had diabetes, the type of diabetes medication and any other medication you are taking and if you have any other medical problems. It is strongly recommended that target ranges are developed for each individual person in accordance with their needs and risks. Speak with your doctor and diabetes healthcare team about your individual target ranges.

TYPE 1 DIABETES[1]	
Target levels	4–8 mmol/L fasting and before meals Less than 10 mmol/L 2 hours after starting meals

TYPE 2 DIABETES[2]	
Target levels	6–8 mmol/L fasting and before meals 6–10 mmol/L 2 hours after starting meals

[1] Target ranges recommended by the National Health and Medical Research Council (NHMRC) 2011
[2] Target ranges recommended by the National Health and Medical Research Council (NHMRC) 2009

People with type 2 diabetes who are not at risk of hypoglycaemia from taking insulin or diabetes tablets that make the pancreas produce more insulin could aim for a blood-glucose level as close to the normal range as possible.

Risk of hypoglycaemia for both type 1 diabetes and type 2 diabetes	Less than 4 mmol/L – if taking insulin or certain types of diabetes tablets that make the pancreas produce more insulin. If you are unsure about what type of diabetes tablets you are taking, check with your doctor if the risk of hypoglycaemia applies to you.

A testing timetable

You'll need to work out a testing schedule with your doctor. Use these guidelines as a place to start. Check with your doctor or diabetes educator what is an acceptable blood-glucose level for you to strive for, how often you need to test and, more importantly, how to do the test accurately.

SITUATION	SUGGESTED TEST SCHEDULE
You have type 1 diabetes and take insulin.	Four times daily, before meals and at bedtime.
You have type 2 diabetes and take no insulin or medication.	One to two times daily, when you get up in the morning and 2 hours after a main meal.
You have type 2 diabetes and take insulin.	Four times daily, before meals and at bedtime.
You have type 2 diabetes and take medication.	One to four times daily, depending on control, when you get up and 2 hours after main meals.

occasionally, in the middle of the night or at different times of the day to gain added insight into your blood-glucose patterns.

Type 2. If you have type 2 diabetes, it's tougher to generalise about your testing needs. If you're managing your diabetes with healthy eating and physical activity alone, your blood levels are probably fairly stable and you may need relatively little testing – maybe twice daily, when you get up in the morning and 2 hours after a main meal. (Avoiding more frequent testing is a good reason to try to manage your diabetes through lifestyle changes.) Once you understand your blood-glucose patterns, you may find that they don't change very much, and your doctor may suggest that you scale back your testing even further – perhaps to three or four times a week.

If you're taking insulin, your testing schedule will probably need to mirror the pattern a type 1 person follows: four times daily, maybe more, depending on your situation. If you're taking diabetes medication, you should test at least twice a day. You may need to test more often, especially at the beginning, when your doctor will want to track how the drug affects your blood glucose.

For women with gestational diabetes. If you have GDM or have diabetes and then become pregnant, keeping blood-glucose levels tightly controlled is especially important for both you and the baby. This means you'll probably have to test your blood often, usually fasting (before breakfast) and 2 hours after each meal.

Five steps to success

It's natural to want to see your blood-glucose levels fall into a healthier range as soon as you start treatment. But while it's good to set ambitious goals, you also want to be realistic. Failing to hit your ideal blood-glucose goals may leave you feeling frustrated and even depressed, which can sap your motivation. To remove the failure factor:

1 Start with no specific goals in mind. Instead, gather the numbers to show you and your doctor, dietitian or diabetes educator where your blood glucose normally falls and work from there.

2 If your typical range is excessively high, don't feel you have to aim for ideal numbers right away. An unrealistic goal may erode your self-confidence and sense of control for the long term.

3 Work with your doctor or diabetes educator to set goals that are an improvement for you.

4 As you achieve greater control and start bringing your average blood-glucose levels down, consult with your doctor or diabetes educator to set new goals, gradually working your way towards healthier numbers.

5 Don't expect to be perfect. Sometimes you'll get disappointing readings for no apparent reason.

Take-charge tips

Outside of your regular blood-glucose testing regimen, it would pay to do some extra self-monitoring at certain times to protect yourself from dangerous blood-glucose highs and, especially, lows. Consider doing additional tests:

○ when you are unwell or stressed

○ before you drive and every 2 hours on a long drive

○ when you make a change in your eating plan, such as eating more or less food than usual at certain times of day

○ when a significant change is made in your insulin treatment

○ when you take medication to treat something other than diabetes

○ before you go into a meeting or other stressful situation

○ when you start a new exercise program.

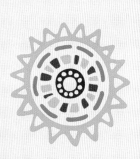

The Tao of testing

The job of self-monitoring is not great fun. New devices promise to make the task more pleasant someday in the future, but for the moment, some people find it tough getting around the inevitable fact that you need to draw blood, and to do it you need to prick yourself – usually in the finger – with a sharp instrument. Most people with diabetes find that the process eventually becomes a no-big-deal routine. Here's how to do it.

1 Wash your hands before you prick your finger. This is important as anything on the skin (such as sugar residue from handling food) can give a false high reading. Dry your hands thoroughly after washing, since excess moisture can also affect your results.

2 Put the test strip into your blood-glucose meter (if it's not built in), which, with most current meters, will turn it on. Wait for the signal that it's ready for a drop of blood.

3 Prick your finger with a pinlike device called a lancet to draw a drop of blood. If you want to prick yourself at other sites instead, that's fine. The forearms and ear lobes can be used as alternatives, although different sites can give different results. Most people find the fingertips easier, and if you are concerned about a hypo, the most reliable.

4 Apply the droplet of blood to the test strip. Most meters have capillary action strips, which draw up the blood and start the meter counting down only when sufficient blood is obtained.

Foreign policy

In Australia, New Zealand and some other countries, such as Canada, the concentration of glucose in the blood is measured in millimoles per litre, which is referred to as mmol/L. However, in the United States of America, a system of milligrams per decilitre is used and is referred to as mg/dl. If travelling in the US and your blood-glucose meter breaks, you may need to consult a doctor to check your blood glucose. A result of 80 would clearly come as a terrible shock, so it is useful to know how to make the conversion.

Simply divide the mg/dl number by 18. Therefore, your reading of 80 mg/dl is actually a healthy 4.4 mmol/L. For example, average blood-glucose goals convert this way:

Before eating:
80 to 120 mg/dl = 4.4 to 6.6 mmol/L

After eating:
less than 180 mg/dl = less than 10 mmol/L

At bedtime:
100 to 140 mg/dl = 5.5 to 7.7 mmol/L

5 Check your reading on the digital display and write down the number. You might overlook this step, but it's probably the most important. If you're trying to develop a record and identify patterns in the rise and fall of your blood-glucose levels, all the trouble you took to get the number in the first place isn't worth anything if you don't then record it, and the possible cause of variation, for future reference. Even if your meter has a memory function, it's a good idea to keep your own record. After all, anything can break. While these are general guidelines, each meter is slightly different, so follow your meter's instructions in order to ensure an accurate test result.

Four essential testing tools

It may sound odd to say so, but there's never been a better time to have diabetes. One reason is that there have never been more tools to help you monitor and manage your condition. The first self-monitoring tests didn't appear until the 1970s, and they consisted of test strips that indicated blood-glucose levels by changing into a colour that you had to compare to a colour chart for your result.

Anyone who's wallpapered or painted a room and found they misjudged the sample swatch will appreciate that a lot of guesswork could very well go into matching test-strip colours

WHAT the STUDIES show

Are the blood-glucose records you share with your doctor on the level? One study in which meters with hidden memory were used found that the numbers patients write down in diaries at home are often lower than the real results. Inaccuracies can easily occur if you forget to write down numbers immediately and have to recall them later on. But there's also a natural tendency to want to make a good report to your doctor. Researchers suggest that some people with diabetes feel guilty if they don't meet their blood-glucose goals or fail to test as often as they need to and fudge the numbers to make them look better. But being honest does the most good in the long run. Discrepancies present a flawed picture of your condition and defeat the purpose of keeping careful records.

to colour charts. Fortunately, there's now a better way. In fact, there's an array of devices to choose from. Don't be daunted by having to sort through them. Instead, rest assured that the basic task is not very difficult and with the range of choices and perhaps the guidance of your doctor or diabetes educator, you should be able to find equipment that will meet your specific needs.

Looking at lancets
Technically, the lancet is the sharp instrument that punctures your skin, while the hand-held

Figuring out features

Manufacturers try to make every meter convenient, but what's handy for you might be an obstacle for somebody else. Here's how several major features compare:

MAIN FEATURE	PROS	CONS
Built-in memory	Allows you to track your results over time. Some units also automatically average your numbers.	Some meters store as few as 10 readings – not enough if you test four times a day and see your doctor only once a month. Aim for at least a 100-reading memory.
Download capability	Can feed your readings directly into your doctor's database or into diabetes-management software, which can generate useful graphs and charts. One meter even uploads to your iPhone.	Unit may not be compatible with your doctor's software. May cost more than simpler meters and the program and cable may cost extra.
Capillary-action test strips	Soaking blood up into the test strip is easier than dropping blood down onto it.	For some people, the occasional blood overload can be messy but does not affect the result.

unit that holds the lancet is called a lancing device or finger pricker. Lancets are disposable both for sanitary reasons and because they can become blunt. Some experts recommend that they be thrown out after each use to ensure that you always use a sterile one, but many people with diabetes think this is wasteful – not to mention expensive – and reuse their lancets about four to six times. (An obvious point, that's nevertheless worth making, is that to avoid being infected you never use somebody else's lancet.)

Many glucose meters come with a finger pricker or even build them in, but you're not wedded to what the meter manufacturer provides. Instead, you need to find an instrument that's comfortable for you. (Theoretically, you can use lancets by themselves, but a finger pricker is not only easier to manipulate with either hand, it's also less painful. The reason is that finger prickers are spring-loaded so that penetration is very quick.) Because your skin may not be as thick as, say, the calloused hands of a construction worker, most devices allow you to make at least one or two adjustments to how deep the lancet penetrates your skin.

A final word to the wise: whichever unit you buy, you'll need to continually resupply your stock of lancets. Lancets are not always interchangeable from one device to the next, and costs can vary, so check out lancet price and availability before you invest in a finger pricker. Contact your state or territory diabetes organisation in Australia or discuss this with your doctor or diabetes educator.

Buying a blood-glucose meter

Meter technology and features change rapidly, and the range of choices can be bewildering, but variety means you should easily be able to find a unit that matches your needs and preferences.

Most modern blood-glucose meters work by detecting minuscule electrical currents created by the enzyme reactions, with the strength of electron flow depending on the amount of glucose present in the blood. The results are then displayed on the meter's digital readout.

To sort through the multitude of blood-glucose meters that are on the market and find one that's right for you, check first with your doctor or diabetes educator. They may be able to steer you towards a particular unit based on their experience of various meters and manufacturers, reports from other patients with diabetes or compatibility with their own record-keeping systems. Other features now available in certain meters include no-strip testing, no coding, bolus calculators for people with type 1, pre- and post-meal markers and much more. As with the table above, some people will benefit from these new features while others may not, depending entirely on individual needs and lifestyle.

Also find out if your health fund or health insurance offer a rebate on available meters. Your diabetes association also offers a wide range of blood-glucose meters for purchase plus demonstration in their use. Special rates may apply for those with a concession, pension or community services card. Contact your diabetes association for further information (see page 24). Meters can also be purchased from many societies and pharmacies. In New Zealand, Pharmac funds specific meters and test strips. Make sure you are shown how to use the different meters available so that you can choose the one that suits you best. When evaluating the choices, you should consider a number of factors, including:

Meter miscommunication

When your blood gets sent to a pathology lab to be tested, they separate the plasma from the blood cells and test only the plasma glucose concentration, and this is what is reported in your blood test results. Until recently, most blood-glucose meters have given readings for whole blood glucose, that is, plasma plus blood cells. Because red blood cells have a lower concentration of glucose than plasma, this reading is usually 10 to 15 per cent lower than the laboratory value. Most of the new meters now available, however, are calibrated to be 'plasma equivalent', which means they should give a reading similar to the laboratory value, while still using a whole blood finger prick sample. Knowing which method your meter uses will help you to compare your home-based readings with those from the pathology tests your doctor orders.

Take-charge tips

Being a 'good bleeder' is a blessing (strange as it sounds) that not everyone shares. If you find that getting blood out of your finger is akin to getting it out of a stone, try these steps to get the juice flowing better:

○ Before testing, do some light physical activity or take a warm bath to boost circulation to your fingertips. Or, if your hands are cold (which indicates low blood flow in your fingers), fill a basin with hot water and let your hands soak for a few minutes.

○ If you have an adjustable lancet, set it for deeper penetration. There's no point trying to save yourself pain with a low setting if you have to repeat the prick to get blood.

○ Swing your arms to force blood toward your fingers, then dangle your arms at your sides and shake your hands.

○ After pricking, don't try to squeeze blood out right away. Instead, hold your hand below the level of your heart and relax for a moment to let blood pool at the lancing site.

Note: For people who have toughened skin, through working as a builder or on a farm, some finger prickers have an adjustable head with depth indicator that makes them suitable for both tough and sensitive skin.

Ease of use. Meters come in different sizes and shapes and you'll want to choose one that is comfortable for you to use. Some require bigger drops of blood for an accurate result than others, which may be an issue if you have poor circulation. If you have vision problems, look for a meter that features larger displays.

The information you need. How much you need to know may depend first of all on which type of diabetes you have. If you have type 1 or type 2 and are taking insulin or medication, you'll probably be taking more readings than if you have type 2 and control your diabetes through healthy eating and physical activity.

If you're testing a lot, you may want a meter that has a built-in memory to help you keep track of the dozens of results you'll accumulate between visits to the doctor. Some allow you to mark readings as before or after a meal. Most also have data ports that allow you to download this information into diabetes-management software on a personal computer and one uploads to your iPhone or iPad. On the other hand, if you're testing only a couple of times a day or even less, these bells and whistles may be superfluous.

Practical details. Points that seem trivial at the outset can become more important to you the more you use your blood-glucose meter. Some units, for example, use standard batteries that you can find in any pharmacy or supermarket, while others take less common (and often more costly) batteries that may be harder to find. These units usually last for thousands of readings, but how many thousands will vary from one model to the next. Meters vary in size and many can fit into a small bag. Other additional features such as alarms, a back light for testing in the dark and strip-free testing can also be helpful.

Cost. Consider the initial outlay when buying a meter, as prices can vary depending on features. Some health funds will pick up the cost of a meter, but even so, manufacturers routinely offer discounts, rebates and trade-ins to get a unit into your hands. It is also wise to consider the cost of other necessary equipment such as lancets. Most blood-glucose meters come in kit form with strips and the lancet device (finger pricker) included. A further financial consideration when buying is the not-insignificant ongoing costs for meter mainten-ance, such as batteries, control-test solutions (if not supplied free by the manufacturer) and the cost of the test strips themselves. Meters generally come with a lifetime warranty. Contact your state or territory diabetes organisation in Australia (see page 24 for contact details) for more information about the cost of different meters currently available on the market and the features that they offer. Also ask about whether there are any special offers available.

Replacing test strips

Test strips are an ongoing expense that equates to a significant amount each year, especially if you're testing four or more times a day. However, in Australia their cost is heavily subsidised under the National Diabetes Services Scheme (NDSS), which is funded by the Federal Government to assist people with diabetes in managing their disease. Under the

Take-charge tips

You can't completely avoid the nip of the finger pricker's tip, but you can minimise the discomfort if you:

○ Use mild soap and warm water instead of alcohol to cleanse hands before testing. Mild soaps dry your hands less and ease stinging, especially if you tend to use the same site. Warm water brings more blood to your fingertips, making it easier to extract a drop.

○ Use an adjustable lancing device so that you can set the penetration depth to match the toughness of your skin.

○ Prick on the sides of your fingers towards the tip, where there are fewer nerve endings but plenty of blood vessels.

○ Finish up by putting a little bit of hand lotion on the prick site to soothe your skin and keep it moist and pliable.

NDSS, strips are the same price for all meters. To register, contact your state or territory diabetes organisation in Australia (see page 24 for contact details).

Once you've started using your system, be aware that test strips have a limited shelf life; using them past their expiry date can give you inaccurate readings and many meters now have a built-in safety mechanism to prevent out-of-date strips from being used. When you buy replacements, you'll find them packaged in different ways – usually in packages of 50 or 100, depending on the meter.

Logbook enlightenment

Most self-monitoring systems provide a logbook in which you can record your results. Recording your blood-glucose levels so that you can track patterns is one of the main reasons you self-monitor. You may be able to get new pages by contacting the meter manufacturer, using the contact details in your instructions. If you don't like the log that comes with your meter, your doctor, diabetes educator or diabetes organisation may have one that meets your needs better by including space to write about medication, insulin or other tests. Or you can simply use a diary to record your numbers (although logbooks provide ready-made columns that may prove more convenient and legible). Whatever kind of log you use, the crucial thing is to get your numbers down on paper – including the date and time of each reading. Don't settle for just numbers, though. Remember, you're looking for patterns and associations, making yourself the subject of a little scientific study – and good scientists take

lots of notes. Write down anything unusual about what you eat and drink, how active you are, if you are unwell or if you are under a lot of stress. These are the observations that a glucose meter can't store in its memory.

Take your logbook with you whenever you go and see your doctor, dietitian or diabetes educator, so that together you can assess fluctuations in your blood-glucose readings and discuss whether adjustments need to be made to your treatment. If your doctor queries a particular reading, for example, 'Was anything unusual going on 2 weeks ago Friday?', your logbook might provide valuable clues.

Five steps to reliable results

To do their job, glucose-monitoring systems need to be accurate, but even more important, they need to be consistent. (Even if your readings are off by a certain amount, if you know this and the degree of error is always the same, you can still get a good sense of your blood-glucose levels.) Here's how to make sure you're getting reliable results:

1 **Calibrate.** Each batch of test strips you buy may have slight chemical variations from other batches, and these can affect your readings, so you need to match your meter to each set of strips before using them. Some meters do this automatically; others need to be calibrated every time you open a new box of strips. Check the directions for either your meter or your test strips to learn how.

2 Check your strips. If your readings seem strangely inconsistent from one day to the next or out of tune with how you feel, you may have a faulty batch of test strips. Check the expiry date to see if they're too old and examine individual packages for damage. Check to make sure the strip is the right one for your meter. Storing strips away from heat, air and moisture is also important.

3 Do a self-critique. Could it possibly be that the problem lies with you? Review the meter's directions and think about your technique. Is there anything you're doing that could throw off results? Have you washed your hands before starting the test? Are you placing the strip into the meter facing the right way? Are you putting the same amount of blood onto the strip each time you test? (Insufficient blood will give a falsely low reading with some meters so it's important to be as consistent as possible with the size of the drop of blood you place on the strip.) Check whether you are using the right type of strip for your particular meter, as this may also have an adverse effect on the accuracy of your blood-glucose reading. If you change meters, make sure that the strips you may have left over from the old meter are still good for the new one.

4 Check the meter. Maybe your meter just needs a 'freshening-up', although most meters no longer need cleaning as blood does not come into contact with the meter. Also, most meters now have a low-battery warning signal.

5 Call the manufacturer. If your metering results seem chronically out of whack and you can't resolve the problem on your own, call your unit's customer service hotline. In some cases, manufacturers will replace unsatisfactory meters at no charge.

Advances in testing technology

Self-monitoring technology has come a long way over recent years, but even so, it's hard to be satisfied with a routine that's painful, no matter how much you might get used to it. Manufacturers have long sought ways to take the sting out of self-testing procedures and have recently made several advances. These improvements don't eliminate the need for regular self-testing, but they can reduce the number of finger pricks you need for self-monitoring or make them more comfortable.

Home testing remains the most effective tool in diabetes management and in avoiding long-term complications. It is the most immediate way of knowing your blood-glucose levels at any time of the day and your diabetes team needs this information to continue to guide you in effectively managing your diabetes. By being responsible for keeping track of your blood-glucose levels you may well feel a sense of 'being in control' and further develop the team approach to the management of your diabetes. Despite all the positives, however, manufacturers continue to work hard at overcoming the discomfort and inconvenience that surrounds the home-testing procedure.

Less-sensitive sites. Some meters require less blood than the globule you extract from your fingertip using a standard lancet, thanks in part to siphon-style (also known as capillary) test strips that you can touch to the blood. Because you don't have to squeeze out a big drop of blood, the finger prickers that come with some meters allow you to obtain blood from other places, such as the forearm or thigh, that are less sensitive than the fingertips. But it is important to know that testing at alternative sites may give results that are different from the blood-glucose levels obtained from the fingertip. The reason for this is that blood-glucose levels in the fingertips show changes more quickly than those at alternate testing sites. This means that alternate site testing is less accurate, particularly at times when your blood glucose is changing more rapidly, such as after a meal, following exercise or when you are experiencing hypoglycaemia (a low blood-glucose level).

No-prick meters. A continuous glucose monitor (CGM) is a device that measures glucose levels every 1 to 5 minutes continuously throughout the day and night. Two types are currently available. One gives a 'real-time' read-out allowing you to see what your glucose level is from minute to minute. The other one you wear for a few days and take back to your doctor, who can download the results to get a better picture of your blood-glucose control and any day to day fluctuations.

This type of monitoring can help in finetuning your blood-glucose control, particularly if you are having difficulties determining the reasons for fluctuating levels. While these devices are now available in Australia they are expensive, particularly the ongoing cost of sensors, and are not covered by private health insurance or government subsidies, making the cost prohibitive for most people to use from day to day. Hopefully this will change in the future, as research has shown that they can help people with type 1 diabetes to achieve better blood-glucose control while reducing the risk of hypoglycaemia.

Highs and lows: why they happen and how to fix them

You wouldn't need to monitor your blood-glucose levels throughout the day if not for the inconvenient fact that they change. Figuring out what makes them go up and down is key to keeping them under control.

Food: the blood-glucose source

Glucose from food makes blood glucose go up within an hour or two of eating a meal, but the extent and speed of the rise can depend on what you eat and how much – and also on how insulin resistant you are. Testing will help you gauge your responses to different foods.

✅ **Adjust your meal plan.** If the meals you've worked out with your dietitian fail to keep your blood glucose under control, you

Treating hypoglycaemia

If monitoring reveals that your blood glucose has dropped below 3.5 to 4 mmol/L, your glucose level is too low. This is called hypoglycaemia, or 'hypo' for short. This can occur if you are taking some types of diabetes tablets but is mainly a side effect of taking insulin. Don't wait for symptoms such as mental confusion, rapid heartbeat, sweating or double vision to occur before you act – they often don't kick in until blood glucose drops dangerously low. The level at which you experience a hypo may vary so regular testing of your blood glucose is important.

Step 1 Start by taking 15 g of a fast-acting carbohydrate to raise the blood glucose as quickly as possible. Discuss suitable treatments with your diabetes educator or dietitian so you are prepared. Examples of fast-acting carbohydrate are:

- glucose tablets or powder; glucose gels or instant glucose

- jelly beans

- sugar-sweetened soft drink (not diet drinks)

- 2 heaped (3 level) teaspoons of honey

Step 2 Wait 5 to 10 minutes. If your symptoms are still present, your level is still too low and you need more glucose to raise it into the healthy range. Retest and repeat Step 1. You may need to continue to monitor your blood glucose and treat your hypo until your levels reach a healthy range, above 4 mmol/L.

Step 3 You need to have a longer-acting carbohydrate to stabilise your blood glucose unless your next meal is within 15 to 20 minutes. Examples are:

- a dense, grainy bread sandwich

- a tub of yogurt

- a glass of milk

- a piece of fruit

may need to go back to the drawing board. You could be getting too many total carbohydrates in a sitting or eating too many high-GI foods – which raise blood glucose faster and higher than other types of food – at once. Mealtime monitoring will help you determine how your blood glucose changes in response to what you eat, and this will provide your diabetes team with the information they need to guide you to better choices. Your doctor may consider increasing your medications or insulin.

✓ **Be consistent.** Talk to your dietitian about the glycaemic index (GI) – a method of ranking carbohydrate in foods according to their effect on blood glucose. You'll probably be advised to

> **? DID you KNOW...**
>
> While most types of physical activity lower blood glucose, some forms of physical stress, such as illness or even sunburn, can raise it. Be sure to wear sunscreen regularly, especially if you take certain diabetes medications, which can make your skin more sensitive to the sun.

include at least one low-GI food in each meal. The better you manage the glucose going into your body, the better you'll be able to predict, and control, the rise and fall of your blood glucose.

✔ **Limit alcohol.** If you drink, try to have a maximum of 2 standard drinks a day, and always with food. It's also a good idea to aim for a couple of alcohol-free days each week. Alcohol can lower blood glucose, putting you at risk of hypoglycaemia and making it harder to detect hypo symptoms. And mixed drinks may be high in added sugar and kilojoules, which will contribute to weight gain.

✔ **Consider medication.** If your meter readings indicate you're having trouble keeping your blood glucose in line through healthy eating and physical activity, your doctor may increase your oral medication.

Physical activity: the glucose gobbler

Moving your muscles boosts the body's fuel consumption. The result being that glucose

levels tend to drop when you're physically active. Overall, this is a good thing and monitoring can provide insight into ways in which you can use physical activity to lower your blood glucose. Work with your doctor or educator to figure out how physical activity should factor into your overall approach to diabetes management.

✔ **Adjust your medication regimen.** Strenuous physical activity can sometimes lower blood glucose for up to 24 hours afterwards. If you're tightly controlling your glucose with insulin or medication, your post-activity monitoring may suggest that you lower your dosages to avoid hypoglycaemia. Ask your doctor or diabetes educator for specific advice and how to adjust your regimen accordingly.

✔ **Tank up ahead of time.** If you're planning to exercise vigorously, you may want to eat more food earlier in the day or take less insulin to make sure you have enough glucose readily available to fuel working muscles. Aim to work out an hour or two after eating, when blood glucose will be naturally higher. However, if you are taking insulin with a meal, this is when it is acting at its peak, thereby increasing the risk of a hypo.

✔ **Keep well fuelled afterwards.** Depending on how strenuous your physical activity session has been, it might be a good idea to increase your food intake for up to 24 hours after being active, to make sure blood-glucose levels don't fall too low. If weight loss is one of your goals, eating more food won't help you achieve this. Discuss this with your dietitian to establish a suitable plan to help you achieve your weight-loss goals.

✅ **Use activity as medicine.** If you're taking insulin and understand through monitoring how physical activity affects your blood glucose, you may find it possible to use physical activity to reduce your insulin requirements. Talk to your doctor or diabetes educator before adjusting your medication regimen.

✅ **Be alert to the unexpected.** Certain types of vigorous physical activity – weight lifting, for example – that unlock glucose stored in muscles can make blood glucose go up rather than down. Your doctor or diabetes educator can suggest how you might adjust insulin or medication treatments accordingly.

Insulin: finetuning the control

If you're taking insulin, the point is to keep blood glucose within an acceptable range, but hypoglycaemia can occur if your injections take your levels too low. On the other hand, you may experience hyper-glycaemia if your doses are improperly timed. Monitoring can help you figure out how to use insulin to keep glucose levels steady.

✅ **Inject earlier to bring down highs.** People taking a rapid-acting insulin, such as Humalog and Novorapid or Apidra, should inject 15 minutes or less before eating. People taking regular (intermediate- or long-acting) insulin normally inject about 30 to 45 minutes before a meal. But if monitoring shows that your blood-glucose levels tend to be high either before or about an hour after you eat, you may want to add more time between injecting and eating to give the insulin a better chance to bring glucose levels down. You might also do something active for a similar effect.

✅ **Adjust the timing of your insulin.** If your blood glucose tends to be on the low side 30 to 45 minutes before you have a meal, you may want to wait until you're closer to eating before injecting insulin to keep blood glucose from dropping lower. If you take rapid-acting insulin, you could wait until you start or are halfway through your meal before injecting, rather than waiting the usual 15 minutes.

✅ **Add small snacks.** People who take insulin or certain tablets may be advised to eat a small amount of carbohydrate (such as a piece of fruit) around mid-morning and mid-afternoon to help keep blood-glucose levels steady between meals. Ask your dietitian or diabetes educator for specific advice about what's best for you.

Illness: you're low, glucose is high

Illness and the stress that sometimes precipitates it can boost blood-glucose levels by stimulating the release of hormones that work against the action of insulin and cause glucose to be released from storage sites in the muscles and liver. Naturally, you mainly need to treat the illness, but you also need to take some extra steps to keep your blood-glucose levels down.

✅ **Drink more water.** If blood glucose is higher than usual, your kidneys are probably working harder and producing more urine. The result is that you become dehydrated from the unusually high urine output. Keep adequately hydrated by drinking at least a cup of water every half hour.

✅ **Avoid exercise.** Even if you think it might bring your blood-glucose level lower, there's the possibility that physical activity will raise your blood-glucose levels. In any case, it's more important that you rest in order to fight the illness.

✅ **Consider adjusting insulin.** If you're taking insulin, ask your doctor if and when you need to take additional or increased doses while you're sick.

Morning: the dawn phenomenon

You'd think blood glucose would be low when you wake up. After all, you've gone an entire night without food. Often, however, blood glucose is high in the morning. The reason is that your body clock triggers the release of hormones that inhibit insulin so that more glucose is available to the body at the start of the new day. This is natural and not necessarily a problem. But if monitoring reveals that your blood glucose becomes excessively high in the morning, consult your doctor or diabetes educator about what actions you can take.

✅ **Take insulin later.** If you're using insulin and take an evening dose, you may find it works better to inject it closer to bedtime for longer-lasting control during the night.

✅ **Ask about a bedtime snack.** Ask your dietitian if a bedtime snack is recommended.

✅ **Always start the day with breakfast.** Try and always start every day with breakfast, even if your blood-glucose level is high. A high-fibre, low-GI cereal with fruit is an excellent choice for breakfast.

✅ **Be active in the evening.** Because the glucose-lowering effects of physical activity can last for many hours, taking a walk shortly after dinner can help keep your blood-glucose levels under control the following morning.

Getting the whole story

Self-monitoring tells you a lot about how your blood glucose is being controlled, but it doesn't give you the entire picture. Each reading you take is a snapshot that shows what your blood glucose was like at that moment. It could be different 10 minutes later. That's like knowing that a lift was on a certain floor at a given moment when your real concern is that it should operate only within a certain range of floors. You need an indication of where the lift is the rest of the time, too. That's where additional tests can help. The most important of these are:

HbA1c. This test indicates what your average blood-glucose levels have been like over a period of between 2 to 3 months, making it an invaluable tool. Your doctor may recommend that you take this test every 3 to 6 months.

The test provides long-term results, not because it measures blood glucose per se, but because of its effect on a particular type of haemoglobin. Found in red blood cells, haemoglobin is a substance that carries oxygen through the bloodstream and clears away carbon dioxide. During red blood cells' roughly 4-month life span, glucose gradually 'sticks' to haemoglobin in a process known as glycosylation (the HbA1c test is sometimes referred to as a glycosylated haemoglobin test). The build-up of blood glucose in haemoglobin reflects how high your blood glucose has been on the whole during that time.

A caveat: glucose attaches itself slowly, so any wild swings in blood glucose you might experience won't be detected – they'll just show up as tame-looking averages in this test. In other words, the HbA1c test doesn't tell the whole story, either. But together, self-monitoring and the HbA1c test provide a good overall view of your blood glucose.

For many years, results from the HbA1c test were measured on a percentage scale from 4 to 13 per cent, with the recommendation that HbA1c be kept below 7 per cent. In 2011, the method of measuring HbA1c results changed from percentage to the new international units of mmol/mol. The recommended target is below 53 mmol/mol (= 7 per cent). Discuss this new form of measurement with your doctor or diabetes educator to be sure you are completely clear about your results.

Fructosamine. Like the HbA1c test, the fructosamine test looks at how much blood glucose builds up in components of your blood. But it uses proteins as a measure, particularly a protein called albumin. This test isn't used as widely as the HbA1c because the results are substantially similar, with one important difference: the fructosamine test measures blood glucose over a period of 2 to 3 weeks. It's a useful 'bridge' between your short-term home glucose tests and the long-term HbA1c. Your doctor may order a fructosamine test for an intermediate check on your progress if you make a change in your insulin or medication, or if you're pregnant.

Four more important tests

While blood-glucose monitoring is a critical part of diabetes management, it's not the only way to keep tabs on your condition – and your risk of complications. These four tests provide important information about your diabetes and overall health.

Urine ketones. If self-monitoring shows your blood glucose is over 15 mmol/L, it's possible you're at risk of ketoacidosis, the condition in which glucose-starved cells burn fat for fuel, releasing acidic ketones into the blood. You can check for ketones at home, with a urine or blood test, providing you have a blood-glucose meter that also tests for ketones. The results

When to have check-ups

To track your diabetes and its potential complications, you need to have regular check-ups that include the relevant tests outlined below, unless otherwise recommended. In New Zealand, every person with diabetes (type 1 or type 2) is entitled to a free annual review. This includes weight, blood pressure, foot examination, your general health and your plan to stay well, plus a check to see that your regular blood tests and eye checks are up to date.

Every doctor's visit
- blood pressure
- weight

Every 3 or 6 months
- HbA1c (average blood glucose): every 3 months for those with type 1 diabetes

- HbA1c (average blood glucose): every 6 months for those with type 2 diabetes

Every 6 months
- foot examination

Once a year
- cholesterol and triglycerides

- eye examination (the back of the retina). If your eyes are showing no sign of damage, this will occur every 2 years.

- urine microalbumin (kidneys)

indicate whether ketones are present in your body. You should also check for ketones if you experience such symptoms as deep or rapid breathing, nausea or vomiting, fever, or stomach pain. Ketoacidosis is a dangerous condition that occurs in people with type 1 diabetes. If you get a positive result, call your doctor immediately.

Lipids. At least once a year you need to get this blood test, which measures a variety of lipids, or fats, in the blood that can raise your risk of cardiovascular disease. Because people with diabetes have a significantly higher than average risk of heart disease, it's especially important to know your blood-lipid levels. The key lipids you're testing for are:

✸ **LDL, or 'bad', cholesterol.** This waxy substance can accumulate and harden on artery walls, interfering with the flow of blood and eventually causing a heart attack or stroke. When you have diabetes, your LDL cholesterol should be less than 2.5 mmol/L (Australia), or less than 2 mmol/L (New Zealand).

✸ **HDL, or 'good', cholesterol.** This beneficial form of cholesterol helps rid the body of the other form by scouring artery walls and ushering deposits of LDL to the liver and out of the body. High levels of HDL are good. (Don't settle for a test that gives you only total cholesterol, which won't reveal the critical ratio between good and bad cholesterol.) Your HDL should be at least 1 mmol/L.

Numbers to know

Recommended target ranges may differ depending on the individual. Therefore it is important to speak with your doctor and diabetes healthcare team about your individual target ranges.

Recommended blood glucose before eating	4 to 8 mmol/L (type 1) 6 to 8 mmol/L (type 2)
Recommended blood glucose after eating	less than 10 mmol/L (type 1)* 6 to 10 mmol/L (type 2)*
Recommended blood glucose at bedtime	7 mmol/L
Blood glucose that indicates hypoglycaemia for those at risk	4 mmol/L or lower
Blood glucose that merits a ketone test	15 mmol/L or higher
HbA1c target	7 per cent or lower; 53 mmol/mol
Recommended total cholesterol	4 mmol/L or lower
Recommended LDL cholesterol	2.5 mmol/L or lower (less than 1.7 mmol/L in New Zealand)
Recommended HDL cholesterol	1 mmol/L or higher
Recommended triglycerides	less than 2 mmol/L (less than 1.7 mmol/L in New Zealand)
Recommended blood pressure	130/80 mmHg or lower

* 2 hours after starting the meal

Triglycerides. Most of the fat you consume is made up of triglycerides, a type of lipid that cells can store for energy later on. High triglyceride levels make your blood thicker and more likely to clot. Yours should be less than 2 mmol/L (Australia), or less than 1.7 mmol/L (New Zealand).

Cardiovascular disease. Rather than looking at individual risk factors, this assessment calculates your risk of developing cardiovascular disease over the next 5 years based on a combination of risk factors, including sex, age, blood pressure, cholesterol and having diabetes.

Blood pressure. You should have your blood pressure recorded every time you visit your doctor. It indicates how hard your heart is working to pump blood throughout your body. If your blood pressure is high, your heart is working harder than it should, placing too much stress on blood vessels. The complications that can result are similar to those of diabetes itself – including damage to the kidneys, nerves and eyes. Current blood-pressure target levels for people with diabetes are below 130/80 millimetres of mercury (mmHg) or below 140/90 mmHg in the elderly – a 2-part reading that reflects the force the heart exerts against the walls of the arterial blood vessels when contracting (known as the systolic pressure, which is reflected in the high number of your blood pressure reading) and the residual pressure within the arteries between heartbeats (the diastolic pressure, which is indicated by the low number of your complete reading). For people with diabetes who have kidney disease, current target levels are below 125/75 mmHg.

Urine microalbumin. This test can detect kidney damage – a common complication of diabetes – at its earliest stages. The test looks for minuscule quantities of a protein called albumin, which normally remains within the bloodstream but shows up in the urine when the kidneys are having trouble filtering wastes properly. If you have type 2 diabetes, you will have a urine microalbumin test on diagnosis and then annually. If you have type 1 diabetes and were adult at the time of diagnosis, you can wait 5 years after diagnosis before the first test, as it's unlikely your kidneys were silently damaged before that time.

A positive urine microalbumin result may qualify you as a candidate for additional treatment – perhaps with a blood pressure–lowering medication, since high blood pressure can narrow the arteries leading to the kidneys and damage the delicate blood vessels inside them.

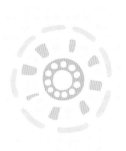

PASSING THE TEST

Maggie, 41, had a family history of diabetes, so she knew she was at higher risk. 'When I noticed I was making frequent trips to the toilet and I was unusually tired for no good reason, I made an appointment with my doctor for a check-up', says Maggie. Not surprisingly (at least to her, then 37 years old), blood tests led to a diagnosis of type 2 diabetes, a prescription for a glucose-lowering drug – and also a wholehearted effort at self-education.

While gathering information from the Internet, Maggie read about the HbA1c test that reveals glucose build-up in haemoglobin over a period of time. 'My doctor hadn't told me about the HbA1c yet – I asked him about it', says Maggie, who considers the test one of her most important tools for controlling her diabetes. Her first HbA1c result was a disturbing 8.9 per cent (75 mmol/mol), well above the recommended level. Having watched her mother suffer with numerous complications, including heart disease, Maggie became determined to control her diabetes. While continuing to monitor her blood glucose each day, her goals focused on improving what, to her, was like a school test and report card all rolled into one: the HbA1c results. 'I started making changes to my eating habits and exercising more seriously.'

A self-professed couch potato, she began using a treadmill and stationary bike, alternating gym days with 30 minutes of walking. She also took a hard look at the number of kilojoules she consumed and decided she was getting too much of some good things. One large daily serving of rice became a smaller portion, and she increased her consumption of coloured vegetables.

'Six months later, my next HbA1c reinforced my work – it was at 5.7 per cent (40 mmol/mol), which is better than normal', Maggie says. 'I get the test every 6 months, and it continues to bolster my efforts.'

Maggie is now something of a crusader for the HbA1c. 'Every time I find out someone has diabetes, the first thing I ask is "What's your HbA1c?" It seems to me that a lot of people just don't know about this test', she says. One of her converts is her husband. He also has diabetes and keeps track of his HbA1c as well. Maggie says she had to buy a bigger handbag for herself and a carry pack for her husband to be sure they always carry a healthy snack as well as their blood-glucose meters and food diaries. 'There are so many tools available to help stay on top of diabetes, and they're affordable. We just don't have any excuses for not using them.'

> *'...there are so many tools available to help stay on top of diabetes...'*

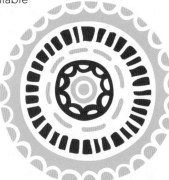

CHAPTER 4
----

eat *to manage* diabetes

Having diabetes is not about never being able to enjoy your favourite foods again. It's about adopting healthy eating principles, which apply to everyone, whether or not they have diabetes. It's also about striking a careful balance. By following a personalised meal plan, you can manage your weight and your blood-glucose levels. Don't think of it as a 'diet', as such, but as a permanent path to better health.

The fact that food is a key part of managing diabetes is no surprise. After all, glucose comes from food, so it makes sense that what you eat plays a role in making your blood glucose go up. But you shouldn't think of food as the problem. Instead, consider it a big part of the solution.

The right eating plan could actually reduce the risk of complications of the disease. If you take insulin or other medication, it could help you reduce your dose. For people with type 1 diabetes, healthy eating can help you better manage your condition.

If you think having diabetes means a no-fun 'diabetic diet' of flavourless meals, and all your favourite foods forbidden, think again. The truth is, a healthy eating plan for a person with diabetes is not very different from a healthy eating plan for anybody else. Although for many years the medical establishment recommended a restricted eating plan for people with diabetes – especially when it came to sugar – research has shown that sugar is not the villain it was once thought to be. The emphasis now is on choices, and some choices are better than others, whether you have diabetes or not. Healthy eating is suitable for everybody, so there is no need to prepare separate meals for you or your family. It is recommended that the bulk of your food come from fruits, vegetables, wholegrain cereals, low-fat dairy products, healthy fats (for example, olive oil, avocado, nuts and seeds) and lean meat or meat alternatives. You don't need to buy special expensive foods.

Your 'eat to manage' game plan

How do you eat to manage diabetes? The goal is to manage blood glucose while getting the right balance of nutrients for good health. But exactly what that means for you will depend on a host of factors. To plot a strategy that will work for you:

✅ **Consult a dietitian.** Your doctor can refer you to an Accredited Practising Dietition (APD) (Australia) or a registered dietitian (New Zealand), who will evaluate your current eating plan and make suggestions based on what, when and how much you like to eat. Don't worry that a dietitian will only give you a list of rules. You may find instead that you have a great deal of flexibility. For example, if your cultural style of eating includes a lot of beans and rice, your dietitian can help make sure those staples remain by, say, limiting the portions that you have per meal, spreading your consumption out over the course of the day or suggesting better varieties. You can access a dietitian through your local hospital or community health service or privately. For people with diabetes in Australia, you may be able to claim a rebate for up to five visits a year from Medicare if your GP refers you under a Team Care Arrangement, but there is usually a gap to pay. You can also claim back rebates from a private health fund if you have 'extras' cover for dietetics. To find an APD or registered dietitian in your area, visit www.daa.asn.au or www.dietitians.org.nz.

✅ **Keep a food diary.** Before you see your dietitian for the first time, keep a log of each morsel – no matter how small – that you eat and drink every day for at least a week. Also write down where you ate a particular food and what you were doing at the time (including exercise). This will help your dietitian find patterns that may reveal the other 'w' – why you eat. If, for example, you often go out with colleagues after work, your dietitian won't want to eliminate this sort of social and business eating, but they may suggest that you nibble on small amounts of pretzels or mixed nuts instead of potato chips. Keeping a record of what you eat and drink will also heighten your own awareness of your eating habits, and help you to find ways you can change.

For your diary, keep a small notebook handy throughout the day so you can jot down what you eat right away. Some people make their notes in digital planners such as their smart phone or iPad, and there are even some websites and apps that can make this easier. If taking notes at every sitting is inconvenient, you can try to reconstruct your food consumption at the end of the day; the record will be valuable even if you forget an item here or there.

✅ **Factor in your blood glucose.** Also show your dietitian your log of daily blood-glucose readings so your glucose levels can be compared to your eating patterns. When you are first diagnosed with diabetes, it is recommended that you test your blood-glucose level at least three times a day. Include fasting readings before breakfast and again 2 hours after meals. Comparing the two will indicate how much your blood glucose tends to rise in response to food, and will help determine when and how much of what you should eat. Some people can manage simply by eating three balanced meals a day and cutting back on the kilojoules in sweets and savoury snacks; others need to follow a more detailed eating plan.

✅ **Put it all together.** Once you and your dietitian have a grasp of your eating and blood-glucose patterns, it's time to decide on recommendations for specific foods you can eat at each meal or snack. This process is part negotiation and part analysis, and it involves other variables that have to be factored in:

❋ **Your weight.** Reaching and maintaining a healthy weight is a key goal in managing your diabetes.

❋ **Activity habits.** Physical activity typically makes blood glucose go down, so how much you do – and when – will affect the amount of kilojoules and carbohydrate you should take in at each meal.

❋ **Insulin use.** If you have type 1, the amount and timing of your insulin injections need to be balanced with the amount of food you eat. If you have type 2 and are using insulin, you'll need to factor this in on top of variables (such as weight and physical activity) that affect insulin resistance.

❋ **Medication use.** What you take, how much and when its action peaks may affect your dietary choices.

❋ **Special considerations.** Be sure to inform your dietitian of results of tests for lipids (such as cholesterol), blood pressure and microalbumin (for kidney function). If you already have high cholesterol and high blood pressure, you will be following a healthy eating plan that includes even less saturated fat. You'll also have to cut back further on salt and eat more potassium-containing foods such as fruit and vegetables. If you have kidney damage, you may have to restrict your protein intake as part of your eating plan.

✅ **Consistency is key.** Once you've developed a plan, you'll keep your blood glucose more stable if you eat about the same amount of food with the same balance of nutrients at about the same times each day. Don't think that you can be 'bad' on some days as long as you're 'good' on others. Eating in erratic patterns only causes blood glucose to seesaw. Instead, try to come up with a healthy eating plan you can live with all the time.

✅ **How's it working?** Self-monitoring your blood glucose will give you, your dietitian and your doctor a sense of how well you're able to manage it with healthy eating. From there, you and your healthcare team can then finetune your plan of attack by tinkering with your meal plan or changing your activity level, insulin dosage or other variables. If you have type 2 and you're having trouble keeping your blood glucose in line through healthy eating and physical activity, you may be a candidate for oral medications or insulin. But if you've managed to lose weight and control your blood glucose through healthy eating and physical activity, your doctor may be confident you can continue without insulin or medication for some time.

Remember: kilojoules count

If you have type 2 diabetes, how much you eat is just as important as what you eat. One of the most significant goals of your meal plan may be to lose weight – if that's what you've been advised to do. To help you accomplish that, your dietitian will want to establish the number of kilojoules you need to eat in one day.

Weight management is essentially an energy-management issue: to maintain your current weight, you must take in only as much energy – measured in kilojoules – as you burn. (One calorie equals 4.2 kilojoules.) If you want to lose weight, on the other hand, you need to take in fewer kilojoules, burn more kilojoules or both.

Dropping kilos is essential for most people with type 2 diabetes because the more fat you carry around your waist, the more your cells become resistant to insulin. When you lose excess weight, your cells' response to insulin improves, and they become better able to take in glucose and remove it from your blood. Just as vital, losing weight reduces your risk of cardiovascular disease by lowering blood pressure and improving your ratio of good to bad cholesterol.

A major US clinical trial published in 2002 clearly proved the importance of weight loss in helping to prevent the development of type 2 diabetes in people with pre-diabetes. Called the Diabetes Prevention Program, it studied more than 3200 adults at 27 medical centres who had pre-diabetes and therefore were at high risk of developing type 2 diabetes. Some of the subjects were given the blood glucose–reducing medication metformin (Glucophage), while others were put in a weight-loss group whose goal was to drop 7 per cent of their excess weight. (A third group got a placebo.) The drug was helpful, reducing the risk of developing diabetes by 31 per cent, but the weight-loss results blew the medication numbers away, reducing diabetes risk by a huge 58 per cent.

Studies suggest that you can make significant gains in blood-glucose control by losing as little as 5 per cent of your body weight. For a person who weighs 79 kilograms, that's 4 kilograms – an achievable goal.

How many kilojoules should you eat?

Everybody's kilojoule needs are different and based on a variety of factors, including age, gender, body weight, metabolism and activity level. Your dietitian will help to develop an eating plan that meets your kilojoule require-ments, but how many kilojoules do you need to eat in order to lose weight? A kilogram of fat contains about 34,700 kilojoules, so it stands to reason that a healthy lifestyle that includes regular physical activity and fewer kilojoules than you are presently taking in will result in weight loss.

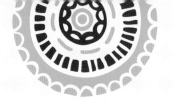

SEVEN DIET MYTHS

Weight loss can be difficult, no thanks to popular misconceptions that have the ring of truth but can actually work against you. Among the more common myths:

1 Desserts are forbidden

The truth is, there's room in your eating plan for any kind of food, especially small amounts of the ones you love most – as long as you control your total energy intake. Denying yourself your favourite foods can lead to binge eating and, ultimately, contribute to your feeling discouraged about your meal plan.

2 You have to lose a lot of weight to make a difference

The closer you can get to your ideal weight, the better, but small, sustained improvements at the beginning of a weight-loss program have the biggest impact on your health. Studies show that losing just 3 to 5 kilograms can improve insulin resistance enough to allow some people with type 2 diabetes to reduce medication or insulin injections.

3 What you eat matters more than how much

Both matter, but research shows that the number of kilojoules in your food is more important than where they come from. For example, a bagel might seem healthier than a small roll, but dense bagels have the kilojoule content of two small rolls. As long as you're not eating too much fat in other foods, the small roll wins.

4 If you exercise, you can eat whatever you want

That's robbing Peter to pay Paul. You can't lose weight if you reduce kilojoules in one way but increase them in another.

5 Skipping meals makes you lose weight fast

Actually, studies show that people who skip breakfast tend to be heavier than people who don't. And skipping meals tends to make you overeat later. If you have diabetes, it's important to keep up a steady intake of small portions of food throughout the day to keep your blood-glucose levels stable and reduce the risk of hypoglycaemia.

6 Carbohydrate is fattening

If you are insulin resistant, your body may find it easier to convert carbohydrate kilojoules to fat than to burn it as energy, but the fact remains that starches (and sugars) are less dense in kilojoules gram for gram than fats. The main issue is kilojoules, so if you load carbohydrate foods with fat – sour cream and butter on a baked potato – or eat them in large quantities (for example, soft drinks) the kilojoule load can add up.

7 You should never eat fast food

Never say never. Fast food can be worked into your meal plan if you choose well. Opt for grilled foods instead of fried, avoid or scrape away high-fat condiments like mayonnaise, and share those hot chips to keep portion size down.

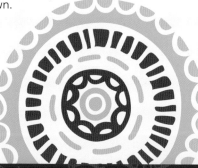

The Recommended Daily Intake provides estimates of the amount of kilojoules required for different people. It is estimated that a man who weighs 70 kilograms has an energy requirement of about 10,400 kilojoules per day. A woman who weighs about 58 kilograms has an energy requirement of about 7600 kilojoules per day. (This is assuming that they are moderately active.)

If your eating plan is designed to help you lose weight, you'll be simply decreasing your energy intake (food) and increasing your energy output (physical activity). The minimum energy intake that provides all of our nutritional needs has been calculated at 5000 kilojoules per day for women, while 6500 kilojoules is recommended for men. A reduction in this level will result in weight loss for most people. However, you must eat a variety of healthy foods at such a low kilojoule intake or you will be placing yourself at risk of developing nutritional deficiencies.

It's also important to distribute your kilojoule intake throughout the day. You may like to take 1000 kilojoules at each meal and the remaining 1000 kilojoules as snacks, which will also contribute to managing your hunger and blood-glucose levels.

What's on the menu?

Surprisingly, all of the foods you eat, from apples to zucchini, fall into only a handful of basic nutrient categories that make up the building blocks of your eating plan. While total kilojoules are a major consideration,

it also matters which building blocks those kilojoules are made of. Why? Because while most food raises your blood glucose within an hour or two of eating, the height and speed of that increase depends on how much and what types of foods you consume.

Food is made up of nutrients that contain kilojoules. Carbohydrate contains 16 kilojoules per gram, protein 17 kilojoules per gram and fat 37 kilojoules per gram. Alcohol is not a nutrient but it contains 29 kilojoules per gram and must be included in the kilojoule content of your eating plan.

Let's first have a closer look at the most commonly encountered of these nutrients – carbohydrate.

Should you cut back on carbohydrates?

That would seem to make sense. After all, most carbohydrates break down into glucose and are the main source of blood glucose, making them an important target of dietary management of diabetes. But carbohydrates are also the body's primary source of energy, so they play a critical part in any healthy eating plan. It is recommended that carbohydrates account for at least half of your total energy intake.

Why so much? It's mainly an energy issue. One gram of carbohydrate contains only 16 kilojoules, while a gram of fat contains 37 kilojoules. That means, gram for gram, you can eat more than twice as much carbohydrate as fat for the same number of kilojoules. A carb-based diet allows you to eat larger quantities of food and therefore a greater variety of foods (both nutritionally and taste-wise) even if you're restricting your total kilojoules.

But shouldn't added sugars be avoided? The answer is yes, but only because they often come in packages that are high in fat and refined starch and low in vitamins and minerals: desserts, confectionery and baked goods, for instance. Otherwise, there's nothing inherently wrong with small amounts of added sugars. Milk contains sugar (lactose) and so does fruit (fructose), and there's no reason to avoid these foods. Starchy carbohydrates include legumes, noodles, pasta, rice, wholegrain breads and cereals, and vegetables such as potato, beetroot, corn, kumara, peas and taros. Carbohydrates are not only the energy powerhouse – many are also rich in dietary fibre and vital nutrients, such as vitamins and minerals.

Counting carbohydrates

Carbohydrates are converted into glucose and released into the blood within an hour or so of eating. So the level of glucose in the blood after a meal is determined partly by the amount of carbohydrate consumed.

One way to control the amount of glucose entering your body is by counting the grams of carbohydrate you take in – information that's available on packaged foods or in carb-counting apps and books. This approach is particularly useful to people with type 1 diabetes, or those with type 2 who must take insulin, because it allows more accurate matching of insulin doses to glucose intake.

To start you out on a carbohydrate-counting plan, your dietitian will advise you of the number of carbohydrates that you need to eat at every meal and snack based on your individual needs and present eating plan. Ideally, carbohydrate should make up 45 to 60 per cent of your daily kilojoule intake. You

Can I eat all the sugar-free foods I want?

You'd think sugar-free foods such as lollies and soft drinks would have less impact on blood-glucose levels than regular lollies or soft drinks. But you can't eat sugar-free foods with impunity.

The reason: Common sweeteners, such as sorbitol and xylitol, may not be sucrose (the technical name for regular sugar), but they do contain carbohydrate, each gram of which can raise blood glucose around half as much as sugar does. Non-nutritive sweeteners such as aspartame contain no carbohydrate or kilojoules, but products that contain these sweeteners (such as yogurt and lollies) usually do. Some sugar-free foods may be high in fat and kilojoules. Read the nutrition information panel to be sure. Some alternative sweeteners can also cause problems such as bloating, pain and diarrhoea if eaten in large quantities, so it's best not to overdo them.

The best advice: Pay no attention to 'sugar-free' claims on the packaging. Look instead at a product's total carbohydrate count.

Getting your fill of fibre

While some food labels list grams of fibre for processed and packaged products, don't worry about 'counting fibre' to get the recommended 30 g per day. It's much better (and easier) to simply work as many grains, beans and fresh fruits and vegetables into your healthy eating plan as you can. Here are some sensible strategies to start out with:

○ **Bump up beans.** Whether dried or tinned, beans and other legumes are among the best fibre sources you can find. For example, half a cup of black beans provides about a quarter of your recommended daily fibre intake.

○ **Hail the whole.** Wholegrain foods contain far more fibre than more processed foods, in which such fibre-containing grain parts as the bran are thrown out. For example, wholegrain bread contains about twice the fibre as bread made with refined white flour.

○ **Preserve the peel.** Routinely thrown away, the peel is often the most fibre-filled part of a fruit or vegetable. You're better off eating apples, carrots and potatoes with the peel still on (make sure that you wash them first if you eat them raw).

○ **Savour stems.** We also often toss out the stalky stems of vegetables such as asparagus and broccoli, but that's where the plant's fibre is most densely concentrated. To make them less tough, chop the stalks into small pieces and cook them a bit longer, adding the broccoli florets slightly later.

○ **Use fibrous fixings.** Products such as bran cereal, oats, barley, some fruits and wheatgerm make good condiments for porridge (which is high in fibre itself), cereal, pureed apples or yogurt. In recipes that call for breadcrumbs, try substituting rolled oats mixed with bran flakes.

then have flexibility in choosing the foods you like in order to hit your target.

Your dietitian can refer you to carbohydrate-counting food lists, apps and books that will help you to better understand what you're trying to achieve when you balance out the carbohydrates in your eating plan. But a general rule of thumb is that one serving of grains, starchy vegetables, fruit or milk contains about 15 g of carbohydrate; non-starchy vegetables, 5 g; and meat and fats, none. But that doesn't mean you can load up on meat or eat the same three carbohydrates at every meal; you still need to aim for variety, low saturated fat and balance. Try to spread your carbohydrate intake evenly throughout the day so that the amount of glucose released into your blood is fairly consistent from one meal to the next.

Why you need fibre

Fibre is an indigestible carbohydrate found in plant foods, such as wholegrain cereals,

> ## ❗ CAUTION
>
> Dried or canned beans or legumes are notorious for producing wind in the intestines, but the effect is temporary and your body will adjust if eating more fibre becomes a habit. Meanwhile, you may feel more comfortable if you add fibre gradually over a period of weeks to give your system a chance to get used to it. Start by adding about 5 g a day (about the amount in half a cup of kidney beans) until you reach the 30-g daily target. Your body will also handle added fibre more effectively if you drink more water. Soaking dried legumes and cooking them in fresh water or rinsing and draining the canned variety can reduce wind production.

grains, fruit and vegetables and should be part of your eating plan for a number of reasons. Soluble fibre (one of two main types, found in oats, barley, some fruits and legumes) mixes with food and water to form a gooey gel that slows digestion and makes blood glucose enter the bloodstream more gradually. In one study, people with type 2 diabetes who got 50 g of fibre in their diet every day for 6 weeks (after starting with 6 weeks of 30 g, the amount recommended for the general population) brought their blood-glucose levels down by about 10 per cent. In addition to lowering blood glucose, soluble fibre helps lower cholesterol, reducing your risk of cardiovascular disease. Insoluble fibre (the other type) improves overall digestive function by helping waste move

through your system. What's more, fibre adds bulk to food, which makes you feel full without adding a single kilojoule.

Factoring in fat

Fat is usually seen as a dietary evil, mainly because it's so dense in kilojoules, and saturated fat is a known contributor to heart disease. But fat also has important roles to play in the body, such as helping to form cell membranes, distributing fat-soluble vitamins and insulating the body against heat loss. A benefit for people with diabetes is that fat slows the digestion process, which means that glucose enters the blood more gradually. As a result, fat plays a bigger role in your diet than you might assume – making up as much as 25 to 30 per cent of total kilojoules.

But the proviso is that the type of fat you eat makes a difference. According to New Zealand researchers, an eating plan for a healthy heart aims to reduce the amount of saturated fat you take in to less than 7 per cent of kilojoules (energy), with less than 35 per cent of kilojoules coming from total fat. Saturated fat is found

Great sources of good fats

- olive oil
- canola oil
- peanuts and peanut oil
- almonds
- avocados

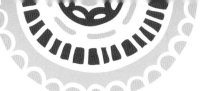

TEN TOP WAYS TO TRIM THE FAT

Fat is a beloved dietary staple because it's both tasty and versatile. It can be creamy, crunchy – and sometimes both at once (think fried ice-cream). But while no one needs to forgo all of fat's pleasures, a lot of the fat that most of us consume comes hidden (and unbidden) in cooking or eating habits that can easily be changed without sacrificing taste.

1 Choose leaner loins
Lean cuts of meat are those that are not 'marbled', which refers to the numerous white streaks of fat. Select meat with no visible fat or choose lean cuts such as 'heart smart'.

2 Chill out
Trimming obvious fat from meat before cooking quickly carves off lots of saturated fat. To make the job easier, put the meat in the freezer for 20 minutes first; this will firm it up for closer cutting and make marbled fat more visible. When preparing soups or stocks, chill stock overnight, then skim the congealed fat from the surface.

3 Salt-reduced snacks
Salty snacks such as potato and corn chips can have as much saturated fat content as beef. For special occasions, choose lower-fat, salt-reduced chips or fresh-cut vegetables with salsa.

4 Switch to skim
Whole milk gets almost half its kilojoules from fat, while low-fat milk has less fat and fewer kilojoules. If you don't like the taste of low-fat milk, blend varieties to start with, progressively adding low-fat milk as you get used to it. And use low-fat milk in recipes.

5 Use sprightly spreads
Try lower-fat versions of cream cheese and other spreads or use lower-fat alternatives such as low-fat ricotta, cottage cheese or hummus.

6 Skin your chicken
Most of the fat in poultry is concentrated in the skin, which you could leave on while cooking to keep the meat moist but should remove before eating – especially drumsticks, which have more than twice the fat of chicken breast, even with the skin off.

7 Use non-stick pans
Why use butter or margarine to keep food from adhering to frying pans when non-stick pans eliminate the need? If you still want to coat the pan, use a small amount of olive oil, canola oil or cooking spray.

8 Retire the fryer
Even with healthier oils, frying adds fat kilojoules you can do without. Better bets are baking and grilling, which add little fat and bring out the flavour of beef, chicken, fish and hearty vegetables such as capsicum and eggplant.

9 Mix your meats
When recipes call for mince, use lean mince and bulk up the meat volume by substituting shredded vegetables, such as onions, carrots and zucchini, and tinned beans or lentils to make the mince go further.

10 Repair the recipe
When baking foods such as muffins, try using only half the amount of fatty ingredients such as margarine and oil and substituting an equal amount of puréed apple or prunes.

WHAT the STUDIES show

Staggering your food intake throughout the day not only helps keep blood glucose on a more even keel, but it also appears to lower cholesterol, according to a study at the University of Cambridge in England. Researchers surveyed more than 14,000 people about how often they eat meals and snacks and matched responses to results of cholesterol tests. They found that those who ate more than six times a day had total blood-cholesterol levels about 4 per cent lower than people who ate only three times a day, and about 5 per cent lower than those who ate only once or twice a day.

in animal-based foods such as meat and eggs and in dairy products such as butter and cheese, and tends to raise levels of LDL ('bad') cholesterol and is associated with an increased risk of cardiovascular disease, thus magnifying the metabolic problems that worsen diabetes. What's more, foods that contain saturated fat are often loaded with cholesterol, which can also raise LDL levels.

But if you eat only small amounts of saturated fat (easily recognised because it usually stays solid at room temperature), where should the rest of your fat kilojoules come from?

The answer is monounsaturated and polyunsaturated fats, neither of which raises your levels of bad cholesterol. Monounsaturated fat is especially recommended because it actually raises levels of good cholesterol, making it the best source of fat in your healthy eating plan. (Polyunsaturated fat, found in such foods as corn oil and safflower oil, ranks second.)

According to some research, monounsaturated fat may also help reduce insulin resistance. These fats are so good for you that the research says either monounsaturated fat or low-GI carbohydrates can be eaten in place of saturated fat. In fact, either one can make up as much as 60 to 70 per cent of your total kilojoules. This allows you some latitude when planning your meals, especially if you have a diverse eating plan. For example, a person who eats an Asian diet may prefer an eating plan high in carbohydrates such as noodles or basmati rice, while someone who eats a Mediterranean diet may want more kilojoules from foods such as olive oil. Both are suitable. But remember that even monounsaturated fat is rich in kilojoules, so don't go overboard, especially if you're trying to lose weight.

Last but not least: protein

Getting the right amount of protein isn't difficult if you're already managing your fat and carbohydrate balance – protein will account for the rest of your kilojoules. You need protein to build and repair tissues and ensure the proper functioning of hormones, immune-system cells and hardworking enzymes throughout the body. But it doesn't have to be the major dietary staple many people assume it should be. In fact, for most people with diabetes, only 15 to 20 per cent of kilojoules should come from protein. You can easily get all you need in just a few servings of protein-rich foods, such as meats, fish, poultry, dairy items and plant foods such as legumes, nuts and soy products. Smaller amounts are also found in vegetables and grains.

Many Australians and New Zealanders eat more protein than is necessary, which raises issues when you have diabetes. One concern is that because the body excretes excess urea from protein, eating more protein than you need makes your kidneys work harder. Diabetes already increases your risk of kidney damage, and some doctors believe that eating too much protein can lead more quickly to kidney complications.

When you do eat protein, about a third to half of it is converted to glucose for energy – far less than carbohydrates. Protein is digested and metabolised slowly compared to carbohydrates, causing a negligible rise in blood glucose.

The low-carbohydrate controversy

Not everyone agrees with the generally accepted recommendations about what your eating plan should look like. In fact, proponents of a number of popular diets argue that the picture is upside down for people with diabetes. If carbohydrates produce the largest and fastest increases in blood glucose, the argument goes, it doesn't make sense to eat more of them than of anything else. What's more, critics note, eating a lot of carbohydrates can contribute to obesity (as can eating too much of anything).

But if you take this message to heart and cut back on carbohydrates, what should replace them? The answer, inevitably, is protein or fat, particularly monounsaturated fat. Proponents of alternative eating plans say that, contrary to popular opinion, people with diabetes can lose weight on such eating plans and keep blood glucose more stable. The popularity of the low-carbohydrate approach suggests that it works for some people – or at least appeals to their desire to eat more bacon, eggs, meat and other favourites. But the consensus in the medical community is that you should view these diets cautiously, with an eye to matching your unique needs.

Who should go low carbohydrate. Low-carbohydrate eating plans are either higher in protein or higher in fat. When considering fat intake, some studies have suggested that eating more monounsaturated fat may be beneficial for people with diabetes, while others have shown that some people with high-GI, high-carbohydrate eating plans develop high triglyceride levels and lower HDL levels. By including more monounsaturated fat and less carbohydrate, the triglycerides were decreased and HDL cholesterol increased.

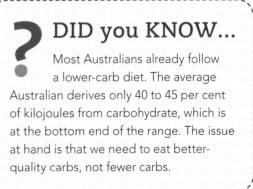

? DID you KNOW…

Most Australians already follow a lower-carb diet. The average Australian derives only 40 to 45 per cent of kilojoules from carbohydrate, which is at the bottom end of the range. The issue at hand is that we need to eat better-quality carbs, not fewer carbs.

The type of carbohydrate is also important. Research suggests that high-carbohydrate eating plans that are high in fibre and contain more low-GI carbohydrates do not raise triglycerides or lower HDL. It would appear from these data that the argument for low-carbohydrate eating plans has not been tested sufficiently, and so low-carbohydrate eating plans are not recommended.

When considering the impact of low-carbohydrate compared with higher-carbohydrate eating plans on weight loss, it would depend on kilojoule intake rather than the type of food eaten. Research comparing low- and high-carb diets has shown that both can be effective. It is the reduction in kilojoules and the ability to stick to the diet long term that predicts success.

Dangers of low-carbohydrate diets. Low-carbohydrate diets may also pose a number of problems:

- ❋ **They're more difficult.** Even a so-called high-fat diet doesn't give you free rein with the doughnuts and bacon. Instead, you're supposed to get more fat from foods such as nuts, avocados and olive oil, still keeping unhealthy saturated fat at less than 10 per cent of total kilojoules. In the meantime, foods containing carbohydrate that you might otherwise be able to enjoy are forbidden. With any 'diet' that's promoted in the media, how much weight you lose depends entirely on your total kilojoule intake compared to how many kilojoules you burn up and how active you are.

- ❋ **They can be nutrient-poor.** If you cut back on carbohydrate foods rich in fibre, vitamins and minerals, you may find it difficult to get all the nutrients your body needs.

- ❋ **They're less proven.** The generally accepted guidelines got that way – that is, generally accepted – from years of research that led experts to conclude that these are the best dietary approaches to managing diabetes. Popular low-carbohydrate diets draw on some of this research, but they don't have the necessary scientific consensus backing up their conclusions.

- ❋ **They may be dangerous.** While the question of whether high-protein eating plans promote the development of kidney damage is unresolved, many people with diabetes already have undiagnosed kidney damage that would make extra exertion by these organs potentially harmful.

Getting enough vitamins and minerals

If you eat a wide variety of foods, you will be getting all of the nutrients that you need. Vitamins and minerals are required for many of the essential chemical reactions that take place in your body, including those that involve kilojoule (energy) metabolism, cell growth and repair, and nerve and muscle function.

Vitamins. Vitamins can be described as fat-soluble and water-soluble. The fat-soluble ones include vitamins A, D, E and K. These are stored in the body, so it is possible for

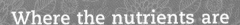

Where the nutrients are

This gives you some indication of how important it is to eat a variety of foods to meet some essential vitamin and mineral requirements.

Vitamin C
Citrus fruits, tomatoes, spinach, capsicum, broccoli and strawberries

Magnesium
Leafy green vegetables (such as spinach), whole grains, dairy products, brown rice, apricots and bananas

Vitamin E
Nuts, such as almonds, Brazil nuts and peanuts, as well as whole-wheat flour

Vitamin B12
Red meat, poultry, seafood and dairy foods.

an excessive intake to result in signs of toxicity. It is extremely difficult to overdose on vitamins if you stick to a healthy eating plan, but it becomes a possibility when vitamin supplements are taken as well.

Water-soluble vitamins. The water-soluble vitamins include vitamins B1 to B6 and B12, folate, biotin and vitamin C. Water-soluble vitamins are not stored in the body so toxicity symptoms are less likely to occur than with fat-soluble vitamins. It is important to constantly replenish your intake of these

vitamins by eating a variety of healthy foods that are a rich source of each vitamin.

Minerals. This group includes calcium, magnesium and iron. As with vitamins, it's best to obtain minerals from food rather than supplements. Taking large doses of certain minerals can impede the body's ability to function properly.

People with diabetes need to include a variety of foods to obtain all the nutrients required by them. For example, leafy green vegetables, whole grains, dairy products, brown rice, apricots and bananas contain significant amounts of magnesium.

Before considering taking any dietary supplements, discuss it with your doctor, diabetes educator or dietitian.

What about salt?

There's one mineral you may need less of: sodium – better known as salt. High blood pressure is common among people with diabetes, and studies suggest that eating less sodium can help control or reduce blood pressure. Avoid using table salt and choose low-salt or no-added-salt tinned or packaged foods. For added flavour, try relying more on herbs and spices in your cooking. To balance your salt intake, eat more potassium-containing food such as fruit and vegetables.

What's the glycaemic index (GI)?

How fast or slow your blood glucose goes up after eating can depend on what you put in your mouth, and in the 1980s, Canadian researchers developed a system to rate the glucose-raising effects of specific foods. It's called the glycaemic index.

GI numbers are based on a comparison point of 50 g of glucose, which is given a value of 100 – a high effect. Carbohydrate foods with a high glycaemic index (equal to or greater than 70) have a greater effect on blood glucose, and foods with a low index (equal to or less than 55) have a lesser effect. Many people find glycaemic-index lists (available from your dietitian or on the Internet) helpful when choosing which foods to eat during meal planning.

Studies have shown that people with diabetes who follow a low-GI eating plan have lower blood glucose than those who eat higher-GI foods, along with lower triglycerides and LDL. A common way to include low-GI foods in your healthy eating plan is to take at least one low-GI food at each meal.

When reading lists of low-GI foods you will see some foods that should not be eaten frequently. For example, chocolate is high in kilojoules and saturated fat but it has a low GI, so a low-GI value alone is not a replacement for healthy food choices. Look for the GI symbol for all-round healthy low-GI choices.

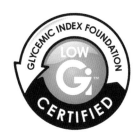

Glycaemic index

Scientists have calculated glycaemic indexes for thousands of foods. Here's a sample of values for a range of different foods, from high to low GI:

Jasmine rice	99
Baked potato	86
Cornflakes	77
Watermelon	76
Dark rye bread	76
Doughnut	75
Sweet potato	61
Raisins	61
Porridge	58
Special K™	54
Peas	51
Banana	51
Doongara rice	50
Sweet corn	48
Spaghetti	44
Fettuccine	40
Whole carrots	39
Apple	38
Kidney beans	36
Fresh apricots	34
Skim milk	32
Peanuts	23
Soy beans	18

Understanding the GI

Everybody responds to food differently. Your blood glucose will not rise to the same extent as the next person's, even if you eat the same food. By itself, this isn't a big problem because GI numbers are still useful once you understand what they mean to you personally. Importantly, the GI of a food itself can change depending on how much it's been processed, what you eat along with it and how it's prepared. Mashing, chopping or puréeing a food (which make it easier to digest) raises its glycaemic index – as can over-cooking it. Even ripeness can make a difference in some cases. For example, a green banana has a GI of 30, while an overripe one's value is 51 (but both are still low GI).

If you eat a high-GI food (a bowl of cornflakes) with a low one (skim milk), the overall glycaemic effect is a balance of the foods together (although the overall GI of the meal is not low). The most important thing is to establish how different carbohydrates and their glycaemic indexes affect you.

Making the most of food exchanges

Another tool your dietitian may bring into play is the food-exchange system, which looks beyond carbohydrates at the healthy eating plan as a whole, organising foods into several groups – generally breads and cereals, fruits, vegetables, milk, meat and protein-based substitutes, fats and sweets. While food exchanges are designed for people with diabetes, many nutritionists find them valuable for anyone trying to manage kilojoule intake, reduce the amount of fat and eat a balanced diet.

The idea behind the exchange system is that every item within a given category is nutritionally equivalent to every other item on that same list – providing roughly the same amount of carbohydrate, fat, protein and kilojoules. Using the portion sizes laid out on the lists is important for making the system work. But the big advantage is that you have a lot of flexibility in choosing foods within each category, as long as they add up to the nutritional budget allowed in your meal plan. Fortunately, portion sizes for many of the groups tend to be similar, which helps give you an intuitive grasp of how much you should eat. One bread exchange, for example, is usually measured in slices (as are many vegetable exchanges). One meat exchange is generally about 30 g – much smaller.

The exchange system strives to give you a range of nutrients from a variety of foods. Still, using the exchange system requires guidance. Your dietitian can help you figure out how many exchanges from each group you should eat.

You may find that the groupings themselves may take some getting used to because they're organised according to kilojoules and nutrient content rather than sources. For example, cheese is in the lean meats and protein-based substitutes as well as the dairy products exchange lists. Starchy vegetables such as corn, green peas and sweet potato are in the breads

Ranges of exchanges

Some exchange lists are subdivided into groups that specify exchanges of, say, very lean meats and substitutes (separate from high-fat meats), or non-fat milk products (separate from whole-milk products). Foods within each category are nutritionally equivalent in the exchange system.

Breads and cereals
- 1 slice wholemeal bread
- ⅔ cup cooked lentils
- ⅓ cup cooked pasta
- ½ cup corn
- 1 small sweet potato

Vegetables
- ½ cup cooked carrots
- ½ cup cooked green beans
- 1 cup raw radishes
- 1 cup raw salad greens
- 1 large tomato

Fruits
- 1 small banana
- 1 small pear
- 25 small grapes
- 6 teaspoons raisins
- ½ cup fruit cocktail

Lean meats and substitutes
- 30 g skinless chicken breast
- 30 g canned tuna (in water)
- 30 g lean meat
- 1 egg

Non-fat and very low-fat milks
- 1 cup skim milk
- 1 cup plain non-fat yogurt
- ¾ cup non-fat, fruit-flavoured yogurt (containing non-nutritive sweetener)
- ½ cup evaporated non-fat milk
- 30 g reduced-fat cheese

Other carbohydrates
- 1 x 5 cm-square brownie
- 2 small biscuits
- 1 tablespoon 100% fruit spread
- ½ cup gelatine
- 5 vanilla wafers

and cereals (in some exchange lists), due to the significant quantity of carbohydrate they are made up of. Some people find that this system provides flexibility with their healthy eating plan, and the consistent intake of nutrients can also encourage better control of your blood-glucose levels.

Is alcohol off limits?

There are plenty of reasons to avoid drinking excess alcohol, starting with the obvious: inebriation and addiction. But assuming you're a responsible drinker, is there room for alcohol in your diet if you are a person with diabetes? Most of the experts agree that the answer is a qualified yes. Alcohol may even have some benefits in terms of preventing the cardiovascular problems associated with diabetes.

A Harvard University study published in the US in 2002 found that women who have a few alcoholic drinks over the course of a week stand an almost 15 per cent lower chance of developing high blood pressure than women who don't drink alcohol at all. Other studies in both men and women have shown that alcohol raises HDL ('good') cholesterol and thins the blood slightly, protecting against cardiovascular disease.

The National Health and Medical Research Council in Australia recommends that women and men have a maximum of two standard drinks per day. It is also strongly recommended that you have two alcohol-free days every week.

Drawbacks of drinking

Firstly, the line between healthy and unhealthy drinking appears to be very thin. In the Harvard study, women who had more than about 1½ drinks a day had a 30 per cent higher risk of elevated blood pressure than non-drinkers did. Furthermore, alcohol's effects on the body are of particular significance when you are a person with diabetes. The main threat is hypo-glycaemia. Alcohol is processed in the liver, which also stores and releases glucose. The result is that wine, beer and spirits hinder the liver's ability to release glucose, which can lead to hypoglycaemia as much as a day after you

drink. Moreover, symptoms of hypoglycaemia can be similar to those of inebriation, making the danger harder to spot.

Another important consideration is that alcohol has 29 kilojoules per gram – almost as much energy as fat – but provides no nutrition, making it a poor choice if you're trying to lose weight. And if you're taking medication, alcohol may be totally out of the question.

Should you drink? Discuss it with your doctor. If you get the okay, follow these guidelines.

✓ **Eat something.** Food slows the absorption of alcohol into the bloodstream, allowing the liver to process glucose better while handling the alcohol. Also try to nurse your drink over a couple of hours to further ease the burden on your liver.

✓ **Sidestep the special stuff.** In addition to their kilojoules from alcohol, sweet wines and liqueurs pack extra amounts of carbohydrate.

What is a standard drink?

One standard drink contains 10 g of alcohol, which is equivalent to:

- 285 ml of ordinary-strength beer
- 425 ml of low-alcohol, or 'light', beer (less than 3 per cent alcohol)
- 100 ml of wine
- 30 ml spirits
- 60 ml fortified wine, such as sherry

Likewise, regular soft drinks and other sweet mixers added to distilled spirits can boost the carbohydrate and kilojoule quotient.

✅ **Exchange cautiously.** As a rule, doctors and dietitians would prefer that you do not drop a nutritious item from your healthy eating plan to make room for alcohol.

Making weight loss work

Knowing what your ideal eating plan should be is one thing. Putting it into practice – especially if you're trying to cut kilojoules – quite another. Anyone who's tried to lose weight can attest to the fact that it's easy for the best-laid eating plans to go awry – at least temporarily. Not to worry. This is a long-term project, and occasional lapses are to be expected. In the meantime, here are a few smart strategies to help you peel off those unwanted kilograms.

Control the kilojoule crunch

Researchers have recently noticed what seems to be a curious trend. In more recent years the proportion of fat in the dietary intake of the average Australian and New Zealander has actually gone down, even as rates of obesity have risen dramatically and continue to rise. Does this mean that fat isn't the villain we've all been led to believe it is? No. The explanation is that while the percentage of fat in the diet may be dropping, the sheer amount of fat and kilojoules we consume is going up because, generally speaking, people in both Australia and New Zealand are eating substantially larger portions of everything.

Controlling your kilojoule intake is the bedrock of all weight-loss plans. But how can you stay on course with your healthy eating plan when food is abundant and the temptation to overindulge is strong? Start by making a few small adjustments to your dining and snacking habits. For instance:

⊛ **Keep food off the table.** If you portion out servings on individual plates at the stove or kitchen bench and don't set food out on serving plates, you'll be less tempted to take more once your plate is empty.

⊛ **Don't eat from packets.** It's easy to lose track of how much food you've eaten if you're nibbling straight from the packet. Instead, portion out dry biscuits, pretzels and other snacks on a plate to give yourself a visible sense of what you're consuming.

⊛ **Downsize your dishes.** Smaller plates and bowls tend to make portions appear larger.

⊛ **Take it slow.** It takes about 20 minutes for the brain's appetite-control centre to register that there's food in the stomach. To wait it out, put down your fork between each bite and take small sips from your drink.

⊛ **Work for your food.** Eating foods that require some effort – peeling an orange, cracking open nuts or cutting up meat, for example – slows you down even more, giving food a chance to make you feel full.

- **Socialise outside the kitchen.** People seem to congregate in the kitchen, but you'll be less tempted to pick at food if you move the action to the living room.

Shop smarter in 10 easy steps

You came, you saw, you shopped. But then you got home from the supermarket and started unloading fatty, starchy snack items and processed sandwich meats. What went wrong? You fell back into the habit of being an average shopper rather than a person with a dietary purpose. In an enticing palace of eating designed to lead you astray, here's how to stay on track:

- **Make a list.** The meal plan you develop with your dietitian will help you figure out which foods you should be buying. Before you

Simple substitutions

Cutting kilojoules is surprisingly easy when small changes add up to big savings. Here's how a variety of foods measure up – and what you can save by making sensible choices.

INSTEAD OF	TRY	DIFFERENCE
1 cup toasted muesli (670 kJ)	1 cup regular Special K™ (480 kJ)	190 kJ
1 doughnut (1045 kJ)	1 bran muffin (375 kJ)	670 kJ
1 cup whole milk (700 kJ)	1 cup non-fat milk (520 kJ)	180 kJ
1 tbsp butter (420 kJ)	1 tbsp fat-reduced margarine (218 kJ)	202 kJ
1 tbsp butter (420 kJ)	1 tbsp low-fat cream cheese (150 kJ)	270 kJ
1 can regular cola (645 kJ)	1 can diet cola (16 kJ)	629 kJ
90 g light tuna in oil, undrained (1050 kJ)	90 g light tuna in water, undrained (380 kJ)	670 kJ
100 g regular minced beef (1230 kJ)	100 g lean minced beef (710 kJ)	520 kJ
1 slice salami (315 kJ)	1 slice pastrami (190 kJ)	125 kJ
100 g batter-fried chicken breast (795 kJ)	100 g roasted skinless chicken breast (605 kJ)	190 kJ
1 scoop vanilla ice-cream (655 kJ)	100 ml low-fat frozen yogurt (350 kJ)	305 kJ

Alternative sweeteners

While it is no longer necessary to eat alternative sweeteners and low-kilojoule foods, there is still a place for them in certain circumstances. There are two groups of alternative sweeteners: non-nutritive sweeteners (also known as 'artificial' or 'intense' sweeteners) and nutritive sweeteners.

Non-nutritive sweeteners are essentially kilojoule-free and therefore have no effect on blood-glucose levels.

Are non-nutritive sweeteners safe?
Yes. Those available in Australia and New Zealand have been thoroughly tested and approved by Food Standards Australia and New Zealand (FSANZ). For women who are pregnant or breastfeeding, Acesulphame K, Alitame, Aspartame (e.g., Equal®) and Sucralose (e.g., Splenda®) are recommended.

Can you cook with non-nutritive sweeteners?
As heat can change the taste, they are best added after you have finished cooking. Only Splenda®, Hermesetas Stevia®, Equal Stevia® and Equal Spoonful® can be added during cooking or baking, without affecting the taste.

Nutritive sweeteners are usually not kilojoule-free and have different effects on blood-glucose levels. Products containing nutritive sweeteners may be labelled as 'carbohydrate modified'.

Advantages
By including low-kilojoule foods and drinks that contain non-nutritive sweeteners (e.g., soft drinks, cordials and jellies) you can add variety without affecting your blood-glucose levels.

Small amounts of nutritive sweeteners will not greatly affect blood-glucose levels and can increase your food choices.

Disadvantages
Some 'diet' products containing alternative sweeteners may still be high in saturated fat and are therefore not suitable to include in your menu plan (e.g., 'sugar free' (carbohydrate modified) chocolate).

Many nutritive sweeteners have a laxative effect and can cause diarrhoea.

The bottom line
Taken in moderation, alternatively sweetened products can add variety and enjoyment to a low saturated–fat, high-fibre eating plan by increasing your food choices. To check the effect sweeteners or sweetener-containing foods may have on your blood-glucose levels, do a blood-glucose test just before eating and test again 2 hours later. You may like to repeat this on a few occasions just to make sure the blood-glucose result is actually due to that specific food.

shop, write down what you need to reduce the chances of buying what you don't need.

✅ **Limit your trips.** Make your shopping list long so that you have to make only one or two trips to the supermarket per week. Besides being more efficient, doing this provides less opportunity to make impulse buys.

✅ **Avoid shopping on an empty stomach.** When you're hungry, you're more likely to grab high-fat and starchy snacks and desserts.

✅ **Follow the walls.** Limit browsing to the outside edges of the supermarket, where you'll find the freshest, healthiest foods: raw produce, low-fat dairy products, fresh lean meats and fish. Venture into the interior aisles only when you're after specific foods, such as pasta and dried beans, to avoid picking up extra items not included in your eating plan.

✅ **Pay attention to portions.** Those biscuits look great – and hey, eating them only costs you 12 g of carbohydrate. But check the serving size: one little biscuit. Eating 'them' – say, three biscuits – brings your total carbohydrate count up to 36 g, which is more than a baked potato. Serving sizes have increased over the years and often 'add-on' benefits such as 'for an extra dollar you can have more cola and more popcorn' is a trap to suggest you are obtaining value for money. What's more important: the dollars you supposedly save or the extra kilograms and poor blood-glucose control?

✅ **Ignore the pictures.** Golden sunshine glowing on freshly harvested grains – an image of health that means nothing. Look at the side of the box instead for the facts, and choose foods that are high in fibre, low GI and low kilojoule.

✅ **Grade your grains.** Want high-fibre bread? Look for the words 'wholegrain', '100 per cent whole wheat', or 'stone-ground' on the label. Often the amount of fibre is listed on the nutrition information panel. Breads labelled simply 'wheat' may not contain whole grains. True wholegrain bread contains at least 2 g of fibre per serving.

✅ **Watch the language.** Beware of foods labelled 'no sugar added' – the wording is carefully chosen because the product may be high in natural sugar and total carbohydrate. You'll find the real story on the nutrition information panel, under 'Carbohydrate' and 'Sugars'. Look at the saturated fat and the kilojoule content. If high, it's not suitable for a person with diabetes.

✅ **Add some zest to your life.** Instead of creamy condiments, load up on such herbs and spices as basil, chives, cinnamon, cumin, curry, garlic, ginger, horseradish, nutmeg, oregano, paprika, parsley and Tabasco sauce. They're so low in carbohydrates, fat, protein, salt and kilojoules that they're considered 'free' items in healthy meal planning.

✅ **Keep your eye on the cashier.** It's no accident that supermarkets pile their impulse items next to the registers. Keep a couple of items from your basket in your hands to stop you reaching for the tempting items on display.

Physical activity: your secret weapon

To shed a kilogram a week, you need to subtract 14,700 kilojoules from your current total, or 2100 kilojoules a day. But that doesn't necessarily mean you have to eat 2100 fewer kilojoules. Instead, you can eat 1050 fewer kilojoules and burn the other 1050 through physical activity. In fact, studies show that combining healthy eating with physical activity is the surest way to lose weight and keep it off for good. Burning additional kilojoules allows you to eat more and still meet your weight-loss goals.

Recent research finds that you need at least 30 minutes of moderate physical activity on most days. You can break up your activity into 10- or 15-minute sessions and still get results. And it's not a matter of engaging in vigorous activity every day.

Exercise – especially strength training – offers another big bonus: a faster metabolism. A kilogram of muscle burns about 180 kilojoules a day, whereas a kilogram of fat burns fewer than 9 kilojoules a day. So by building up your muscle mass, you can turn yourself into a virtual kilojoule-burning machine. Researchers have found that middle-aged adults who worked out with weights three times a week for 6 months built enough muscle to raise their resting metabolism by 330 to 660 kilojoules a day – the equivalent of a 20- to 40-minute work-out.

Turn to Chapter 5 for more information on how – and why – you need to be physically active when you have diabetes.

Attitude makes the difference

Some researchers say that losing weight and following a meal plan are as much a psychological challenge as a physiological one. And one of the primary tasks is accepting that your health can improve – but maybe not by tomorrow.

Eating plans that promise quick results seem to be everywhere. But it's counterproductive to expect change to happen quickly. While it's true that some eating plans can take kilograms off fast, few can guarantee that the weight will stay off. For that to happen, you need to view dietary change as a permanent adjustment in the way you live. Many weight-reduction eating plans rely on prescriptive eating that does not offer food choices and doesn't include behavioural methods to increase healthy eating. You may eat poorly because you're cooking for one or you're bored. Addressing these needs and developing alternative behaviours to manage these feelings is a good start to meeting the psychological challenge of instituting a healthy eating plan.

Accepting good eating habits as a permanent part of life protects against a number of other attitude snags that can hinder your progress. If you see your eating plan as a temporary measure you take until you drop a certain number of kilos, you'll tend to think of yourself as either 'on' or 'off' your eating plan. That promotes a sense that healthy eating demands special willpower and that eating a food you like or a special treat means you've cheated. You'll have better results if, after you make a mistake, you quickly move on to make better choices next time.

DIVIDE (MEALS) AND MANAGE (DIABETES)

It sounds strange, but Carolyn Glosup, 57, can thank her diabetes diagnosis for making her a fitter, healthier person than she was several years ago. 'I weighed about 125 kilograms, my back hurt and I often felt dizzy, so I used a tripod cane to get around', she says. Carolyn was treated for a double ear infection but continued to feel faint when standing up, so her doctor looked for another cause – and found that her blood-glucose level was over 16 mmol/L.

'The day my doctor said I'd have to go on insulin, I went right out and found a dietitian. My mother had been diagnosed with diabetes but wouldn't stay on a healthy eating plan. She'd eat savoury snacks instead of a decent meal. She needed at least one injection a day, plus a urine test every morning and four finger pricks throughout the day. She hated it, but wouldn't do anything about it. I knew I didn't want to get to the point where I'd hate my lifestyle, so something drastic had to happen.'

Back then, Carolyn skipped meals but would drink many cups of sugared iced tea throughout the day, then dig into a huge meal just before bedtime – an eating style that wreaked havoc with her blood glucose and piled on the weight. 'I'd have a big steak equal to about three burger patties, sometimes crumbed and fried chicken – and I loved the skin', she says. Today, Carolyn divides three square meals so she's eating several times a day. Breakfast might be a bowl of cereal, followed in a couple of hours by a slice of toast. Lunch is a sandwich and dinner is usually lean beef or chicken that's been grilled or baked – not to mention skinned – and a balance of vegetables. 'My husband and I went from four loaves of bread a week to less than one', she says. She still drinks plenty of tea – but it's sweetened with sugar-free lemon-lime soda.

Carolyn refers to her new eating habits as 'food modification' rather than a diet, and it's led to other improvements in her life: her blood glucose is usually around 7 mmol/L and she's lowered her blood-pressure and cholesterol levels. She's lost 44 kilograms – and the cane. 'I walk on a treadmill for 30 minutes every day or just chase my dog around. I used to wear baggy track suits all the time, but now I live in jeans. My husband says I look fantastic. And he's doing well, too, having lost 4 kilograms and improved his blood-pressure and cholesterol levels as well.'

'But the best part is that I feel good, I'm managing my diabetes and I know I'm doing the best that I can.'

> '... I'm managing my diabetes and I know I'm doing the best that I can ...'

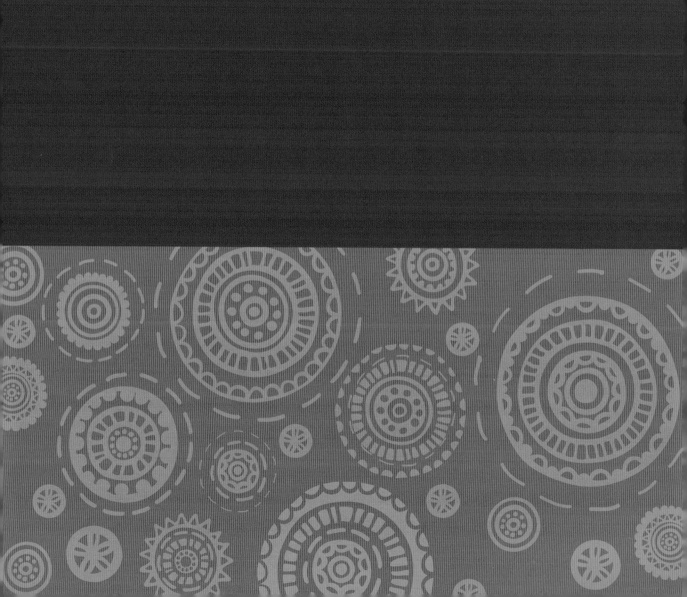

exercise *is* medicine

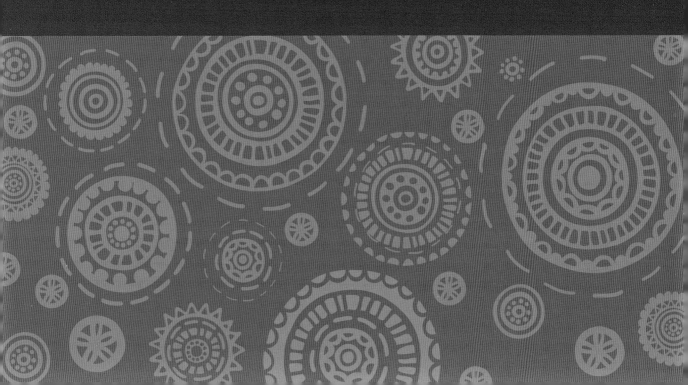

Increasing your activity levels trims fat from your body and helps you to tip the scales in the right direction – two key ways to control diabetes. But there's more: physical activity is also powerful in its ability to bring down blood glucose by helping the body to utilise insulin more effectively. That makes physical activity one of the most effective ways to control diabetes, not to mention feel more energised and reduce your risk of a heart attack or stroke. Adding regular physical activity sessions to your schedule doesn't have to take a lot of time or effort. It can even be fun.

I nactivity and excess abdominal fat are key features of type 2 diabetes in most people, but the good news is that you can change both. Even if there is increased risk in your family, adopting healthy eating habits and increasing regular physical activity will take you a long way towards reducing your waistline and improving your health. With consistent lifestyle changes, some people may decrease their diabetes medication and in certain cases may even no longer require it. However, even if your medication stays the same, you will find your general health and wellbeing will improve in many ways.

Research has demonstrated that just sitting less may improve your blood-glucose levels. So set the alarm to take 5 minutes to move out of every hour at work or home, watching TV, reading, etc. Do a few knee bends, rise up on your toes ten times every hour; not only will this help reduce blood-glucose levels, it will reduce joint stiffness and improve concentration. Further increasing regular physical activity and planned exercise adds even greater impact by enhancing insulin sensitivity in muscle, resulting in greater benefits to your glucose control.

The metabolic engine

Exercise is a metabolic booster rocket because it improves the transport of molecules that open a gate that directs the glucose into the muscles. If you have type 2 diabetes, this is the reason you feel more energetic when you exercise.

Glucose, the fuel needed to make energy, moves from the blood into the muscle engine. In other words, muscle is the major site for glucose clearance from the blood, and muscle contractions act as a glucose 'pump', with or without insulin. The more the pump works, the better the effect. As muscle glucose storage goes up, blood glucose goes down, resulting in greater energy to enjoy life and leisure time activity.

A matter of fat

Better management of diabetes is not only about glucose control but also about lowering fat in the blood vessels and other organs. Body cells in a glucolipotoxic (glucose and fat) environment don't work well, so reducing both excess glucose and blood fats is important for good health.

Another reason why exercise improves the symptoms of diabetes is via its effect on body composition, specifically by decreasing fat deep in the abdomen as well as in the muscles, and also by increasing the amount of good quality muscle. The deep abdominal fat cells secrete substances that interfere with the actions of insulin and promote insulin resistance. This is why reducing abdominal fat is a high priority. With inactivity, more fat accumulates in the muscle, too. Not only does this have a negative effect on muscle strength, if this fat is not burned for energy it just sits there creating a very toxic environment for the muscle cells. The good news is that exercise reduces these excess fat deposits in the abdomen and muscle, and the result is more energy and a healthier, stronger body.

Short- and long-term effects

The benefits of exercise are both short term and long term. The effect of a bout of exercise lasts about 2 days for its blood glucose–lowering effect, so activity must be at least every second day. However, the longer-term benefits of exercise increase with changes in fat and muscle to last over time. Better glucose metabolism and fat burning then have a positive effect on the heart, blood vessels, kidneys, liver, nerves and brain.

Waist not weight

Sometimes exercise is dismissed because of relatively small or no effects on weight; however, if you increase muscle, lose fat and your weight is the same, this is a great success. If your waist girth goes down even when you weigh the same on the scales, this is also an achievement because it indicates abdominal fat loss. Exercise with 'waist loss' is the key to improved diabetes management, but in the longer term, there

WHAT the STUDIES show

The DO IT study compared weight loss using diet alone, exercise alone and a combination of the two. After a year, those who exercised more and ate less lost the most weight. A year later, the 'combined' group was still ahead of the 'diet only' group who regained most of the weight they had lost. This is a good example of the sustained benefits of combined improved eating and exercise habits.

should be more fat loss and this would result in an appropriate 'weight loss'.

Reducing kilojoules only by eating less will reduce your weight via fat loss and muscle loss but exercise is the only way to maintain muscle while you are losing fat. Resistance exercise such as weight lifting is the only form of exercise that increases muscle. So with exercise, metabolism can improve without weight loss, simply via the added effects of the muscle pump, but further gains can be achieved when fat decreases (especially in the abdomen) and muscle increases. A number of excellent scientific reviews demonstrate that people with type 2 diabetes who have the most abdominal fat actually have a greater rate of abdominal fat loss with exercise. Research consistently demonstrates that the combination of healthy eating, aerobic and resistance exercise is the best recipe for preventing or managing diabetes.

The most important step is to move – in ways that you enjoy, in ways that don't hurt and in ways that can progress.

Added bonus

Exercise can also help to lower blood pressure, important for reducing the risk of stroke, heart and kidney disease. Together, increasing muscle and decreasing body fat improve joint pain and symptoms of arthritis, minimising discomfort when moving about in the world. Exercise and reduced abdominal fat also improve sleep and this in turn promotes better glucose control by decreasing a big contributor to daily stress and lethargy. Exercise isn't only good for your physical health, it helps people

to cope with the emotional difficulties of life, dealing with a chronic disease and symptoms of depression.

Inactivity is associated with dementia, and both high glucose levels and the inflammation related to the deep abdominal fat cells in many people with type 2 diabetes appear to be linked to a higher risk of Alzheimer's disease. With exercise, muscles produce many anti-inflammatory substances and some of these are the ones that are lacking in people with Alzheimer's disease and depression. The take-home message is that moving is good for mood and memory.

What type of exercise?

Exercise and Sports Science Australia (ESSA) recommend exercise based on health status. For those with low risk to their health, accumulating a minimum of 210 minutes of moderate activity or 125 minutes of vigorous intensity exercise each week is a great goal. This should consist of a combination of aerobic (e.g. walking, bicycling, swimming) and resistance training at moderate to high intensity (30 minutes on 2 to 3 days each week) for the best results. However, whatever exercise you decide to do, first discuss it with your doctor to be advised of any precautions.

Aerobic

Extensive research on aerobic exercise has consistently demonstrated positive effects on diabetes symptoms. Working at an easy level has benefits, while working harder has more, but it depends on general health, preferences and limitations. It's very important to start slowly and progress so that you feel good. (The motto 'No pain, no gain' is wrong, outdated, ineffective and risky.)

Aerobic activity can be walking, bicycling, dancing, boxing, swimming or rowing, among others. Modification may be required for those people with heart, circulatory or respiratory diseases, but exercise is an important part of therapy for these conditions and most people intuitively feel a level of exertion that is right for their body.

Resistance training

A relatively new area of research has been the effect of resistance training (weight lifting) on symptoms of type 2 diabetes. A review of studies on resistance training showed that it improved glucose control and insulin sensitivity, generally decreased the percentage of body fat, increased muscle but did not change weight. Because strong muscles provide the ability to be active and those with type 2 diabetes lose muscle at a faster rate compared to others of the same age, this confirms the importance of maintaining muscle with resistance training to maintain physical function. Ideally, weights should be moderate to heavy but modified for pain conditions and joint disease with the advice of an experienced exercise physiologist.

Combined training

Although the evidence for the effects of combined aerobic and resistance training is

Extra safety precautions

Exercise places healthy but mild stress on the body, so it is recommended that people with diabetes take a little extra care when exercising. Consider these tips.

○ Discuss your activity plans with your doctor, who may want to review your diabetes management before you start.

○ Always wear comfortable clothes.

○ Never hold your breath while you're exercising.

○ Protect yourself from the sun and try to exercise during the cooler parts of the day.

If you have diabetes, you are advised not to exercise if:

○ your blood-glucose levels are above 15 mmol/L;

○ you are feeling unwell;

○ you have been drinking alcohol; or

○ you feel breathless or experience any pain during exercise.

still evolving, this is now the recommended exercise prescription for good health as well as for type 2 diabetes prevention and management. It appears that including both every week adds further benefits over just one type of training alone.

Exercise and hypoglycaemia

Exercise is effective in lowering blood glucose, and now with oral medications, hypoglycaemia (when blood glucose is too low) is rarely a problem. However, on some types of medications or combinations of medication this may occur. When diabetes is managed with insulin, depending on if it's fast or slow acting or a combination of both, hypoglycaemia may be more likely to occur. An insulin pump has a different management strategy. Your health care practitioners can assist in planning to minimise hypoglycaemic events.

- Know the signs Confusion, shaking, light-headedness or difficulty speaking all indicate that you should stop exercising immediately.

- Have a snack handy When your blood glucose is too low, you can quickly bring it back up with a high-carbohydrate snack, such as a couple of glucose tablets, 4 to 6 jelly beans or a glass of regular soft drink or juice.

- Use the buddy system Try to walk or work out with someone who could lend a hand in an emergency.

- Carry identification Even if you're just strolling through your neighbourhood, carry ID with your name, address and phone number, plus emergency information, such as how to reach your doctor and the dosages of your medication or insulin.

- Ask for a nutrition review If you are having regular hypoglycaemia events, consider asking for an additional nutrition review by your dietitian.

- Check your blood glucose levels Always check them before and after physical activity.

Action stations

Walking is a great form of exercise; it costs nothing and you can do it just about everywhere. Increasing the total number of steps you take each day is a good start but developing a habit of walking is essential to enjoying the long-term benefits.

Many people with type 2 diabetes carry excess weight and may find it hard to walk due to arthritis, breathing difficulties or diabetes complications such as heart problems or peripheral neuropathy. In these circumstances, stationary bike riding and weight training can be achievable options. These types of exercise can be done at home or in a group setting and can be adapted to suit all forms of physical limitations. A skilled exercise physiologist with experience in exercise specifically designed for diabetes can provide guidance and support.

Resistance exercise can be with body weight, resistance bands, hand weights or equipment. The key is to progress by increasing the resistance gradually. Some muscles may improve in strength much quicker than others and changes may be required where there is joint pain. There are very few medical reasons to avoid resistance training exercise; however, retinal pressure or injury, some joint disease, nerve inflammation and some surgical issues may require modifications. Talk to your doctor and physiotherapist.

In referring you to an accredited exercise physiologist, your GP should communicate any health details relevant to exercise participation as the types, intensity and volume of exercise you take will need to be considered in light of any risk factors you may have.

Exercise and hypoglycaemia

Exercise and medication can sometimes act as a 'double dose' in lowering your blood glucose. This is less likely with the current types of tablets but the way this happens depends on your individual response to exercise and medication, the type and timing of your medication (insulin and/or tablets), the type, intensity and duration of exercise you take as well as what you ate at your last meal.

If you have experienced hypos or are 'hypo-unaware', always have hypo treatment with you when exercising and make sure someone is with you who knows how to help you should you need it. Check your blood-glucose levels before starting your exercise, and again when you have finished. Then record your levels so you and your doctor can assess your individual responses. This information helps you to organise your exercise program. Recording your blood-glucose levels is also advisable when you change either the type or dose of your medication or the type, intensity and duration of your exercise program.

Exercise and hypotension

Many people with type 2 diabetes take medication to lower their blood pressure. Exercise also lowers blood pressure and after stopping exercise or moving from a seated to standing position, you may experience some dizziness for a few seconds. This is usually not a problem as it results from the combined effect of exercise and medication lowering blood pressure and slowing the pump of blood against gravity from the legs to the brain. This should only be transient but being aware of it can prevent a fall. There is no reason not to take medication or not to exercise but seek medical advice if this effect is sustained.

WHAT the STUDIES show

The Lift for Life program used resistance training in various communities in Melbourne. After 8 weeks, men and women aged 45 to 93 years had an average 1.9 cm decrease in waist circumference but those who remained for 24 weeks lost an average of 4.9 cm. All experienced greater leg and arm strength as well as improved agility, and these factors make moving so much easier. There is no age limit to improving your health. In fact, the older you are, the more you need muscle strength to move safely and effectively.

Help!

I know physical activity helps me, but I can't get motivated to go out for a walk. Call it the threshold barrier. Taking that first step is always the hardest. Sometimes, with life so busy, you don't even think about exercise. At other times, you know you should, but lack the willpower. Here are some steps that can help.

○ Put your walking shoes by the door at night so you will see them first thing in the morning. They will remind you that getting out there is a priority for the day.

○ Have a destination in mind. Going to the shop, post office, newsagent or café makes walking seem more purposeful and time-worthy.

○ Book walking time on your calendar. Once you have booked the time, stick adhesive reminder notes on the fridge and doors to spur you on – a technique shown to work in studies.

○ Enlist a friend to walk with you or, if that's not possible, to call and ask if you have walked. A sense of accountability is one of the best motivators for exercise.

○ Find an article of clothing that fitted you when you weighed 10 per cent less or a photo of yourself at the time. Display it prominently as an inspirational reminder of your goal.

Where to begin

The first step in your activity plan is to decide what you like and when you can do it, keeping in mind that the best time to exercise is when your blood-glucose levels are likely to be at their highest (usually within 2 hours of starting a meal). But remember that if it is not always possible to choose the best time, it should still happen.

Walking is an ideal way to start your body moving. A walking program can start with as little as 5 minutes, gradually increasing each week. A minimum of 30 minutes brisk walking is recommended. The intensity can gradually increase by adding a fast walk for 30 seconds every 5 minutes, progress to 45 seconds, then 60 seconds every 5 minutes.

Walking in a park might provide stairs where a few step-ups and step-downs can stimulate oxygen and blood flow. If you enjoy exercising with others, join a walking group, an exercise or dance class. Some prefer to go it alone; others exercise with a friend to stay committed!

Be prepared for obstacles to your plans such as change of seasons. For those with diabetes, complications such as foot pain, numbness or burning may require some modifications to their exercise programs. Leisure time activity should be around friends, family and fun.

Life plan

Gradual progression and small changes over time are most likely to support long-term

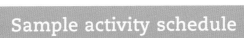

Sample activity schedule

Use this schedule as a guide to starting a new exercise program

	WEEK 1	WEEK 2	WEEK 3	WEEK 4
Mon	Walk 10 minutes	Walk 15 minutes	Walk 20 minutes	Walk 25 minutes
Tue	Walk 10 minutes + resistance exercises 1 x 10 repetitions	Walk 15 minutes + resistance exercises 2 x 10 repetitions	Walk 20 minutes + resistance exercises 3 x 10 repetitions	Walk 25 minutes + resistance exercises 3 x 10 repetitions
Wed	Walk 10 minutes	Walk 15 minutes	Walk 20 minutes	Walk 25 minutes
Thu	Walk 10 minutes + resistance exercises 1 x 10 repetitions	Walk 15 minutes + resistance exercises 2 x 10 repetitions	Walk 20 minutes + resistance exercises 3 x 10 repetitions	Walk 25 minutes + resistance exercises 3 x 10 repetitions
Fri	Walk 10 minutes	Walk 15 minutes	Walk 20 minutes	Walk 25 minutes
Sat	Any activity	Any activity	Any activity	Any activity
Sun	Leisure activity	Leisure activity	Leisure activity	Leisure activity
	WEEK 5	**WEEK 6**	**WEEK 7**	**WEEK 8**
Mon	Walk 30 minutes	Walk 35 minutes	Walk 40 minutes	Walk 45 minutes
Tue	Walk 10 minutes + resistance exercises *heavier weight 3 x 10 repetitions	Walk 15 minutes + resistance exercises *heavier weight 3 x 10 repetitions	Walk 20 minutes + resistance exercises *heavier weight 3 x 10 repetitions	Walk 25 minutes + resistance exercises *heavier weight 3 x 10 repetitions
Wed	Walk 30 minutes	Walk 35 minutes	Walk 40 minutes	Walk 45 minutes
Thu	Walk 10 minutes + resistance exercises *heavier weight 3 x 10 repetitions	Walk 10 minutes + resistance exercises *heavier weight 3 x 10 repetitions	Walk 10 minutes + resistance exercises *heavier weight 3 x 10 repetitions	Walk 10 minutes + resistance exercises *heavier weight 3 x 10 repetitions
Fri	Walk 30 minutes	Walk 35 minutes	Walk 40 minutes	Walk 45 minutes
Sat	Any activity	Any activity	Any activity	Any activity
Sun	Leisure activity	Leisure activity	Leisure activity	Leisure activity

* For resistance exercises, 3 x 10 = 10 repetitions of the exercise, followed by a rest of 30 to 45 seconds, repeat this another two times to equal 3 sets of 10 repetitions

Follow each exercise session with stretches.

> **! CAUTION**
>
> It is advisable to speak with your doctor to rule out health conditions that may require extra caution and modifications to exercise. Both aerobic and resistance exercise can lower high blood pressure so exercise shouldn't be avoided unless blood pressure is very high or not controlled with medication. Your doctor may advise you to have some tests to rule out heart disease, and under most conditions exercise will be part of the medicine to improve cardiac health. In general, there are few reasons to avoid exercising. Even with back pain, movement often improves symptoms and helps cope with chronic pain. Nerve damage in the feet requires care but stimulating nerve cells and nourishing them with improved blood flow from exercise may assist in preserving function.

changes so be patient and accept that it can take time to change old habits and create new ones. While muscle soreness with any new activity is normal, it usually lasts no more than a couple of days. Gradually increasing the duration, frequency and intensity of your exercise allows your body to adapt slowly and helps to reduce the risk of muscle and joint injuries. While exercise can often reduce pain, in some circumstances it may make it worse. Professional advice from a physiotherapist and an exercise physiologist is important in preparing for increased activity, or if pain occurs as a result of exercise. The best way to find out how well your exercise program is helping is to ask yourself these questions:

- Do you feel more energetic?
- Are you less stiff in the joints?
- Are you coping better with stress?
- Are your blood-glucose levels nudging down?
- Are you sleeping better?
- Are you actually enjoying exercise?
- Are your clothes a bit looser around the waist?

Commitment and motivation

Sometimes you may need to talk to someone – a friend or a health professional – to renew your commitment. If you like routine, establishing the process enables the pattern. Some people enjoy variety, so changing the type and environment of exercise you do each week might be a key to success. If you like to work towards specific goals, then measuring the duration of exercise or the increase in strength might be motivating tools, or using a heart rate monitor or a pedometer. Everyone is different and there are different challenges at each stage.

✦ **First stage** Old habits replaced with new.

✦ **Maintenance** Sustaining the changes and adapting to barriers (e.g. seasons, illness, work changes or family commitments).

✦ **Habit** Exercise is part of your life; perhaps it needs to be revved up a bit.

✦ **Achievement** Progressing the exercise and leisure time activity for further benefits through life stages.

STEPS TO SUCCESS

Maria Holland, a 34-year-old participant in the DO IT study, remembers the moment she realised what exercise could do to bring down her blood-glucose levels. 'One night after dinner, I tested my blood glucose and it was 12.4 mmol/L,' she says. 'Then I went for a 20-minute walk and took a reading again, and my glucose level was down to 7.4 mmol/L. I'd never done a before-and-after comparison before, and it was a eye-opener to see how big a difference I could make just by walking.'

That was incentive enough to make 20-minute walks part of her routine just about every day. 'I felt that I could start with 20 minutes', she says. 'I was capable of exercise, but until then, I just didn't do it.' Two weeks into her walking routine, however, she started to feel a definite change of attitude. 'Exercise is one of those things you don't always feel like doing, but if you do it anyway, you feel good afterwards', says Maria. 'I started to feel that I wanted to do more.' By the third or fourth week, 'I became almost addicted to it,' she says. 'If I didn't go out for a walk, it just felt wrong.' Maria quickly worked up to 30-minute walks and would even go as long as an hour if she had the time. Fortunate to live in a safe neighbourhood, she would often take peaceful, quiet walks through residential streets at night.

> '… it was an eye-opener to see how big a difference I could make just by walking …'

Just as important, Maria started finding ways to work more steps into her day. At the hospital where she worked as a nurse, for example, if she had to climb three flights or less she would take the stairs instead of the lift. At home, she took over the task of mowing the lawn from her husband. And whenever she took one of her children – aged 14, 12 and 3 – to football practice, she would walk the perimeter of the field instead of sitting and waiting.

Within 2 months, Maria's blood glucose dropped to normal, healthy levels – something that medication had been unable to accomplish before she exercised – and she shed 30 kg during the study. Since then, she has lost a further 13.6 kg. Part of the secret, she says, is that walking helps her to stick to her eating plan. 'If I eat a cupcake, I think of all the exercise it would take to burn it off', she says. 'It's a mindset you get into that keeps you motivated.'

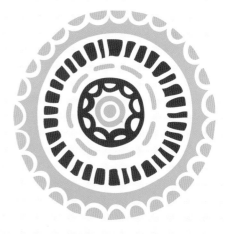

Strengthening and toning

You can perform the entire Strengthening and Toning Routine in about 10 minutes, so there are no excuses for not making time for it. To make it even easier, you can do only the upper body sequence, the lower body sequence or the core body sequence, then do a different sequence tomorrow. Each of them takes just 3 minutes.

UPPER BODY: **Wall push**

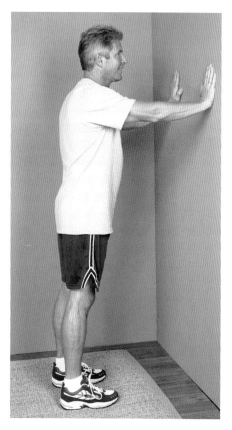 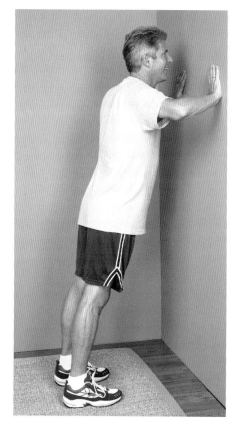

NOTE: *Only perform this exercise if comfortable for the shoulders and wrists.*

Progression: Move feet further away from the wall.

1 Facing a wall about an arm's length away, stand with your feet directly under your hips. Lean forward and place your palms against the wall with your elbows slightly bent. Keep your shoulder blades back.

2 Inhale as you slowly bend your elbows, bringing your chest closer to the wall. Do not arch your back. Exhale and slowly press back to the start position. Keep your core tight throughout. Do this 10–15 times.

BENEFIT
Strengthens the chest and triceps muscles in a single movement.

UPPER BODY: **Bent-arm row**

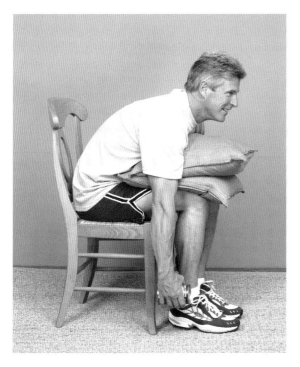 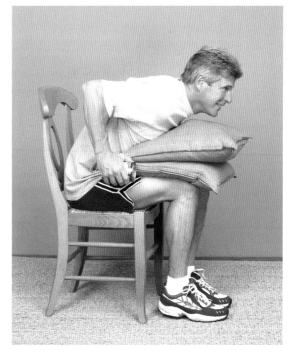

1 Sit on a chair with a large pillow on your lap for support. Grasping a full can of soup or a light hand-weight in each hand, lean forward, keeping your back as straight as possible. Let your hands hang towards the floor, but do not allow your shoulders to drop.

2 Exhale as you raise your elbows towards the ceiling, keeping them close to your body. Hold for 1 second, then inhale as you return to the starting position. Do this 10–15 times.

NOTE: *Keep your chin tucked in.*

Progression: Increase the weight in each hand.

BENEFIT Works the middle and upper back and, to a lesser extent, the biceps.

LOWER BODY: **Wall slide with raised arms**

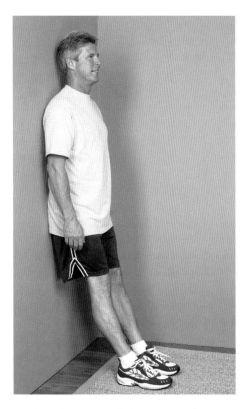

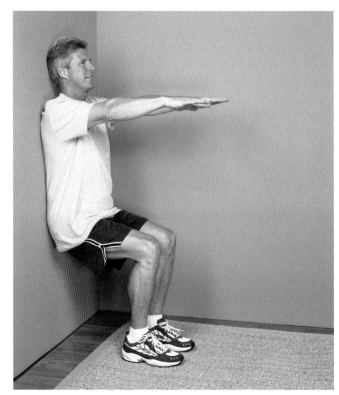

1 Place feet in parallel position in line with hips. Keep knees and toes in line. Maintain this alignment during the lowering. Make sure the knees do not roll inwards.

2 If comfortable for the knees, lower until your thighs are parallel with the floor. If uncomfortable for the knees, go only a half or quarter way down. Lower for 3 counts and inhale. Rise up to starting position squeezing the buttock muscles for 1 count and exhale.

BENEFIT Works the large muscles of the hips and buttocks for improved walking performance. To increase intensity, hold a full can of soup in each hand.

CORE BODY: **Dry swimming**

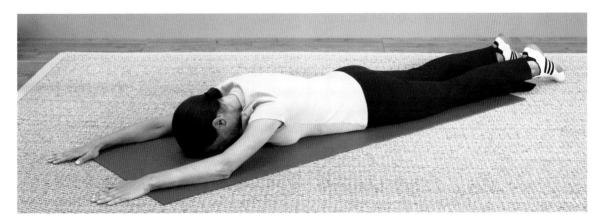

1 Lie face down on a mat or rug with your arms and legs stretched out straight, like Superman in flight. It may be more comfortable to put a small folded towel under your forehead.

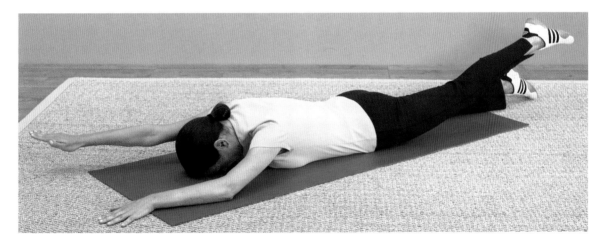

2 Keeping your neck relaxed (don't lift your head), tense your abdominal muscles, then raise your right arm and left leg and hold for 1 second. Slowly lower both limbs and repeat with the other arm and leg. Repeat for 30 seconds. Stop if you feel any back pain while doing this exercise.

BENEFIT Good for back muscles if comfortable. Strengthens the lower back and bolsters the muscles that run along the lower part of the spine, improving posture and preventing lower-back pain.

CORE BODY: **Baby lift**

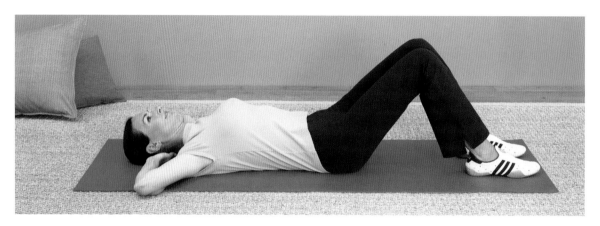

1 Lie on your back with your knees bent, your feet flat on the floor and your hands behind your head, if comfortable, with your elbows out to the sides.

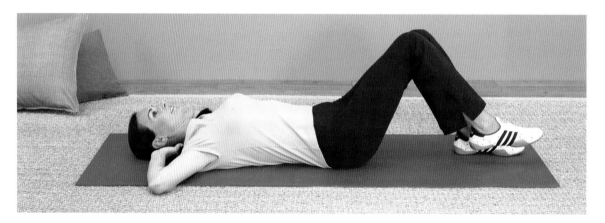

2 Inhale and contract your abdominal, side and back muscles to control the natural curve of the lower back. Keep it in position with the leg raises, then raise your right foot about 3 to 5 cm off the floor. Hold for a count of 4 (breathing with each count: out 1, in 2, out 3, in 4), then lower your foot to the floor as you exhale. Repeat with the left leg.

NOTE: *Place your arms where comfortable.*

BENEFIT Like traditional sit-ups, this exercise works the abdominal muscles, but it focuses on the control and stability of the spine.

Body basics for balance and mobility

Even as you go through your usual routine, you can add more movement to your day. Do one of these exercises while you're brushing your teeth, sitting in the car, standing in a queue, sitting at your desk or waiting for the kettle to boil.

AT THE SINK: **Tree pose**

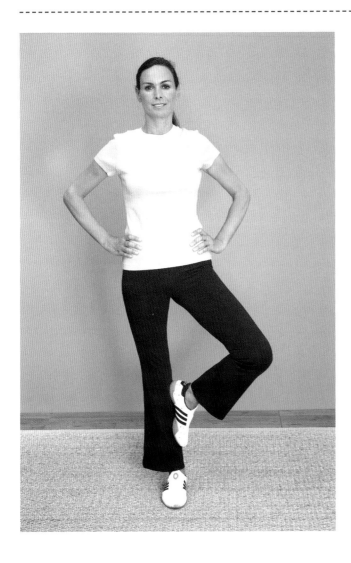

Stand up straight with your legs together. Slowly raise your left knee to the side, resting the bottom of your left foot against the inner calf of your right leg. Balance there for a count of 15, keeping your right knee unlocked. Pull your stomach in for support, check that the hips are in line, not twisted or tilted sideways, and keep your back straight and your chin up. Think about 'growing tall' through the top of your head. Repeat on the other side.

BENEFIT Trains the support muscles of the lower leg, back and abdomen for balance and control.

AT THE SINK: **Calf raise**

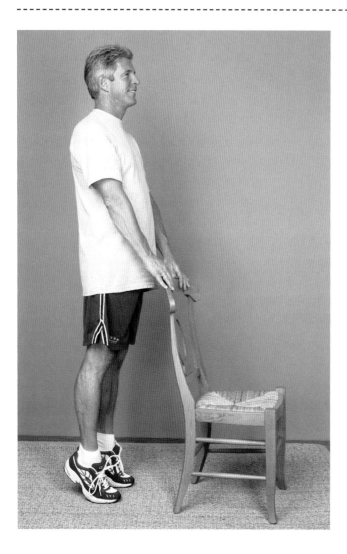

Stand with your feet directly under your hips, with your arms resting comfortably at your sides or, if you need help with balance, your hands on the sink (or the back of a chair). Slowly rise on your toes and hold for 10 seconds, then slowly lower yourself back down. Do this 6–10 times.

Progression: Perform this exercise one foot at a time.

BENEFIT Strengthens the calves and shins, which improves agility and balance and helps you to push off with your toes when walking.

STANDING IN A QUEUE: **Standing abdominal squeeze**

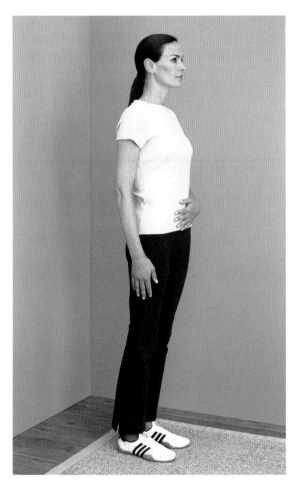 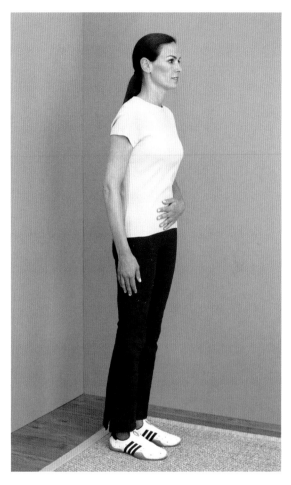

1 Stand with your feet hip-width apart. Keeping your neck, shoulders and arms relaxed, breathe in and out. Then gently pull in your stomach using your abdominal muscles, as if a belt were being tightened around your mid-section.

2 Hold this and breathe normally for 60 seconds. Do this 3–10 times.

> BENEFIT Doing this exercise while standing strengthens muscles that support your back against the strain of extra weight in your stomach.

STANDING IN A QUEUE: **Buttock toner**

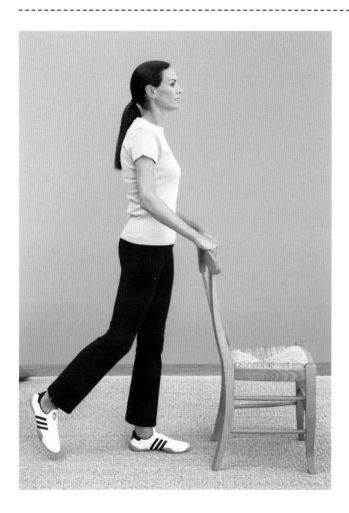

Stand up straight with your feet hip-width apart, your arms at your sides (or on a chair if you need help with your balance) and your shoulders relaxed. Squeeze the muscles of your buttocks together as tightly as you can, hold in your stomach and move your right leg about 5 cm behind you with your foot off the floor. Do not arch your back. Hold for 10 seconds, then change legs. Do this sequence 3–10 times with each leg.

BENEFIT Works the powerful muscles in your buttocks, which are involved in virtually every movement your body makes.

AT YOUR DESK: **Upper back push-down**

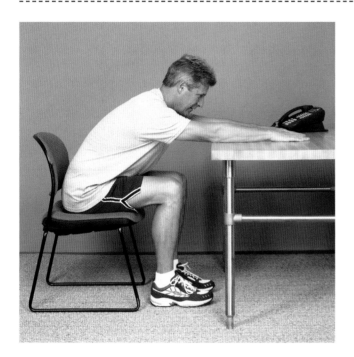

Sit at your desk, preferably in a chair without wheels. Position the chair 60 to 90 cm from the desk and keep your feet flat on the floor. Inhale and bend forward, extending your arms straight onto the desktop, with your palms down and your fingers spread apart. Exhale and press down with your hands and forearms as hard as you can while holding in your abdominal muscles. Hold for 30 seconds. Do this 4 times.

NOTE: *Perform only if comfortable.*

BENEFIT Stretches the back and shoulders, and is good for posture, tension relief and healthy joints.

IN THE CAR

Steering wheel lift press

While you're waiting at a red light, grasp the bottom of the steering wheel with your palms up. Inhale and then, while you're exhaling, push up on the wheel with your palms as hard as you can. Hold, breathing normally, until the light turns green.

BENEFIT Works the biceps, the primary load-bearing muscles of the arms.

Abdominal squeeze

While you're waiting at a red light or stop sign, gently breathe in and out, allowing your diaphragm to descend so that your stomach pushes out. Then don't breathe in but gently draw in your abdominal muscles as if you are trying to pull your navel back towards your spine. Hold this and breathe normally for up to 60 seconds.

BENEFIT Improves posture and tones the stomach to support your back and make you look slimmer.

AT YOUR DESK: **Overhead press**

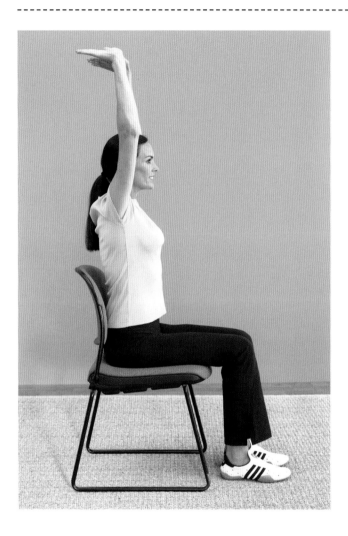

Sit up straight with your back firmly against the back of your chair and your feet flat on the floor, about hip-width apart. Raise your arms over your head with your palms flat and your elbows facing to the sides. Inhale and press up as if you were going to push the ceiling with your hands. Hold for 10 seconds, breathing normally. Repeat.

> BENEFIT Stretches the shoulders and improves mobility.

AT YOUR DESK: **Thigh toner**

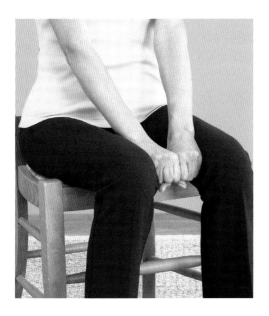

Sit up straight. While drawing in your stomach muscles, curl your hands into fists and place them between your knees. Squeeze your fists with your thighs and hold for 30 seconds. Repeat.

> **BENEFIT** Strengthens and firms those difficult-to-isolate muscles in the inner thighs.

AT YOUR DESK: **Palm clasp**

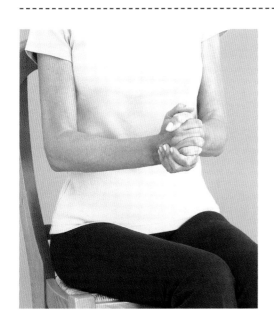

Sit up straight and grab one hand with the other. Press your palms together hard for 5 seconds, then release. Do this 4 times. You can also do this exercise while waiting at traffic lights or watching TV.

> **BENEFIT** This any-time, anywhere exercise works the chest and arms.

IN THE KITCHEN: **Knee raise**

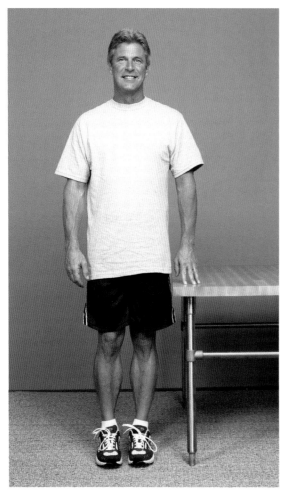

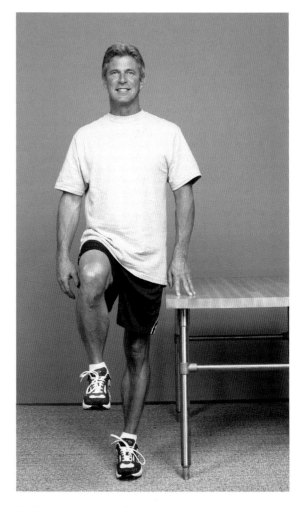

1 While waiting for water to boil, stand sideways near the kitchen counter. Place your left hand on the counter for balance.

2 Keeping your trunk upright, transfer all your weight to your left leg and raise your right knee to hip level. Hold for 5 seconds, then lower your foot to the floor. Repeat with the other leg. Do this 5 times with each leg.

BENEFIT By removing the hands for support, this exercise challenges the muscles that coordinate balance and support for walking.

IN THE KITCHEN: **Biceps curl**

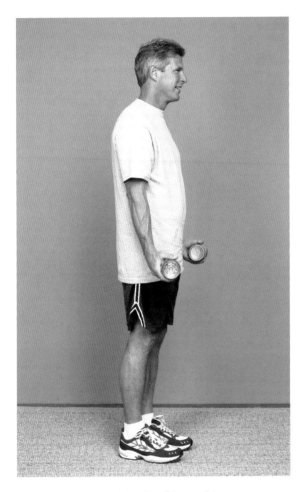

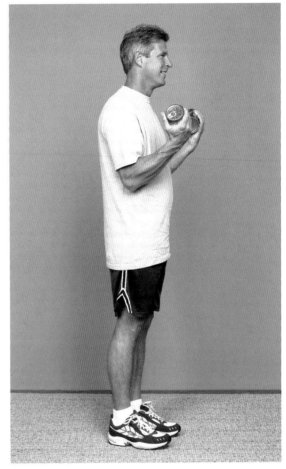

1 Stand with your feet shoulder-width apart, holding a full can of soup in each hand by your sides, palms facing forward.

> BENEFIT Works the biceps, which are important for pulling, such as yanking up weeds in the garden, and lifting, whether it's a bag of groceries or your grandchild.

2 Exhaling, curl your forearms towards your chest, keeping your elbows close to your sides. Keep your abdominal muscles tensed and don't allow your lower back to sway. Hold for 1 second. Inhale and return to the starting position. Do this 10–15 times. If it's too easy, find a heavier object to lift.

Progression: Increase the weight in each hand.

Stretching exercises

This yoga-based routine stretches out the kinks and improves blood flow. It works as a morning wake-up routine, too. Do the whole routine, slowly and gently, and don't pause between movements. You'll become more flexible the more you practise this.

Mountain pose

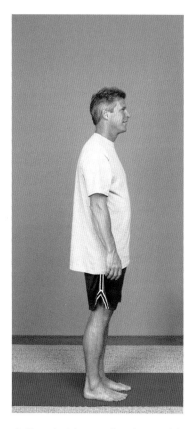

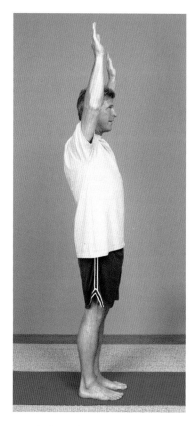

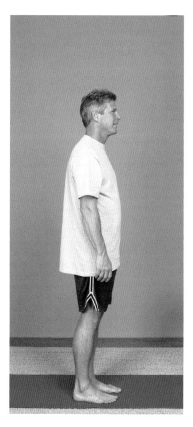

1 Stand with your feet hip-width apart, your back straight and your knees flexed.

2 Inhaling, slowly raise your arms to the sides and continue until they are over your head, with your palms facing forward. Exhaling, slowly lower your arms.

3 Repeat.

Standing side stretch

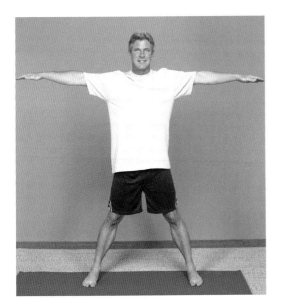

1 Stand with your feet 60–90 cm apart – wider than hip-width – and raise your arms to the sides to form a T.

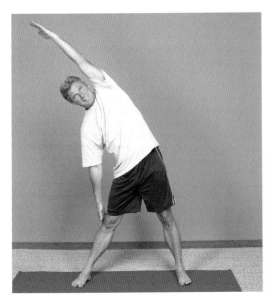

2 Exhaling, bend to the right and grasp your right leg with your right hand just below the knee, while bending your left arm slightly over your head so your left elbow moves closer to your ear.

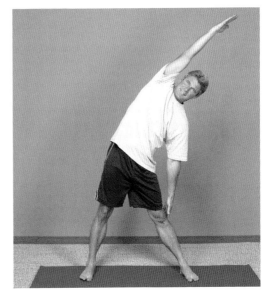

3 Inhaling, return to the starting position and repeat on the other side. Do this 3 times.

Touchdown tilt

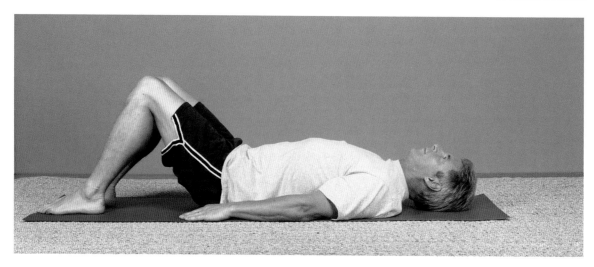

1 Lie on your back with your knees bent and about hip-width apart, with your arms at your sides and your hands on the floor, palms down.

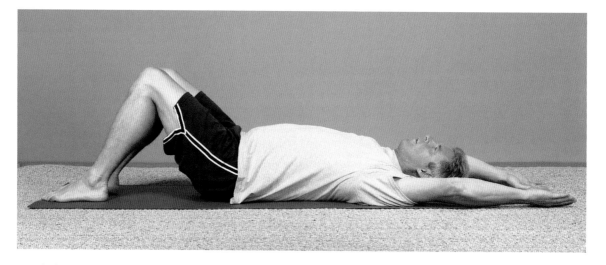

2 Inhaling, raise your hands over your head. Let your back arch slightly and touch your hands on the floor above your head or, if it's more comfortable, rest them by your ears with your elbows bent. Exhaling, bring your arms back to your sides and flatten your back gently towards the floor. Do this 3 times.

NOTE: *Perform only if comfortable.*

Lying twist

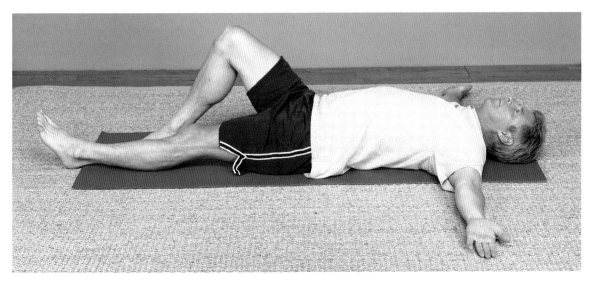

1 Lie on your back with your right knee bent so that your foot is on the floor near your left knee.

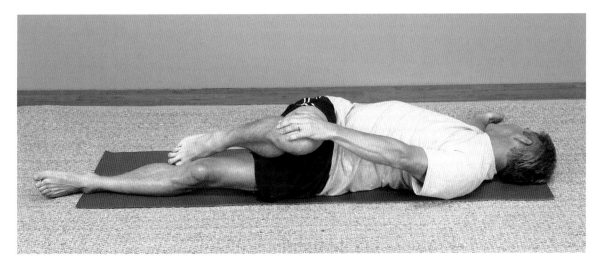

2 Exhaling, turn your head to the right and use your left hand to gently pull your right knee towards the floor on the left. Inhale and return to the starting position. Repeat on the other side. Do this 3 times.

NOTE: *Perform only if comfortable.*

Upward raised legs

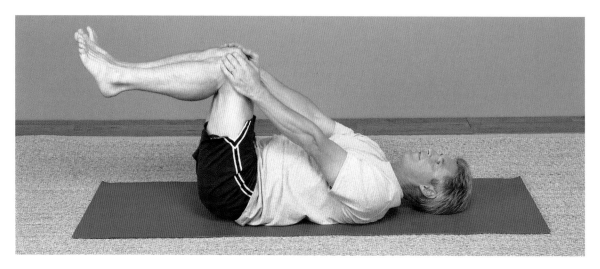

1 Lie on your back and use your hands to pull your knees towards your chest, keeping them slightly apart.

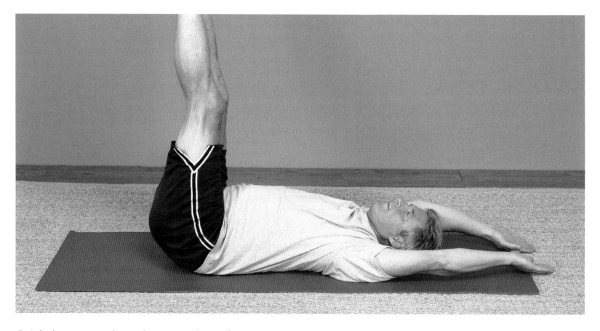

2 Inhaling, extend your legs straight up from your hips so the bottoms of your feet point towards the ceiling. At the same time, extend your arms above your head to touch the floor, keeping your chin tucked into your chest. (Place a small pillow under your head if it's more comfortable.) Exhaling, return to the starting position. Do this 3 times.

Relaxation pose

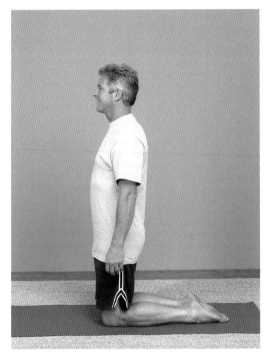

1 Kneel on a rug or mat with your knees slightly apart and your arms at your sides.

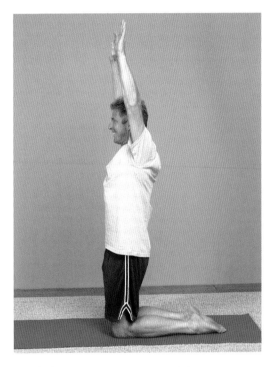

2 Inhaling, raise your arms straight over your head. (If that feels uncomfortable, raise your arms in front of you at a 45-degree angle.)

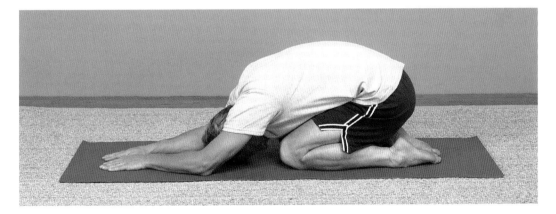

3 Exhaling, bend forward at the waist and lower your extended hands and forearms to the floor, moving your hips back so that you are sitting on your feet. Hold for 30 to 60 seconds. Do this exercise once only.

Cat pose

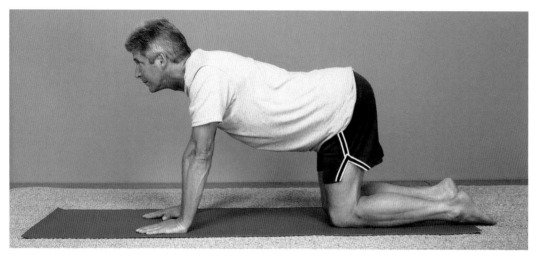

1 From the Relaxation Pose, get on your hands and knees. Inhaling and keeping your weight distributed evenly on your arms and legs, raise your chin and arch your back so it makes a gentle U-shaped dip towards the floor. Move at your pelvis, sticking your bottom out.

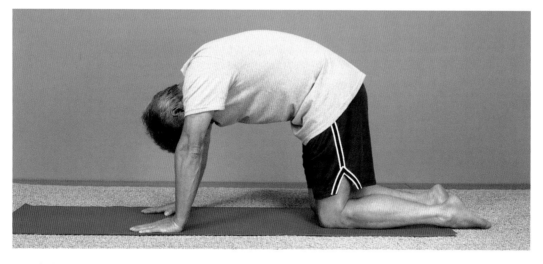

2 Exhaling, lower your head, tuck in your bottom and tilt your pelvis to round your spine, starting with your lower back and progressing through your middle and upper back. At the end of the pose your head should be slightly lower than your hips. Do this 3 times.

NOTE: *Perform only if comfortable.*

Good ways to get going

Different types of activity have different benefits. Your goals are to move your body, pump up your heart rate – and have fun doing it. What you choose is a matter of preference, though some aerobic activities may be more appropriate for you if you have any limitations or complications. Here's what some of the most popular forms of physical activity have going for them.

Walking

Benefits It doesn't cost anything and you can do it virtually anytime, anywhere – down your street, at the shops or in a park. Walking is a low-intensity activity, which makes it a good starting point for any activity program, but if you pick up the pace (especially on hills), it delivers a solid cardiovascular work-out. If you have joint problems or pain, establish a minimum amount that you can cope with and very gradually increase where possible (it might be one minute each week).

Tips Always wear supportive, well-fitting shoes. Try to walk for at least 10 minutes at first, then gradually lengthen your walks as you feel more comfortable. Keep the pace easy until you hit the 20- to 30-minute mark, then start cranking up the intensity. Aim for a pace of about 8 kilometres per hour. A simple device called a pedometer, available at sporting-goods stores and some Australian pharmacies or, in New Zealand, the Diabetes Supply Scheme, can keep track of your pace for you.

Jogging

Benefits It's as convenient as walking. Because it's more intense, you can get a better work-out in less time. It also feels (and looks) more serious than walking, which can bolster your sense of accomplishment. Wear supportive, well-fitting shoes.

Tips A good way to progress to a running program is to set out for a walk/jog. Start out by walking briskly, then progress into a run. When you feel winded, walk again. As you become better conditioned, you'll find yourself jogging more and walking less. If your joints start to bother you, rest for a day or two or go back to walking. To minimise the risk of injury, avoid hard pavement and opt, whenever possible, for soft but even surfaces, such as smooth expanses of grass or running tracks.

Swimming

Benefits By taking the load off joints, swimming is one of the exercises least likely to injure you, especially if you're overweight. If you have existing neck or shoulder problems, you will benefit from professional advice about swimming strokes and technique to assist in preventing further discomfort. It's also highly aerobic, depending as much on heart and lung capacity as muscle power.

Tips Start at a leisurely pace with strokes that feel comfortable for your breathing. When your aerobic conditioning improves, you can start holding your breath more. Make it a goal to do a certain number of laps without stopping. You might also decide to take a water-aerobics class if one is offered at a leisure centre or gym near you.

Water running

For those who find that the arm actions of swimming aggravate their neck, shoulders or back, water running with a buoyancy belt is a great option. It's hard work and very effective and can progress in distance and intensity.

medications & surgery

Less than a century ago, there was not a single treatment for diabetes. Then came insulin and the first medications for type 2 diabetes. Now, new treatment options offer unprecedented flexibility, with shorter- and longer-acting forms of insulin to choose from and an assortment of medications that can be mixed and matched to meet your own specific needs. Meanwhile, new devices delivering insulin without needles are being developed, and surgery, though not entirely risk-free, offers a worthwhile solution for some.

You're eating properly, you're active – but your blood glucose is still too high. What now? Healthy eating and physical activity go a long way towards controlling blood glucose, but there will still be times when you'll need extra help. For people with type 1 diabetes, insulin is essential to survival. People with type 2 can benefit from insulin, too, but injections may still be a long way down the road if you can get a grip on glucose with tablets.

In the not-so-distant past, the medical options for controlling diabetes were limited. Initially, there was just insulin and, starting in the 1950s, a single class of oral medications (known as sulfonylureas) that could help bring down blood glucose. From the mid-1990s new classes of medications emerged. Now if you have type 2 diabetes, you can choose from several types of oral and injectable medications – all of which combat high blood glucose in different ways. This has vastly expanded your treatment options, not only because each type of medication represents an advance in itself but because the various types can be used together in dozens of different combinations that best suit your individual needs.

It's important to note, by the way, that diabetes tablets are not simply oral forms of insulin. Acids in your digestive tract would break insulin down and render it useless before your body could use it, which is why insulin has to be injected instead of swallowed. Tablets and injectable medications for type 2 diabetes don't work for people with type 1 diabetes because such medications often rely on the ability of the pancreas to produce at least some insulin – which simply doesn't happen with most type 1 patients. In fact, being able to use these medications as a first line of medical therapy is a key distinction between type 2 and type 1 diabetes.

Medications have helped millions of people with type 2 diabetes lead healthier and more fulfilling lives, but they're not a cure for type 2 diabetes any more than insulin is a cure for type 1. And you can't put aside your eating plan or regular physical activity just because you're taking medication. If anything, the reasoning goes the other way: if your doctor prescribes medications, achieving better glucose control with healthy eating and physical activity may get you off medication or reduce your need for additional medication or insulin over time.

> # ! CAUTION
>
> Diabetes medications that boost insulin output share a common side effect: they can cause hypoglycaemia – actually, a sign that they're doing their job. To keep glucose levels from falling too low, take the medication exactly as prescribed and don't make up a missed dose by taking twice as much next time. Avoid skipping meals, and carry a carbohydrate-containing snack in case you ever need a quick hit of glucose. Also remember that the consumption of alcohol significantly increases the risk of hypoglycaemia.

When do you need medical help?

Whatever the miracles of medication, for those with type 2 diabetes, controlling blood glucose naturally with healthy eating and physical activity will always top your doctor's orders. Medications, after all, often have side effects. Yet sometimes doctors put people on medication right after diagnosing type 2 diabetes. What makes you a candidate for medication?

It all begins with your blood glucose. Remember that a diagnosis of diabetes kicks in when oral glucose tolerance test results are 11.1 mmol/L or more and you're trying to bring them down to around 7 mmol/L. Beyond that, your long-term HbA1c test results need to come in below 53 mmol/mol (previously 7 per cent).

There are no hard-and-fast rules about when to start taking medication because everybody's body is different and each case must be treated individually. But doctors tend to follow some rough guidelines, as outlined below.

Deciding who needs medication

Generally, doctors will advise that you try to bring blood glucose under control with healthy eating and physical activity alone as long as your fasting glucose is around 8 mmol/L or less. If your HbA1c number is holding at around 7 per cent, there's a good chance that initially you'll manage with just lifestyle changes. If this number creeps up to 7.5 or above, you'll probably need extra help. Still, at this level your doctor will usually advise that you try healthy eating and physical activity alone for a 3-month trial period. Then, if your HbA1c number is still above 7 per cent, you'll probably need to take medication.

If you start off with fasting blood-glucose levels higher than 8.5 mmol/L or your HbA1c results hit 8 per cent, your doctor may put you on tablets from the start, particularly if you are experiencing symptoms of high blood-glucose levels. But that doesn't mean you'll stay on them forever. Often, medications are used to gain immediate control over blood glucose until healthy eating and physical activity have a chance to produce results. After that, it's possible you may be able to stop taking tablets. However, your blood-glucose levels will need to be checked regularly, and most people with type 2 will eventually need medication and possibly insulin. Your doctor will advise you about all of this.

Blood-glucose numbers aren't the only factor that dictates whether you need medication. For example, let's say your numbers suggest that healthy eating and physical activity alone would help you, but you're not overweight (true of 10 to 20 per cent of people with type 2) or you're already eating healthily and are active. In each case, it's unlikely that eating one less biscuit or exercising an extra 10 minutes will make a significant difference, so your doctor may prescribe medication sooner than they would someone with similar numbers who is overweight and sedentary.

You may not be given tablets if you have other health problems that make them a poor choice for you. For example, metformin, one of the most popular diabetes medications, can cause a potentially fatal build-up of lactic acid in the blood (a condition called lactic acidosis) in people who have kidney, heart or liver disease, and it shouldn't be taken by these people.

Bringing in insulin

Even after you've started on medication, your doctor will keep a sharp eye on your blood glucose. If one prescription isn't working adequately, other medications or combinations may be advised. You might go through five or six different regimens before insulin is prescribed. Once it's clear that medication, healthy eating and physical activity aren't doing enough to keep your blood glucose under control, an evening or bedtime dose of insulin may be added to offset the glucose released by the liver at night.

For some people with type 2 diabetes, it makes sense to go straight to insulin therapy. Doctors may advise this strategy when their patients don't tolerate oral medications well, have diseases of the kidneys or liver, or have a greater need for insulin due to injury, infection or severe stress.

People with type 2 diabetes often don't need as many injections as people with type 1 because the body is still able to manufacture insulin (or use the insulin it produces) to some extent. But the longer you have type 2 diabetes, the less your body can do on its own, and the more likely you are to need insulin. This doesn't mean that you have failed in your efforts to control your diabetes – just that your diabetes has progressed to a point at which other types of therapy can't help you as much as they need to.

The medication line-up

There are six classes of tablets currently available in Australia and New Zealand for lowering blood-glucose levels and two classes of injections. Some make the body produce more insulin, others make cells better able to take in glucose or slow the release of glucose into the blood, and still others do several things at once.

Choosing which medications to use can be a complicated business, and you'll need to trust your doctor to help you make the right choices. But you, too, need to learn about their effect so you can discuss decisions and understand your options if the medications you're prescribed don't work well for you.

Bear in mind that medication works best in people who have had diabetes for less than 10 years. That's because medications build on the body's ability to produce some insulin, but this ability tends to dwindle as diabetes progresses. You can also expect medications to become less effective the longer you take them. That's why it's good to have choices; often your doctor can add a different medication to your regimen.

Sulfonylureas: the old and the new guard

Sulfonylureas are the granddaddies of diabetes medications. Some of them have been around for almost 50 years and are still among the most widely prescribed treatments. For many years, there were four sulfonylureas, referred to

? DID you KNOW...

The sulfa-drug class includes antibiotics that were new to battlefields during World War II. When a French army doctor noticed that the antibiotics made some patients act as if they had low blood glucose, he wrote about it to a colleague, who began experiments that showed sulfas could bring down blood glucose in animals. From these discoveries, the first oral medications to treat diabetes, the sulfonylureas, were developed and made available in the decade after the war.

as first-generation medications. More recently, second- and third-generation medications have been added.

All sulfonylureas bring blood glucose down in the same way – they bind to beta cells in the pancreas and stimulate them to produce more insulin. They differ from each other mainly in how much of them you need to take, how often you take them, how quickly they work and how long they last. For example, the second-generation medications are far more powerful than their first-generation counterparts, so much lower doses are required. They are also less likely to interact with other medications.

Side effects. The main side effect of sulfonylureas is hypoglycaemia (low blood-glucose levels). However, this can be avoided by eating regularly, not missing meals and having an extra snack if more active than usual. Less common side effects include an upset stomach or skin rashes. Let your doctor know if these problems persist. Some people are allergic to sulfa medications (which include sulfonylureas and some antibiotics), so, though these effects are rare, be on the lookout for skin rashes, hives or swelling, especially of the airways. Your doctor will not prescribe sulfonylureas if you have liver or kidney problems or if you're pregnant.

Mighty metformin

Since its introduction, metformin has become a best-selling diabetes medication – and it's no wonder when you look at the amazing diversity of effects packed into each tablet. Metformin reduces the amount of glucose released from storage sites in the liver. This keeps blood-glucose levels low not only after eating but between meals and during the night as well. It also hinders the absorption of glucose from the food you eat. By itself, metformin will not cause hypoglycaemia because it doesn't make cells draw glucose out of the blood. And because it attacks the problem from a completely different angle, it makes the perfect companion to sulfonylureas. Combining these two medications is one of the most common forms of diabetes medication therapy.

Another plus is that people often lose weight when taking metformin, though it's not clear why. It may reduce the appetite by irritating the gastrointestinal tract or by giving food a strange taste (often with a metallic tang). Whatever the reason, this gives metformin an advantageous edge for type 2 people who are overweight and trying to lose weight through lifestyle changes anyway.

And there's more. Metformin brings down LDL ('bad') cholesterol and triglycerides (while raising 'good' HDL cholesterol) and may make muscles more insulin sensitive. It works so well, in fact, that it cuts the risk of diabetes in people with impaired glucose tolerance by 31 per cent, according to a major US study called the Diabetes Prevention Program involving more than 3000 participants.

Side effects. Metformin sounds like a miracle medicine, but it's not perfect. The most common side effects are digestive problems, including loss of appetite, nausea, bloating, flatulence and diarrhoea. These side effects often disappear after several weeks and are less likely to crop up if you start on low doses and take the tablet with food. Some people find it causes headaches, but this is not common. You should not take metformin if you have kidney disease, severe liver disease or congestive heart failure, as these are conditions in which this particular medication can promote lactic acidosis, which is a potentially fatal build-up of lactic acid in the bloodstream. Drinking a lot of alcohol while you're on metformin can also promote this dangerous condition, so be completely up-front with your doctor about your alcohol intake when you're both considering this medication.

And always use caution if you're trying not to become pregnant, as metformin may improve fertility (probably because insulin resistance, which the medications help correct, makes you less fertile), and can render hormone-based contraceptives less effective.

Sensitivity training for cells

Another class of medications gets the difficult-to-pronounce award for its scientific name: thiazolidinediones. Despite the long-winded name, the idea behind these medications is relatively simple. They attack high blood glucose from a third angle – by boosting the insulin sensitivity of cells so that the cells are better able to take in glucose and clear it out of the blood. This makes the medications especially useful for keeping blood glucose down immediately after a meal, so your doctor may add it to your regimen if other medications fail to do this. If you have type 2 and use insulin, these medications (usually taken once a day) may also allow you to reduce your dose.

Side effects of thiazolidinediones can include gaining weight and retaining extra fluid in the body. Thiazolidinediones (sometimes called glitazones) must not be taken if you have liver problems or heart failure or you are taking tablets to get rid of extra fluid in the body. They should also not be taken by women who are pregnant or breastfeeding. Rarely, some thiazolidinediones have been associated with liver dysfunction so if they are prescribed, your doctor will arrange a blood test every few months to monitor your liver function.

Don't expect instant results: it takes several weeks and even as long as 3 months for muscle and fat cells to fully respond to these medications. Like metformin, however, they may bring down cholesterol and triglyceride levels and won't cause hypoglycaemia.

Side effects. It's no surprise that metformin is more popular than thiazolidinediones. These medications make many people gain excess weight and often cause swelling from water retention, especially around the ankles. They may also cause digestive problems such as nausea and vomiting, yellowing of the skin and headaches. As with most medications, you should not use thiazolidinediones if you're pregnant or breastfeeding. And always use caution if you're trying not to become pregnant, as thiazolidinediones may improve fertility (probably because insulin resistance, which the medications help correct, makes you less fertile), and pioglitazone can render hormone-based contraceptives less effective.

The glucose stopper

The medication acarbose (Glucobay), which is technically known as an alpha-glucosidase inhibitor, works to prevent enzymes in the intestines from breaking down carbohydrates into glucose, leaving the carbohydrates to be digested later by bacteria lower down in the intestine. This slows the release of glucose into the bloodstream and restrains the rise in blood glucose that typically follows a meal. Most commonly taken at the start of each meal, this medication may be a good choice if you have trouble keeping blood glucose steady after eating, especially if thiazolidinediones don't work well for you. Hypoglycaemia isn't a problem with this medication unless you combine it with other medications, such as sulfonylureas. If you do experience a bout of hypoglycaemia while on this medication, however, it's important to treat it by taking glucose tablets, as regular table sugar (sucrose) will not work.

Side effects. Because it leaves carbohydrates to be fermented by bacteria in the lower gastrointestinal tract, this medication produces a lot of flatulence, bloating and other digestive problems, including stomach pain and diarrhoea, and some people find this medication intolerable for just those reasons. In many cases, however, these effects will ease up over time. It helps to start on a low dose and gradually take more as your body adjusts. Still, this medication is not a good choice if you have a pre-existing gastrointestinal condition such as irritable bowel syndrome or ulcerative colitis or if you suffer from liver or kidney disease.

Me-too meglitinides

Though chemically different from sulfonylureas, the medication in this category, repaglinide (Novonorm), works the same way as the old stand-bys do – by wringing more insulin out of the pancreas. One difference is that repaglinide takes effect more quickly than sulfonylureas, so you can take it with your meal (or up to half an hour beforehand) to keep your blood-glucose levels down after eating. And its effects are short lived so this medication offers flexibility for people with erratic eating patterns, such as shift workers.

Side effects. Like sulfonylureas, this particular medication can cause hypoglycaemia, but because it is specifically designed to work when your blood glucose is already higher after eating, this tends to be less of a problem than with the older oral medications. Take it just before meals to reduce the risk, and limit alcohol as it can increase the chances of a hypo.

You might also experience nausea, some minor weight gain, itching and skin flushing, but these side effects are usually mild. However, you should not take repaglinide if you are pregnant or breastfeeding, and you should also avoid it if you have known liver or kidney damage.

Dipeptidyl peptidase-4 (DPP-4) inhibitors

Sitagliptin (Januvia) and Vildagliptin (Galvus) are relatively new medications that increase the body's ability to lower blood-glucose levels when they are elevated. They do this by increasing the levels of hormones that increase the production and release of insulin from the pancreas and reduce the production of glucose by the liver. They are prescribed only when diet and exercise plus the use of either metformin or sulfonylureas has been ineffective in lowering blood-glucose levels.

Side effects. Because they only work when blood-glucose levels are raised, they are unlikely to cause hypoglycaemia on their own but may do so if taken in conjunction with a sulfonylurea. Common side effects include a runny nose, sore throat, cough, discomfort when swallowing, headache and nausea or stomach upsets. If you have kidney disease you may need a reduced dose of the medication. They are not suitable if you are pregnant or breastfeeding.

Incretin mimetics

Exenatide (Byetta) and Liraglutide (Victoza) work by mimicking the effects of the body's own incretin hormones, which help to control blood-glucose levels after meals. They do this by stimulating the pancreas to release more insulin, reducing the release of glucose from the liver, slowing down the digestion of food and increasing the feeling of fullness after eating. Unlike other medications for type 2, which are in tablet form, these newer medications are taken by injection. They may be prescribed with metformin, a sulfonylurea or both.

Side effects. These medications don't usually cause hypoglycaemia if taken with metformin but can if taken along with a sulfonylurea.

They can cause digestive upsets including nausea, vomiting and diarrhoea, and some people may develop allergic reactions. They shouldn't be taken by people with kidney or digestive diseases and as they slow down stomach emptying, they can affect some medications that need to pass through the stomach quickly. These incretin mimetics are not suitable for women who are pregnant or breastfeeding.

Dodging medication interactions

Before your doctor prescribes medication for you, first discuss the name and nature of any other medications you're taking. Also make sure doctors treating other conditions know that you have diabetes. Many medications can make diabetes worse by raising blood-glucose levels. Others can lower blood glucose and may need to be factored into your diabetes medication dosage. The effects can vary from mild to major changes in blood-glucose levels. Watch out for:

Medications that may raise blood glucose

- Blood-pressure medications: beta-blockers, calcium channel blockers, minoxidil, thiazide diuretics

- Medications for HIV: megesterol acetate, pentamidine, protease inhibitors

- Antipsychotics: lithium, phenothiazines

- Tuberculosis medications: isoniazid, rifampin

- All corticosteroid medications

Medications that may lower blood glucose

- Pain relievers: aspirin, acetaminophen

- Blood-pressure medications: alpha blockers, angiotensin-converting enzyme (ACE) inhibitors

- Infection fighters: cibenzoline, gancyclovir, mefloquine, pentamidine, quinine, quinolones, sulfonamides and tetracyclines

- Antidepressants: doxepin, MAO inhibitors, tricyclics

Common combinations of oral medications

Sometimes the combination of two medications is better than just one on its own, especially if the two work in different ways. Here are some of the combinations your doctor might consider when deciding on your medication regimen, especially if one medication alone does not sufficiently control your blood glucose. When you take a combination of medications you'll be asked to watch carefully for any side effects.

⚛ **Metformin plus a sulfonylurea**

Why you might use it: To make the pancreas produce more insulin while keeping baseline blood glucose low. It's the most popular – and probably the most effective – medication combination for diabetes.

What to watch out for: Hypoglycaemia, gastrointestinal troubles (mild diarrhoea, nausea and bloating).

⚛ **A sulfonylurea plus a thiazolidinedione**

Why you might use it: If first-line sulfonylureas begin losing their ability to prod your pancreas into stepping up insulin production, it can be beneficial to bring in either rosiglitazone or pioglitazone to boost your body's insulin sensitivity.

What to watch out for: The dual action of producing more insulin and making cells more receptive to it makes you especially susceptible to hypoglycaemia.

⚛ **A sulfonylurea plus an alpha-glucosidase inhibitor**

Why you might use it: Using acarbose to keep glucose from being absorbed can help keep blood glucose low after meals if the sulfonylurea medication can't accomplish this on its own.

What to watch out for: Digestive discomfort, hypoglycaemia. Keep glucose on hand in case you do have a hypo, as table sugar (sucrose) won't work effectively.

⚛ **Metformin plus an alpha-glucosidase inhibitor**

Why you might use it: Not every medication combination has been subjected to a detailed research study. However, this particular combination has, and results show the two medications together are better than metformin on its own at keeping blood-glucose levels under control, especially after eating.

What to watch out for: Mainly flatulence, bloating and other effects from bacterial breakdown of carbohydrates.

⚛ **Metformin plus a thiazolidinedione**

Why you might use it: This combination may be useful if sulfonylureas have lost their effectiveness, particularly if being overweight has made you insulin resistant.

What to watch out for: Digestive problems.

⚛ **Metformin, a thiazolidinedione and a sulfonylurea**

Why you might use it: If you're taking metformin plus a thiazolidinedione, or metformin plus a sulfonylurea, and your blood glucose is still too high, a third medication may be added to your regimen. **What to watch out for:** Hypoglycaemia.

There are currently three diabetes medicines available that combine two different drugs into a single tablet. These may be prescribed as an alternative to taking these medications separately. They include:

- ✳ **Glucovance:** a combination of glibenclamide (a sulfonylurea) and metformin.
- ✳ **Avandamet:** a combination of rosiglitazone and metformin.
- ✳ **Janumet:** a combination of sitagliptin (Januvia) and metformin.

Side effects and precautions for these medications are similar to those of the single medications.

There are many diabetes medications available, each group working in different ways and in varying dosages. You and your doctor will decide what's best for your individual needs, and together assess how well you respond to what you take so your doctor can finetune your regimen if necessary. Regardless of which medication is chosen for you, expect to start on a low dose and move to higher doses the longer you stay on that particular medication.

As new medications become available or medication options change, it is important to discuss with your doctor whether one of these latest options might be suitable for you in managing your diabetes more effectively.

Insulin: who needs it?

Insulin is considered to be one of modern medicine's true breakthroughs. When it first became available, there was only one kind of insulin, still known today as 'regular' insulin, though nowadays there are many more insulin options.

Whether it comes from a vial or from insulin-producing cells in the pancreas, everybody needs insulin, of course – not just people with diabetes. But if your pancreas isn't doing what it should, you need to take over its job yourself. That's not only a task for people with type 1 diabetes. In fact, a number of people with type 2 diabetes need insulin as well, usually because the beta cells of the pancreas can't manufacture enough insulin to meet the body's needs (even with medication) or cells become more insulin resistant.

Normally, the pancreas pumps just the right amount of insulin necessary to help cells take up the glucose in your blood. Though a healthy pancreas constantly makes subtle adjustments, there are two basic insulin patterns you need to mimic artificially whether you have type 1 or type 2:

- ✳ A continuous, low-level baseline of insulin to keep blood-glucose levels stable between meals (this is sometimes referred to as basal insulin).
- ✳ Extra bursts of insulin (known as boluses) when blood glucose rises above this baseline level, especially after a meal.

Insulin at a glance

Insulin falls into five basic categories, with the following characteristics:

TYPES OF INSULIN	DESCRIPTION	TYPES AVAILABLE IN AUSTRALIA
Rapid acting	Rapid acting insulin starts acting within about 15 minutes (so should be taken just before a meal), peaks at 1 hour and lasts 3 to 5 hours.	• Novorapid® (Insulin Aspart) • Humalog® (Lispro) • Apidra® (Insulin Glulisine)
Short acting	Short-acting insulin starts acting after about 30 minutes (so should be taken about 30 minutes before a meal), peaks at 2 to 4 hours and lasts up to 6–8 hours.	• Actrapid® • Humulin® R
Intermediate acting	Intermediate-acting insulin starts working after about 90 minutes, peaks between 4 and 2 hours and lasts up to 16 to 24 hours. It is generally taken once or twice per day in the morning and evening.	• Protaphane® • Humulin® NPH • Hypurin Isophane
Long acting	Long-acting analogs are a more recent addition to the market. They have no peak, giving a relatively flat baseline insulin dose for up to 24 hours, although some people will still need two injections per day.	• Lantus® (Insulin Glargine) • Levemir® (Insulin Determir)
Mixed	Mixed insulins contain a mixture of rapid-acting or short-acting insulin with intermediate-acting insulin in different combinations. For example, 30/70 has 30 per cent short- or rapid-acting and 70 per cent intermediate acting.	• Novomix 30 • Humalog Mix 25 and 50 • Mixtard 30/70, 20/80 and 50/50 • Humulin 30/70

If you have type 1 diabetes, you'll typically take doses of different insulins throughout the day to cover all your needs. If you have type 2 diabetes, the number of doses you take (and the type of insulin you use) will vary according to how well your pancreas is functioning.

Choosing the right insulin

Insulin has improved in both quality and variety over the years, starting with the way it's made. Until recently, most insulin was extracted from animals, such as cows and pigs, and purified for use in humans. It worked well for most people with diabetes, but other people had allergic reactions to it, such as redness, itching, swelling or pain at the injection site. Today animal insulin has been replaced with human insulin whereby human DNA with insulin-making instructions is inserted into bacteria to make them manufacture an insulin that has the same structure as human insulin.

What matters most about insulin, however, is how it behaves. There are insulins available on the market today that differ in how fast they start working, when their action peaks and how long they stay active. Insulins are organised into five categories based on how long their effects last.

Short-acting insulin. Regular insulin is now officially classified as 'short acting'. This means that it starts to work quickly but then doesn't last very long. It's possible to use short-acting insulin to provide a burst of blood-glucose control when you need it, particularly in time for a meal. Regular insulin kicks in after 30 to 60 minutes, peaks in 3 to 4 hours and then lasts for a total of 6 to 8 hours.

Rapid-acting insulin. Are you someone who doesn't want to wait half an hour to eat while your injection takes effect? No problem: the newer rapid-acting insulins have been chemically altered to work even faster. Lispro (Humalog), Insulin Aspart (Novorapid) and Insulin Glulisine (Apidra) start to lower blood glucose in about 5 to 20 minutes, peak in 60 to 90 minutes and last 3 to 5 hours – a pattern closer to what you would experience after eating if you had a healthy, functioning pancreas. Besides allowing you more freedom to eat when you would like, rapid-acting insulin is less likely than regular insulin to cause hypoglycaemia because it doesn't stay in your system after the glucose from your meal is used up.

Peakless long-acting insulin. These new insulins have a relatively constant action with no pronounced peak over 24 hours. In other words, they more closely mimic the pancreas's background insulin production by holding insulin levels steady over the long haul. Insulin Glargine (Lantus) is designed for once-a-day use while Insulin Determir (Levemir) is usually taken twice a day.

Intermediate-acting insulin. The effects of these particular insulins fall in between short-acting and long-acting insulin. These insulins have either protamine or zinc added to delay their action. Intermediate-acting insulins available with protamine added are Protaphane, Humulin NPH and Hypurin Isophane (beef). Cloudy in appearance because of the additives, these insulins start bringing blood-glucose levels down after approximately 1.5 hours, peak in 4 to 12 hours and last for 16 to 24 hours. They are specifically designed to give you good half-day insulin coverage and are often used in combination with short-acting insulin.

Ins and outs of insulin therapy

The type of insulin you take, and when and how you take it, is a choice that you and your doctor will make, depending on a number of factors, including the type of diabetes you have, your blood-glucose levels, your usual eating and exercise patterns and other lifestyle factors.

Insulin comes in many different forms. This includes:

- long- and intermediate-acting insulins, which are usually taken once or twice a day and provide a 'background' dose of insulin
- rapid- and short-acting insulins, which are taken with meals to cover the rise in blood-glucose level that occurs when we eat
- mixed insulins, which are a combination of the two.

Type 1 diabetes

These days most people with type 1 diabetes take a long-acting basal insulin once or twice per day (morning and/or evening) and rapid-acting insulin before meals (and sometimes with snacks). This is known as MDI (multiple daily injections) or a basal-bolus regime. The other option is to use an insulin pump, which delivers a small dose of rapid-acting insulin continuously across the day with extra 'bolus' doses given when you eat.

The key to making your insulin regime work for you is to be able to closely match your food (in particular your carbohydrate intake) and insulin. This can be done in two ways:

- By giving set doses of insulin with each meal and eating the same amount of carbohydrates at each meal, from one day to the next. If you have a fairly regular routine and eat similar meals from day to day this may be a simple option for you. You will need to be able to work out the amount of carbs you are eating, generally using carb portions or exchanges (see page 100). Your doctor may also want you to have a correction dose if you are high before a meal. In the past this is the way most people were taught to balance their food and insulin.

- By adjusting doses according to the amount of carbs you are eating – this is often called flexible insulin therapy. If you would prefer to be eating to your appetite rather than having to eat according to your insulin, this can be a much better option. Your diabetes team will help you to work out how much insulin to have for the amount of carbs you eat (your insulin to carb ratio) and how to correct for high and low BGLs (your insulin sensitivity or correction factor) and other factors such as exercise. Insulin adjustment is used in both flexible insulin therapy and if you use a pump. The difference between a pump and flexible insulin therapy is that the pump only uses rapid-acting insulin and gives you the ability to set varying basal rates for different times of the day. Because our background insulin needs can vary across the day this gives an extra level of finetuning and can be particularly useful for those who find they tend to go low overnight but get a large rise in blood-glucose levels first thing in the morning.

While multiple daily injections and insulin pumps are the most common ways to treat type 1, some people may use different insulin regimes. This could include:

- long-acting insulin once or twice daily, in the morning and/or evening, and short-acting insulin (rather than rapid-acting) given three times per day before meals
- A mixture of short-acting and intermediate-acting insulin taken twice-daily, at breakfast and dinner
- An intermediate-acting insulin taken once daily at bedtime with short-acting or rapid-acting insulin given before each meal.

Type 2 diabetes

If you have type 2 diabetes and your blood-glucose levels are higher than desirable despite a healthy lifestyle and regular medication, your doctor may recommend the addition of insulin. You may start by just taking insulin once per day, either a long-acting basal insulin or a pre-mixed insulin, which is usually taken at night or in the morning depending on when your BGLs are the highest. At this stage you may still continue to take your oral diabetes medications.

Over time it is common to need additional insulin to control blood-glucose levels, particularly to help with the rise in BGLs that occurs when you eat. If you are taking a long-acting insulin this may mean adding some short or rapid-acting insulin before one or more of your meals. If you start with a once-a-day pre-mixed insulin this may need to be increased to twice per day (usually before

breakfast and dinner). Some people with type 2 eventually end up taking insulin in a similar way to those with type 1 diabetes, with a long-acting insulin taken once or twice per day and a rapid-acting insulin before meals, which means additional injections (4 to 5 per day) but more flexibility.

A weighty side effect

Intensive therapy gives you tight control over your blood glucose and therefore is the best way to ward off complications. You may, however, have to deal with an effect you hadn't counted on: weight gain. Why? Because close glucose control makes cells better able to use glucose for energy (kilojoules), so the body pours less of it out in urine. This effect can be more of an issue with those people with type 2 who are already struggling to keep their weight down.

The first thing to be aware of with the weight issue is that the benefits of better blood-glucose control far outstrip any harm from a few extra kilograms. Studies find, for example, that even when insulin therapy causes weight gain, cardiovascular risk factors like blood pressure either don't change or, in the case of cholesterol and triglycerides, actually get better. If metformin still works for you, it can help by assisting the insulin you inject to work better and thereby reduce the amount you need. So can increasing your physical activity plan or adjusting your meal plan. Talk to your doctor or diabetes educator.

Calling the shots

Injections can seem scary at first, but most people quickly get used to them. The thin, small-gauge needles available today are specially coated and extremely sharp, so they slide easily into the skin with minimal pain. With a little practice and attention to a few details, injections soon become just another problem-free part of a daily routine for most people.

When it comes to deciding where to inject, you have plenty of options. Any place that you have a layer of fat just below the skin is a good option – the abdomen, the tops and outer sides of your thighs, your buttocks and, less commonly, your upper arms. But the all-around winner is the abdomen, which usually has the most ample folds of fat and absorbs insulin faster and more consistently than other areas do.

It is important not to inject in the same site from one injection to the next. This can make the skin harden, create thick lumps or cause small indentations to form. But neither do you want to move to a new part of the body each time, since insulin is absorbed more slowly in some areas than others, which would make it tougher to keep the effects of your injections consistent. The best solution is to inject in the same general area, but place consecutive injections about a centimetre away from each other, rotating the sites as you go. If you're injecting at several different times of day, you might want to take, say, your morning injections in one area of the body and your evening ones in another, but still rotate them at those times within their designated areas.

Minimising the pain

Fine, sharp needles go a long way towards keeping the injections prick-free, but you can take additional steps to minimise the discomfort caused by having to inject frequently:

✓ Relax. Tense muscles can promote tightness that makes it harder for the needle to penetrate your skin.

✓ Insert the needle quickly. The same way that tearing an adhesive plaster off sensitive skin can cause increased pain or discomfort, so slowness and hesitation make injections hurt more.

✓ Keep the angle of the needle steady as it goes in and out so it's not swivelling around under your skin.

✓ Choose a fresh site with each injection so you're not putting the needle into tissue that's still sensitive from your last injection.

✓ Avoid giving injections in the inner thigh, where rubbing from leg movement can cause soreness at the injection site.

✓ Use a needle only once; they become blunt very quickly and wear-and-tear of the needle can be seen after just one injection.

Injection alternatives

When you think about injections you probably picture a syringe and a big needle. But these days there are other options that are much easier and more convenient to use, with most people using an insulin pen with a very small, fine needle.

Pen injectors. These have largely replaced syringes and are generally an easier and more convenient option. The insulin cartridge is contained inside a pen-like device, and a small needle is attached to the end of the pen to give the injection. The insulin dose is 'dialled up' and the insulin is delivered by pressing the plunger on the end of the pen. Most insulins come in replaceable cartridges to fit inside a pen device, or disposable pens, which are discarded once the pre-filled cartridge is emptied. They are easier and more discreet than a syringe and vial, particularly when injecting away from home, and they can be less intimidating if you are afraid of needles.

Pen needles come in different lengths ranging from 4 mm to 12.7 mm and the choice of needle depends on a number of factors, including your size (a shorter needle is better if you are thin to reduce the risk of injecting into muscle) and the amount of insulin you are injecting (a longer needle is better when large doses are being injected). However, it is now recommended that most people use shorter needles (less than 8 mm) due to the risk of intramuscular injection posed by larger needles.

> ## ! CAUTION
>
> When you're injecting into the abdomen, avoid the area 5 cm around the navel, where tougher tissue can make insulin absorption inconsistent. Also avoid injecting into moles, scar tissue or hard muscles such as the shoulders.

Steps for injecting with an insulin pen

1 Always follow the manufacturer's instructions to ensure the correct technique.

2 Fit a needle to the top of the pen.

3 Re-suspend cloudy insulin if applicable.

4 'Prime' the pen to ensure it is working correctly and there are no air bubbles.

5 Dial up the required dose of insulin.

6 Insert the needle and push down the plunger to administer the insulin dose.

Needle-free jet injectors. These devices send a fine stream of insulin through your skin under pressure, removing the necessity to insert a needle into your body. They are not entirely pain-free and some people find that the jets cause bruising. The jet injector is currently unavailable in Australia and New Zealand, although it can be bought online from the US on the Internet. It is a bulkier and more expensive way of delivering insulin than other methods and has no added advantages, although it can be of assistance for the very few people who have true needle phobia. If you're considering a jet injector, discuss it with your doctor or diabetes educator, and ask if you can arrange to test one before buying.

Insulin pumps. These look like a pager and are worn outside the body (clipped onto a belt or waistband). They deliver rapid- or short-acting insulin constantly through a narrow flexible tube that is attached to a catheter located under the skin, usually on the stomach. The pump is then programmed to give the necessary amount of insulin – generally a small steady dose throughout the day (known as the basal rate) and an extra amount (called a bolus) whenever carbohydrate food is eaten.

Used correctly, insulin pumps can give you tighter control of your blood-glucose levels without multiple injections, can reduce hypoglycaemia and can give more flexibility. To work effectively, however, they require regular monitoring of blood-glucose levels and adjustment of insulin doses. You will need support from a team of diabetes health professionals with experience in pump therapy.

The major disadvantage of a pump is that because it only delivers rapid-acting insulin, if the pump malfunctions, blood-glucose levels will rise quickly, with the risk of hyperglycaemia and ketoacidosis. It is therefore essential to carry a spare pen or syringe in case things go wrong. They are also more costly than injections, although in Australia most

Safe disposal of sharps

Used syringes, pen needles and finger prickers must be disposed of in an Australian or New Zealand Safety Standards-approved sharps container, which is puncture-proof and has a secure lid. These are usually yellow in colour and are available through pharmacies and your state or territory diabetes organisations, and in New Zealand some local branches of Diabetes New Zealand. Another option is to use a BD safe clip. This device clips off the needle section from syringes and pen needles and stores them inside. The remaining part of the syringes can be put into your regular garbage at home. However, finger prickers must be disposed of in a Safety Standards-approved container.

In Australia, procedures to dispose of sharps containers vary from state to state. Many local councils provide inexpensive sharps containers and collect full containers for disposal. You may also be able to collect a new sharps container from your local pharmacy and exchange it when it is full. Ask your state or territory diabetes organisation, local council or your diabetes educator about the safe disposal procedures in your area.

In New Zealand, procedures to dispose of sharps containers vary. Ask your diabetes educator, pharmacy or Diabetes New Zealand branch.

WHAT the STUDIES show

Insulin pumps can be used by people with diabetes of all ages, even toddlers. Whoever is in charge of the small child's care must be responsible for checking blood-glucose levels and injection sites regularly. The benefit of using an insulin pump is more stable blood-glucose levels, and, as a result, better control of diabetes. Still, it involves a lot of hard work and commitment.

private health funds will cover the cost of the pump itself, and the pump consumables are now subsidised under the National Diabetes Services Scheme (NDSS). In New Zealand both insulin pumps and consumables are funded for people who meet certain criteria. To see if you're eligible for a pump, talk to a member of your diabetes team.

Children with type 1 diabetes in Australia under the age of 18 years who don't have private health cover may be eligible for a subsidy under the JDRF Type 1 Diabetes Pump Program to cover between 10 per cent and 80 per cent of the cost. For more details visit www.jdrf.org.au/our-community/insulin-pump-grants/pumps-information.

Syringes. These were the only method available until the 1980s, and, while they have largely been replaced by insulin pens, some people still choose to use syringes. With this method, insulin is drawn up into the syringe from a vial, and then injected. Insulin syringes come in 30, 50 or 100 unit sizes depending on the dose of insulin required. The main advantage of a syringe is the ability to mix two different insulin types, which means fewer injections for those who take two different types of insulin at the same time. They are also less likely to malfunction than a pen. But drawing up the insulin is more time consuming and can be difficult when injecting away from home.

Steps for injecting with a syringe:

1 Prepare the syringe – choose the correct sized syringe and remove from packaging

2 Resuspend cloudy insulin if applicable

3 For a single insulin dose
   a. Inject air equal to the volume of insulin into the vial
   b. Draw out insulin dose
   c. Check for correct amount and no air bubbles

4 For a mixed insulin dose
   a. Inject air equal to the dose of cloudy insulin into the cloudy vial
   b. Inject air equal to the dose of clear insulin into the clear vial
   c. Draw out clear insulin dose
   d. Check for correct amount and no air bubbles
   e. Insert needle into cloudy vial and withdraw correct amount
   f. Ensure total dose is correct.

Is surgery a consideration?

Undergoing surgery is always a big decision because it poses so many risks – of complications during the procedure, problems with anaesthesia and also post-operative pain and disability, to name a few. But what if an operation could dramatically improve your blood-glucose control and reduce your diabetes-related health risks? Surgery may indeed offer solutions for some people.

Diabetes isn't like heart disease or cancer, in which the problem to be confronted is often clearly visible. How do you surgically correct an imbalance that exists at the molecular level within the blood flowing throughout your body? Despite it seeming an unlikely eventuality, new techniques are on the horizon, but at the moment, there are just two ways to address the question of surgical solutions for diabetes.

For type 1: pancreas transplants

The most obvious surgical solution to the problem of diabetes is to get a new pancreas, an option that's mainly considered for people with type 1 diabetes because they can't produce any insulin naturally. A pancreas transplant provides a replacement source of insulin, with the donated organ (or part of one) typically installed in the pelvis just above the bladder. The old pancreas is usually not removed because it can still make digestive enzymes.

When successful, a pancreas transplant can eliminate the need for supplemental insulin, bringing glucose under normal control. Furthermore, there's evidence that the progression of complications such as diabetic retinopathy may be slowed and perhaps even arrested thanks to the new pancreas. But – and you knew this was coming – the pancreas transplant procedure definitely has its drawbacks.

Beyond the very real difficulty of finding transplant donors, the body's immune system is naturally inclined to reject foreign tissue and requires taking potent immunosuppressant medications (such as cyclosporine or corticosteroids), which make you more vulnerable to infection from viruses and bacteria and less able to fight other diseases, including cancer.

Usually, pancreas and kidney transplants (necessary because of kidney failure from damage caused by high blood glucose) are done at the same time and about 80 per cent of people who have such double operations are free of insulin treatment after a year. But as many as 15 per cent of people who have this particular operation don't survive more than 5 years after the surgery (partly because they are quite sick to begin with). When successful, however, the improved blood-glucose control appears to protect the newly transplanted kidney from the recurrence of diabetic kidney failure.

Another transplant operation, islet cell transplants (the islets of Langerhans make up only about 2 per cent of the mass of the pancreas) are now being performed using the procedure based on the findings of a Canadian team of doctors, who changed the anti-rejection medication protocol associated with this particular operation to achieve greater success. The islet-cell recipients no longer require insulin injections, but they still need to take immunosuppressant medications indefinitely. This procedure is thus restricted to those with severe diabetes complications or hypoglycaemic unawareness.

For type 2: weight-loss surgery

Because obesity is so closely tied to diabetes and its cardiovascular complications (especially in people with type 2), some doctors think weight-loss surgery offers a quick way to wipe out a number of big health problems in one fell swoop. Other doctors are more cautious, saying it's unwise to undergo major elective surgery when you can choose far less drastic options to address the issue of losing weight effectively.

The pros and cons of surgery

The good:

- A 2008 Australian study of 60 people with type 2 diabetes found that 73% of those who had gastric banding achieved remission of their diabetes after 2 years, compared to only 13% in the control group.

- A US study of just over 100 people with type 2 diabetes who underwent lapbanding surgery found that after 5 years of follow-up 80% either no longer had diabetes or had an improvement in their diabetes (a reduction in blood-glucose levels and/or reduced use of diabetes medications).

- A study comparing different types of bariatric surgery found that around 60% of those having a gastric band and 80% of those having a gastric sleeve or gastric bypass were no longer taking their diabetes medication after 3 years.

- A Swedish study of 1700 obese individuals who had undergone weight-loss surgery (either gastric banding, a gastric sleeve or gastric bypass) found that their risk of developing diabetes over a 15-year period was reduced by 80% compared to a control group.

The bad:

- A study of close to 4500 adults with type 2 diabetes who underwent gastric bypass surgery found that of the two-thirds of participants who experienced an initial remission of their diabetes, 35% redeveloped diabetes within 5 years.

- Another study found that almost one-third of patients who were followed up 12 years after gastric banding surgery had experienced band erosion and close to half had had their band removed.

- In a Swiss study of people 6 years after having lapband surgery, one-third had complications including band erosion, slippage and catheter/port-related problems.

However, for those who are obese and are unable to lose weight with diet and exercise, weight-loss surgery may be a consideration and is becoming more common in Australia and New Zealand. Known as bariatric surgery, it involves making changes to the digestive tract to reduce the intake and absorption of food, with the aim of improved weight loss and maintenance.

There are a number of different types of weight-loss surgery but the most common are gastric bypass and gastric banding.

Gastric bypass surgery. This involves surgery to make the stomach smaller and allows food to bypass part of the small intestine. By reducing the size of the stomach, you feel fuller more quickly and are only able to eat small amounts of food at a time. Bypassing part of the intestine also results in fewer kilojoules being absorbed.

Laparoscopic adjustable gastric banding. Commonly known as lapbanding, this surgery makes the stomach smaller. An inflatable band is placed around the upper part of the stomach, which, when tightened, reduces the size of the stomach and restricts the amount of food you can eat. The band is filled with saline and more can be added over time to make it tighter to assist with ongoing weight loss. The saline can also be removed if it is too tight.

Gastric sleeve (sleeve gastrectomy). The gastric sleeve is a relatively new procedure that involves permanent removal of around two-thirds of your stomach, significantly reducing your stomach capacity. It is the first stage of gastric bypass surgery (left). While not reversible, the advantage is that it doesn't actually change the rest of your digestive tract: food is still processed in the same way and only the volume your stomach can hold is changed, meaning that nutrients are still absorbed as usual and the risk of deficiencies is lower than with gastric bypass surgery. As well as reducing stomach capacity, the sleeve also reduces the levels of appetite hormones, which helps you to feel less hungry between meals. Weight-loss surgery doesn't replace the need for following a healthy diet and getting exercise. In fact, the success of the surgery depends in part on your commitment to following the guidelines given to you about diet and exercise. It can also come with significant side effects and complications, which need to be carefully considered.

Weight-loss surgery, particularly gastric banding, has become much more common in recent years. According to the Obesity Surgery Society of Australia and New Zealand (OSSANZ) around 13,000 surgeries are carried out each year. While there are no accurate figures it is estimated that gastric banding makes up 45 per cent, gastric sleeves 40 per cent, gastric bypass 10 per cent and other types of surgery 5 per cent.

Despite its increasing popularity, this form of treatment for obesity should be used only as a last resort for those who have not adequately responded to intensive lifestyle measures to control their weight. It is important that people with diabetes considering surgery discuss it first with their doctor. The potential complications and side effects that surgery can incur must be carefully considered before making the decision to pursue this treatment option.

PUMPING UP CONTROL

Wearing an insulin pump is an excellent way to control blood glucose – even if it's not the most attractive fashion accessory, according to Stephanie Peters, 24. 'I heard about the pump a few years ago and gave some thought to getting one while I was at uni, but decided I didn't want that sort of contraption on me', says Stephanie. She changed her mind when she began working full-time.

Stephanie had tried various insulin regimens since she was 10 years old, when she was first diagnosed with type 1 diabetes. 'I had the classic symptoms – weight loss, bed-wetting, constant thirst. My dad found half-filled cups of water all around our home', she recalls.

During her university years, while on a mixture of fast-acting and long-acting insulins, Stephanie found it particularly difficult to keep her blood glucose in check. 'I'd become more active, and I needed to adjust the long-acting insulin at night if I planned to exercise the next day', she says. But she didn't always know when she'd be able to fit in that extra activity – and if she couldn't fit it in after all, her blood glucose would end up too high. On the other hand, an unplanned exercise session might lower her blood glucose too much. 'I often had to eat even when I wasn't particularly hungry or didn't want to take the time out to eat something, and it became inconvenient', she says.

Still, Stephanie couldn't bring herself to plug in a programmable system. 'I wanted to wear formal dresses, not a pump. I had no problem giving myself up to six injections a day – it was just like brushing my teeth.'

Then Stephanie started a new job, and the idea of a pump took on new appeal. 'With work, my life became more scheduled, but also more hectic. Carrying needles around became a pain', she says. 'I knew other people had had good luck with the insulin pump, so my doctor agreed that I should try it out for a couple of days.' More than a year later, she's still wearing it.

> '... I knew other people had had good luck with the insulin pump ...'

The pump replaces most injections, but not monitoring. 'You don't put it on and forget it. It takes a lot of monitoring and you have to be motivated.' For example, she's noticed that her glucose tends to be high in the afternoon, but she can correct it by pumping extra insulin.

Meanwhile, Stephanie has managed to fit the pump into her wardrobe – in fact, a dressmaker sewed a special pocket for it in a bridesmaid's dress she wore recently. 'When I buy clothes, I wonder where the pump will fit and what sort of bra I need. It's an issue and it's still my one complaint', she says.

preventing complications

By itself, high blood glucose doesn't seem that bad. After all, you can have it for years without even knowing it. The problem is the havoc it can wreak on your eyes, kidneys, nerves, heart, arteries, feet – you name it. Controlling blood glucose is the critical first step to keeping diabetes-related complications at bay. But other simple strategies, such as testing regularly, having regular check-ups and taking good care of your feet, can go a long way towards preserving your health.

To manage diabetes successfully, it helps if you can see how the actions you take (or don't take) today will affect you in the future. That's because, ultimately, diabetes makes you look ahead. If you don't control the disease, you can count on serious health problems occurring down the road. But if you take charge today, you can minimise, or prevent, complications tomorrow.

For many people diagnosed with type 2 diabetes, long-term health complications may have already set in. Even though it can take as long as 10 to 15 years for serious damage to occur, cases of type 2 often develop silently over a long period of time, and many people who have just been diagnosed find they already have related health problems.

No matter what your current situation, it's never too late to take steps that will keep you healthier in the days, months and years ahead. And if you have the benefit of an early diagnosis, the chances are good that you can avoid the worst effects of diabetes, which could include:

- higher cardiovascular disease (heart attack and stroke) risks
- kidney disease
- eye disease
- nerve disease
- foot damage
- related complications, such as sexual dysfunction, gastrointestinal problems and infections.

Why complications?

It seems strange that one disease can cause so many other problems throughout the body. After all, kidney disease by itself doesn't cause heart disease, and eye damage doesn't promote nerve damage. Why do these seemingly unrelated problems appear together when you have diabetes? The answer is that they're not unrelated but linked by high blood glucose.

You know from handling sweet foods in your own kitchen that when sugar is more concentrated, it becomes stickier. The same is basically true in your blood. Excess glucose can stick to cells in the blood, making it more difficult for red blood cells to deliver oxygen or white blood cells to fight infection. Sticky glucose can also make it harder for blood to flow through blood vessels, impeding circulation to important areas such as the feet and organs like the kidneys and eyes. When glucose clings to fatty substances in the blood, they may be more likely to adhere to blood vessel walls, gumming them up and leading to blockages that cause heart attacks or stroke.

Because high blood glucose is the common culprit in diabetes complications, the single most important thing you can do to bring down your risks for all of them is to get your blood glucose under the best control you can. Studies show what a difference good glucose control can make.

WHAT the STUDIES show

Diabetes is a significant cardiovascular risk factor that is often clustered with other risk factors. People with diabetes are two to three times more likely to suffer heart attacks than people without diabetes. A recent Australian survey revealed that some 65 to 80 per cent of people with diabetes will die as a result of cardiovascular disease. According to the National Heart Foundation of New Zealand, 40 per cent of all deaths are caused by cardiovascular disease.

- People with type 1 diabetes who maintain tight blood-glucose control can cut their overall risk of complications by half, according to a 1993 US study called the Diabetes Control and Complications Trial. In that study, the risk of eye disease was cut by 76 per cent, nerve damage by 60 per cent and kidney damage by 35 to 56 per cent.
- People with type 2 diabetes who bring blood glucose down gain a 35 per cent reduction in risk of complications with every percentage-point drop in their HbA1c test results, according to the 20-year United Kingdom Prospective Diabetes Study (1998).
- People with pre-diabetes (impaired glucose tolerance) who improved their blood-glucose profile by losing weight with healthy eating and physical activity cut their risk of ever developing diabetes (and complications) by as much as 58 per cent.

This mounting evidence takes the 'Why complications?' question in a different direction – why suffer from them at all when it may be in your power not to?

Reducing your cardiovascular risks

Cardiovascular disease and diabetes often appear together. It isn't entirely clear how the two diseases affect each other, but the most pertinent facts are clear enough: if you have diabetes, you're two to four times more likely than the general population to have heart disease. In fact, heart attacks are what ultimately kill up to 80 per cent of people with diabetes.

The risks are so high that having diabetes can put you in the same danger zone as a person who has already had a heart attack – and is thus likely to have another. Heart attack is just one of several problems to watch out for when you have cardiovascular disease. Most of them come down to two basic conditions, both of which you can take steps to control.

Assessing atherosclerosis

Cardiovascular is an umbrella term that includes both the heart (the *cardio* part) and the blood vessels (the *vascular* part). In a healthy person, a strong heart sends blood through the body via a network of smooth and elastic blood vessels. But problems arise when blood vessels become stiff, narrowed or clogged – a condition known as atherosclerosis.

Atherosclerosis can occur in a number of ways related to diabetes. High blood glucose can slow blood circulation and promote the formation of clots. Being overweight (especially if you are heavier around the abdomen) and having high levels of blood fats such as cholesterol and triglycerides (common with diabetes) can lead to obstructions in blood vessels. Depending on where they occur, these slowdowns in blood flow can trigger a number of different problems.

- When arteries that feed the heart become obstructed, the heart can't pump as efficiently as it should. Initially, this can cause chest pain from angina, a condition in which heart tissue is damaged from lack of nutrients. If a coronary artery becomes completely blocked, the result is a heart attack.

- If blood flow slows down in the arteries that feed the brain, lack of oxygen can cause what's known as cerebrovascular disease, in which areas of the brain become impaired. Often, the condition starts with temporary loss of brain function that can produce symptoms like slurred speech, weakness and numbness. A total blockage can cause a stroke.

- When blood flow to the arteries feeding the legs is impeded, a condition known as peripheral vascular disease develops. A partial blockage can cause temporary pain (called claudication) in the thighs, calves or buttocks. A complete blockage can end up causing gangrene, although this doesn't happen very often, because blood to the legs

Collateral damage

Over time, poorly controlled diabetes can wreak havoc throughout the body. But keeping your blood glucose in line will significantly reduce your risks. What's more, there are other steps you can take to minimise the damage.

SITE	DAMAGE	PREVENTION
Blood vessels	High blood glucose slows circulation, promotes high levels of blood fats such as cholesterol, and encourages the formation of blood clots. Potential result: blockages that can cause heart attack and stroke.	• Lower blood pressure and cholesterol with healthy eating and regular physical activity • Quit smoking • Ask about aspirin and consider ACE inhibitors • Eat heart-healthy foods such as fish, nuts and anti-oxidant–rich fruits and vegetables
Kidneys	Blood glucose gums up delicate capillaries that filter wastes. Kidneys work harder but less efficiently, gradually losing function and ultimately failing.	• Get tested regularly for signs of damage • Bring down high blood pressure • Avoid high-protein diets
Eyes	Diabetes can cause the walls of the smallest blood vessels to weaken, causing tiny balloon-like bulges in the vessel walls. Bleeding from the blood vessels or leakage of fats and fluid into the surrounding tissues can occur. If this leakage of fluid into the tissues occurs at the macula, then it will lead to reduced vision.	• Treat high blood pressure • Get regular eye examinations • Report any rapid changes in sight immediately • Treat high cholesterol • Quit smoking
Nerves	Blood glucose may block nerve signals or interfere with normal nourishment of nerves. The range of effects can include pain, lack of sensation in the body's peripheries, muscle weakness and loss of control over automatic functions like heartbeat, digestion and sexual response.	• Report symptoms to your doctor immediately • Tight control of blood pressure and blood-glucose levels • Quit smoking • Get regular exercise
Feet	A combination of poor circulation and nerve damage can make feet prone to injuries that heal slowly and can quickly become infected.	• Wear good shoes everywhere • Inspect feet daily • Keep feet clean and dry • Change socks frequently • Tell your doctor or podiatrist about any changes

can usually bypass the blockage using other arteries. Still, poor leg circulation, often combined with nerve damage, can lead to serious problems in the feet.

High blood-pressure havoc

High blood pressure can build up silently, just as diabetes can, and the two diseases often develop in tandem. If you have diabetes, you're twice as likely to have high blood pressure than the average person is, and about 60 per cent of all people with type 2 diabetes do. Controlling high blood pressure is critical if you have diabetes because the damage it causes contributes not only to atherosclerosis but also to kidney and eye disease. All told, high blood pressure has a hand in 35 to 75 per cent of all complications that go along with diabetes.

You need a certain amount of blood pressure (the force that blood exerts against artery walls) for good circulation. But too much gradually weakens the heart by making it work harder and damages the lining of blood-vessel walls, making it easier for atherosclerosis to set in. High blood pressure can also weaken arteries in the brain and cause them to balloon out at the point of the weakening, a condition called an aneurysm. The bursting of an aneurysm is potentially fatal.

To avoid problems strive to keep your blood pressure down to at least 130/85 millimetres of mercury if you have diabetes.

Preventing cardiovascular disease

Some of the steps you've already put in place to help to take control of your diabetes can

---

Should you take weight-loss medication?

Slimming down has the double benefit of reducing your risk of cardiovascular disease and controlling high blood glucose, which makes weight-loss drugs sound like an appealing option for people with diabetes.

While it's not possible to lose kilos just by taking a tablet (you still need to exercise and stick to a low-kilojoule eating plan), weight-loss drugs may help if healthy eating and physical activity aren't enough on their own. A recent German study even found that one of them, orlistat (Xenical), lowered blood glucose after eating, reducing the need for glucose-controlling medication.

Still, doctors advise that you approach diet pills with caution. Orlistat, which works by blocking fat absorption in the intestines, can cause a range of unpleasant side effects, including having to defecate more often, faecal incontinence and oily stools. Other weight-loss drugs have been taken off the market because of concerns they may have a detrimental effect on your health. Check with your doctor to see if weight-loss drugs are appropriate for you.

also work well against heart and vascular problems. But you and your doctor may want to try other options as well – including trying out medications that attack a number of diabetes-related problems at once. Here are some of the most important steps to consider:

✓ **Keep up the good work.** By being active regularly and following your healthy eating plan, you stand to lower your risk of cardiovascular complications considerably. For example, by eating more low-GI carbohydrates and fibre (from fruit, vegetables, whole grains, legumes and nuts) and replacing saturated fats (from animal foods) with healthier fats from foods such as fish, nuts, avocado and olive oil, you can reduce the amount of cholesterol in your blood. This will also help you to lose excess weight – a major contributor to high blood pressure and its associated health complications. Eating less salt is also important – avoid adding salt to your food during and after cooking, and try to limit the number of processed foods you consume and only choose those that are salt-reduced. At the same time, regular physical activity helps to strengthen the heart, keep blood vessels supple and it also appears to lower blood pressure even if you're not losing a great deal of weight.

✓ **Don't smoke.** There are plenty of good reasons to give up smoking, but start with the fact that it speeds up or exacerbates just about every process that contributes to cardio-vascular disease, whether or not you have diabetes. If you have diabetes, smoking doubles your risk of having a heart attack and you are

three times more likely to die of cardiovascular disease. Even if you are under 40 years of age, the risk is still high. Smoking reduces blood flow through the arteries by making them even stiffer and narrower, raises blood pressure, contributes to the formation of plaques that can lead to blocked vessels, makes it easier for blood to clot around obstructions and worsens pain from peripheral vascular disease.

People in their 20s and 30s who smoke have more fatty deposits on the walls of their blood vessels than non-smokers of the same age, which leads to blocked blood vessels and eventually to heart attack and stroke. Smoking also slows the circulation in the smaller blood vessels, and people with diabetes are already at an increased risk of poor circulation in their feet and legs. Smoking can also aggravate foot ulcers, foot infections and blood vessel disease in the legs.

If all of those reasons aren't enough to convince you to give up smoking, then perhaps one of the most disturbing of all the smoking statistics might: an alarming 95 per cent of people with diabetes who need amputations are those who choose to smoke. If you need help quitting the smoking habit, call the Quitline (contact details for Australia and New Zealand on pages 274–5).

✓ **Ask about aspirin.** This widely used anti-inflammatory has proven to be a major player in the battle against cardiovascular disease. In addition to relieving pain, aspirin also makes the clot-forming particles in blood, called platelets, less able to stick together. As a result, taking aspirin every day can cut the risk of a

Heeding the warning signs

Cardiovascular emergencies can sneak up on you suddenly, though there's often time to react effectively if you pay attention to warning signals. Call an ambulance immediately if you experience any of the following symptoms:

AILMENT	SYMPTOMS
Heart attack	• Tightness or pain in your chest • Pain or discomfort that radiates from the chest to the neck, shoulders or arms, especially on the left side where your heart is • Dizziness, lightheadedness, sweating, nausea or shortness of breath (don't assume these are signs of hypoglycaemia if you're also experiencing pain)
Stroke	• Weakness or numbness of the face, arm or leg, especially on one side of the body • Difficulty speaking or understanding others • Mental confusion • Vision problems • Difficulty walking or keeping your balance • Severe headache
Aneurysm	• Severe headache, back pain or abdominal pain that won't go away • Dizziness • Blurred vision • Nosebleeds

heart attack by a whopping 60 per cent. One recent US study found that taking one tablet at bedtime can also reduce high blood pressure, though, as with all medications, it can cause unwanted side effects so you should not use it without first seeking medical advice.

Talk to your doctor about whether aspirin is appropriate for you. Many people find that it irritates or causes bleeding in the stomach, though taking coated tablets that dissolve in the small intestine can help you avoid these problems. Still, you should avoid aspirin if you have a stomach ulcer or liver disease. And talk to your doctor about how aspirin affects the performance of other medications you may be taking – including blood thinners and medication for hypertension.

✔ **Investigate ACE inhibitors.** There are many medications to treat high blood pressure, but one class appears to have special benefits to people with diabetes. Called ACE (angiotensin-converting enzyme) inhibitors, they work by blocking a process in which one hormone turns into another that constricts blood vessels. ACE inhibitors are popular for bringing down blood pressure because, compared with other similar medications, they have few side effects other than causing a persistent dry cough in some people. (Newer medications called angiotensin II receptor blockers eliminate that problem.) The bonus is that recent research shows that ACE inhibitors lower the risk of cardiovascular problems in people with diabetes even if they don't have high blood pressure. They also help to protect the kidneys. What's more, a study published in 2000 found that people taking the ACE inhibitor ramipril were 30 per cent less likely to develop diabetes, which suggests that this medication also improves insulin sensitivity.

✅ **Seek help from statins.** People with diabetes often have high cholesterol, which is a risk factor for heart attacks. But many aren't reaping the benefit of cholesterol-lowering drugs called statins. Talk to your doctor about them to see if they are a viable option for you and if they fit into your medication regimen.

✅ **Eat a heart-healthy diet.** Eating a heart-healthy diet means:

✱ Being choosy with your fats to keep your cholesterol levels in check. You don't need to cut out all fat but you do need to avoid or limit foods containing large amounts of saturated fats and trans fats. Saturated fats are found in animal foods and some cooking oils such as palm and coconut oils, while trans fats are found in many processed foods such as commercial biscuits, pastries, fried foods and some margarines. Replace these with polyunsaturated or monounsaturated fats found in plant foods such as nuts, seeds, avocado and vegetables, nut and seed oils such as olive, canola, macadamia, grapeseed or sunflower oil.

✱ Including more omega-3 fats, which protect against heart disease by reducing the risk of blood clots and abnormal heart rhythms, and lowering blood pressure. These are found mainly in fatty fish (for example, salmon, sardines, mackerel) as well as some plant foods, particularly linseeds, chia seeds and linseed oil.

✱ Increasing your intake of soluble fibre from foods such as legumes (lentils, chickpeas and dried or canned beans), oats, oat bran, barley, psyllium, linseeds and many fruits including apples and pears. Soluble fibre helps to remove cholesterol from the blood and also helps with blood-glucose control.

✱ Eating a handful of nuts each day: nuts have not only been shown to lower cholesterol but also contain many other cardio-protective nutrients, and studies have shown a strong link between nut consumption and a lower risk of heart disease. Choose the unsalted variety.

✱ Eating more whole grains such as dense wholegrain breads, oats, barley, quinoa, cracked wheat, buckwheat, brown rice and wholegrain pasta. Eating two to four serves of wholegrain foods a day can reduce the risk of heart disease by as much as 40 per cent, which is equivalent to the effect of the most common cholesterol-lowering drugs.

✱ Including soy products in your diet – research has shown that soy protein can help to lower the levels of total and 'bad' LDL cholesterol. Try switching to soy milk, including tofu in stir-fries, choosing soy and linseed breads and adding soybeans to soups and casseroles.

✅ **Turn to tea.** Certain foods appear to have an especially powerful protective effect against cardiovascular damage. One of these is tea, which numerous studies have linked with better heart health. In one of the most recent research studies, tea drinkers who averaged 2 or more cups a day had a 44 per cent lower death rate after a heart attack than those who didn't drink tea; moderate tea drinkers had a 28 per cent lower death rate. Tea's protective effect is thought to come from its bounty of flavonoids, which are anti-oxidant compounds found in both black and green tea that appear to prevent cholesterol from clogging arteries, discourage blood from clotting and also contribute to keeping blood vessels supple.

✅ **Think about anti-oxidants.** Anti-oxidant nutrients like vitamins C and E counteract a process called oxidation, in which unstable molecules produced by the body's use of oxygen damage healthy tissue. Among their benefits, anti-oxidants make cholesterol less likely to stick to artery walls. Good sources of vitamin C include citrus fruits, tomatoes, berries and capsicum. Vitamin E is found in nuts, avocado, vegetable oils and wheatgerm.

Caring for your kidneys

The first thing to appreciate about your kidneys is that you have two of them, nestled on either side of your spine towards the back of your torso just above your waist. Two is really more than you need – people can survive with only one (assuming it's healthy). But it's a sign of how important the kidneys are that the body builds in such redundancy.

The kidneys are the body's sewage plant, where blood flows to be filtered through a complex of tiny blood vessels called capillaries. Cleansed blood is sent back into circulation while wastes and toxins are taken out and sent to the bladder for excretion in urine. The kidneys are hardworking and efficient, and they tend to keep quiet even when their job becomes difficult – which is when blood-glucose overloads damage the delicate capillaries and structures that filter your blood.

It takes years of blood-glucose abuse to wreck the kidneys, but once the kidneys are damaged, there's no repairing them. Total loss of kidney function ultimately requires dialysis, in which you're hooked up to a blood-cleansing machine for 2 to 4 hours a few times a week. Another option is a kidney transplant.

The kidney-disease countdown

Between 20 and 40 per cent of people with diabetes develop kidney disease, also known as nephropathy. In fact, in Australia diabetes is the second most common cause of end stage renal failure and accounts for 25 per cent of all new cases (40 per cent in New Zealand). Still, research studies show that you can avoid kidney disease, especially if you're alert to what happens as the disease progresses – and you act early. You can expect uncontrolled kidney damage to move ahead in several stages.

✳ First, the kidneys start filtering waste faster in an attempt to clear blood of excess glucose, boosting the glomerular filtration rate or GFR. Some of the structures inside the kidneys begin to get bigger, intruding on space normally used by blood-filtering capillaries, making them less efficient and causing the kidneys to work harder.

✸ After a year or so, the kidneys start becoming less able to filter waste or keep nutrients that should stay in the body from being expelled. Small amounts of a protein known as albumin may become detectable in the urine, a condition known as microalbuminuria.

The blood-cleansing kidneys

The kidneys produce and eliminate urine through a complex system of some two million tiny filters called nephrons. At the top of each nephron, in the Bowman's capsule, is the glomerulus, a microscopic cluster of capillaries. Blood flows at high pressure through the glomerulus, where urea, toxins and other wastes are filtered out and ultimately expelled through the urine. The purified fluid is returned to the blood via the renal vein. Over time, high blood glucose destroys the nephrons.

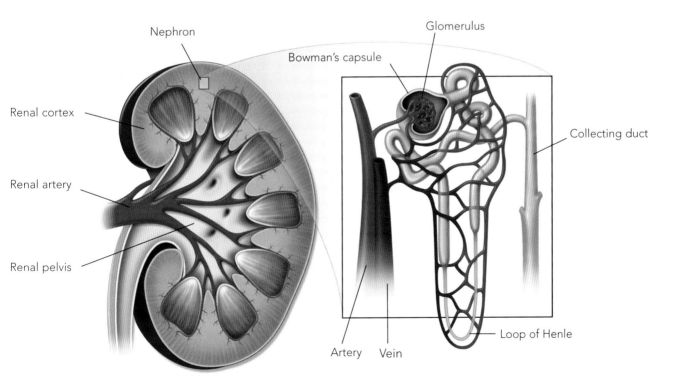

✳ As the kidneys become more damaged, you lose more albumin, whose job is to keep water within the bloodstream. The deficit causes water to build up in the body's tissues, causing such classic symptoms of kidney disease as puffiness around the eyes and swelling of the hands and feet. At the same time, the liver starts to pump out cholesterol and other fats that are involved with manufacturing albumin, boosting your cardiovascular risks. If you have type 2 diabetes, there may still be time to ward off kidney failure at this stage (known as nephrotic syndrome), but it may be too late if you have type 1.

✳ The last two stages are in the realm of kidney failure, in which the body becomes increasingly less able to filter waste. In the first stage of kidney failure, called renal insufficiency, treatment may still be of benefit, but as damage gets worse, you enter end-stage renal failure, when even good blood-glucose control probably can't stave off the inevitable: dialysis or a transplant.

Kicking kidney complications

Closely controlling blood glucose is the single most important way to keep kidney disease at bay. But managing high blood pressure, which can narrow arteries leading to the kidneys and damage the delicate blood vessels inside them, also plays a big role. That means there are plenty of steps you can take to reduce your risk or slow the progress of kidney disease. Some of these cut your chances of developing other complications as well.

✓ **Test regularly.** Hallmark symptoms, such as swelling, fatigue and pain in the lower back, don't usually show up until a lot of kidney tissue has already been damaged – perhaps as much as 80 per cent. But it's possible to detect the early signs of kidney disease well before that with regular tests. Your doctor will order a urine test called microalbuminuria at diagnosis and again every 12 months. Your doctor may also suggest that you be tested for creatinine, a waste product of muscles that a healthy kidney will clear from the blood but a damaged one will leave behind in detectable amounts.

✓ **Treat high blood pressure.** Taking ACE inhibitors to control hypertension benefits the kidneys by relieving pressure that can damage delicate filtering structures and keeping blood vessels flexible. In fact, some studies find that taking ACE inhibitors cuts deaths from diabetic kidney disease in half. Even in people who don't have high blood pressure but have signs of kidney damage, research suggests that ACE inhibitors are beneficial. Anything else you do to bring down blood pressure – especially not smoking – will also benefit your kidneys. Discuss with your doctor the appropriateness of using ACE inhibitors.

✓ **Cut back on protein.** Not everyone agrees that eating less protein will help stave off kidney disease, especially in its early stages. But if this occurs, it is recommended that you talk to your doctor and dietitian. You may be advised to decrease your protein intake. Many of us eat far more protein than we need, leaving the kidneys to excrete the excess waste

– urea – a burden that may accelerate damage. Restricting protein may be helpful if kidney disease progresses even though blood glucose and blood pressure are under control. There is also some evidence that replacing animal protein, particularly red meat, with vegetable protein (for example, soy) can reduce the progression of kidney disease. If concerned, ask your doctor or dietitian.

✅ **Protect against infection.** Having a burning sensation when you urinate, constantly having to go to the toilet and cloudy or bloody urine are signs of a urinary tract infection (UTI), which should be treated with antibiotics. UTIs are common in people with diabetes, partly because damage to nerves that control the bladder can keep you from voiding properly, leaving waste to fester in the body. As a result, the kidneys can be further damaged by the ravages of bacteria. You need to drink 1.8 litres of water a day to prevent UTIs. While some studies have found cranberry juice may help to prevent UTIs in women with recurrent UTIs, other studies don't show a benefit. In many of the studies the subjects failed to continue taking the cranberry juice, particularly over longer periods of time, and this may explain why the studies have not found it to be effective. Cranberry supplements (tablets or capsules) have been found to have a similar effectiveness to antibiotics, which could make them a useful alternative. However, more studies comparing products with standardised amounts of the active ingredient are needed before it is routinely recommended for clinical use.

✅ **Mind your meds.** A wide range of medications, prescription and over-the-counter, can be hard on the kidneys. Among them are ibuprofen (such as Advil and Motrin) and naproxen (Aleve), along with more potent anti-inflammatories available by prescription. Other prescription drugs that can make kidney damage worse include certain antibiotics and lithium. Be sure to check with your doctor whenever you get a new prescription to see if there are any warnings about taking it if you have kidney disease.

Being wise with your eyes

Like the kidneys, the eyes are nourished by small blood vessels that can easily be damaged when you have diabetes. Left alone, this can lead to vision loss – diabetes is a leading cause of preventable blindness in the adult population. But most eye problems can be treated if caught early – and it may be possible to avoid them altogether.

As always, tight blood-glucose control makes a big difference. In the US Diabetes Control and Complications Trial, risk reduction from good blood-glucose control was greater for eye disease (76 per cent) than for any other complication. Still, you can't afford to be complacent about the possibility of eye damage, especially because you typically won't notice it in its earliest stages.

Most eye damage from diabetes takes place in the retina, the light-sensitive area at the back of the eye that registers visual signals and sends them to the brain through the optic nerve. High blood glucose (especially when combined with high blood pressure) can weaken small blood vessels that supply the eyes with oxygen and nutrients, causing them to puff up and rupture like balloons – a condition known as non-proliferative retinopathy. In some cases, leakage and lack of nourishment can directly damage the retina and make your vision blurry, but you may not notice anything at all.

If the damage progresses, you can develop a more severe condition called proliferative retinopathy, in which more blood vessels start to sprout in the retina to make up for blood delivery lost through burst vessels. This only compounds the problem by leading to more

How diabetes affects the eyes

Lining the interior of the eye is the retina, a delicate 10-layer membrane packed with nerve fibres and photoreceptors. Diabetic retinopathy occurs when uncontrolled high blood glucose damages or blocks the tiny blood vessels (capillaries) throughout the retina, cutting off the blood supply to small patches of retinal tissue. The damaged blood vessels also tend to leak, producing swelling within the retina. As retinal damage progresses, new blood vessels sprout and vision may become increasingly blurred. About 25 per cent of people with diabetes have some degree of retinopathy.

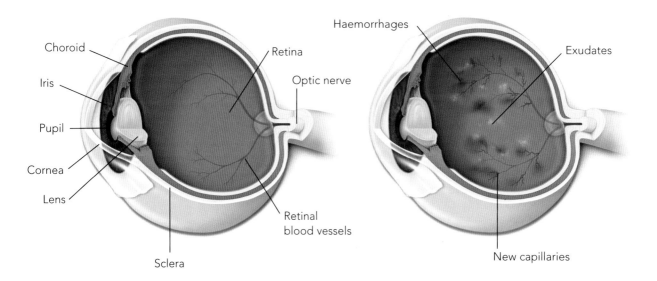

Choroid

Iris

Pupil

Cornea

Lens

Retina

Optic nerve

Retinal blood vessels

Sclera

Haemorrhages

Exudates

New capillaries

ruptures. These can block light to the retina and cause haemorrhages and pressure inside the eyes, which contributes to scar tissue that can eventually cause the retina to start tearing away from the eye (retinal detachment). Retinopathy can also cause macular oedema. In this condition, the central area of the retina (called the macula), which allows you to see sharp detail and colour, swells, causing loss of fine vision.

How to stay a visionary

The key to keeping your sight clear is to keep on the lookout for symptoms that may point to a problem.

✓ **Be alert to changes.** It's easy to dismiss subtle changes in your vision as minor annoyances, but when you have diabetes, you can't assume you need a new glasses' prescription or that your eyes are just getting 'old'. Granted, those may be possibilities – and high or low fluctuations in blood glucose can temporarily affect your vision as well. But you should still call your doctor or eye specialist right away if:

- your eyesight seems blurry
- you experience double vision
- your vision becomes distorted, or straight lines, such as telephone poles, look warped
- spots or lines seem to float in front of your eyes
- your field of vision seems narrower
- you have more difficulty seeing clearly in dim light
- it seems as though a window shade has been drawn over your field of vision.

? DID you KNOW...

Twenty-five per cent of people with type 2 diabetes already have signs of early retinopathy when they're diagnosed. It is rare to find retinopathy within the first 5 years of diagnosis for people with type 1 diabetes. After 8 years, retinopathy is present in 50 per cent of people. After 20 years, all people with type 1 diabetes have some retinopathy, and 60 per cent of people with type 2. Regular eye examinations are critical if issues of prevention and control are to be addressed properly.

- You feel pressure or pain in your eyes
- You have trouble perceiving colours, especially blue and yellow, or making distinctions between similar colours

✓ **Keep regular watch.** You may not be able to see or feel the earliest signs of retinopathy, but an eye specialist can easily pick them up during an eye examination, so it's important to schedule regular eye checks. An eye chart on the wall is not sufficient – go to an ophthalmologist, optometrist or diabetes specialist physician, who will give you a comprehensive examination that includes dilating your pupils to look directly at the retina. People with type 1 diabetes need an eye examination within 3 to 5 years of the onset of the disease and people with type 2 need to have an examination immediately after diagnosis. After that, everyone with diabetes

WHAT the
STUDIES show

Aspirin helps protect your heart, but
there's evidence that it can help protect
your eyes, too. One study found that
people with diabetes had a four-fold
increase in tiny blood clots in the
capillaries that nourish the retina. These
clots may eventually starve the retina of
oxygen and nutrients and trigger the
growth of new, abnormal blood vessels.
Aspirin may protect the capillaries from
clots and help stave off retinopathy.

needs to have their eyes checked once a year,
unless otherwise recommended by an eye
specialist.

✅ **Get help for hypertension.** Easing
your blood pressure can reduce your risk of
retinopathy or slow its progression. Ask your
doctor if, in addition to changing your eating
habits, getting regular physical activity and not
smoking, you need to take medication.

✅ **Evaluate your activity.** Once you learn
you have retinopathy, check in with your doctor
to take another look at your physical activity
program. Certain forms of exercise can be
jarring to the delicate structures within the
eye or may increase the amount of pressure
inside the eye and thus lead to more retinal
bleeding. It may help to see an exercise
physiologist for advice on the most suitable
exercise program for you.

✅ **Discuss surgery.** The best way to prevent
further damage from retinopathy may be to fix
the harm that's already been done. Using a type
of laser surgery called photocoagulation, an
ophthalmologist aims a thin beam of laser light
at the retina to destroy ruptured blood vessels,
seal areas that are leaking and prevent new
vessels from forming. In some cases, laser
surgery can slow the rate of vision loss by
90 per cent or more. Another form of surgery,
called cryotherapy, destroys abnormal blood
vessels by freezing them with a probe – a
technique that is especially useful for those
areas that a laser can't reach, or for people
who still have proliferative retinopathy
after laser surgery. In a third operation,
called a vitrectomy, the eye's jellylike core
(the vitreous humour) is taken out so that
doctors can remove scar tissue from inside
the eye and repair the retina if it has started
to detach.

Nipping nerve damage in the bud

Nerve damage may be one of the most
far-reaching complications of diabetes
because the nervous system controls
or contributes to so much – everything
from your sense of touch (and pain) to
muscle movement, digestion and sexual
function, just to name a few. Fortunately,
you probably have time to prevent nerve
damage, which usually develops after
you've had diabetes for at least 10 to
15 years.

Doctors don't entirely understand how diabetes causes nerve damage, but likely possibilities are that high blood glucose upsets the balance of chemicals that allow nerves to transmit electrical impulses, deprives nerves of oxygen by impeding circulation and damages the nerves' protective coating (called the myelin sheath). Thankfully, diabetes doesn't appear to affect the brain and spinal cord – the components of the central nervous system. Still, the rest of the body's nerves, which carry electrical impulses through what amounts to an intricate network of 'wires', are vulnerable to diabetes-related signal slowdowns, miscommunication or interruptions.

There are three major types of nerve damage, or neuropathy, each of which can affect the body in many different ways. If you develop neuropathy, your doctor will determine which kind it is mostly by your symptoms and where they occur.

Polyneuropathy. The most common type of nerve damage affects multiple nerves throughout the body (*poly* means 'many'), but it mainly affects the long nerves of the peripheral nervous system that run through the arms and legs. You'll often hear this kind of nerve damage referred to as distal symmetric neuropathy because it strikes areas away from the central nervous system (*distal* refers to distance from the centre) and tends to cause symptoms on both sides of the body (symmetric). Polyneuropathy generally doesn't affect movement; it instead disrupts sensation, often causing pain, cramps or tingling in the hands or feet and, later, numbness.

Focal neuropathy. Far less common, focal neuropathy concentrates on a single nerve, or set of nerves, and often affects only one area of the body – which is why it's sometimes called mononeuropathy (*mono* means 'one'). Unlike polyneuropathy, which tends to develop gradually over time, it appears suddenly, often causing numbness or pain, or weakness in the muscles, depending on which nerves are affected. Although it can crop up anywhere, focal neuropathy often causes Bell's palsy, in which nerves lose control over muscles in the face, causing features to droop. Focal neuropathy can cause eyes to cross if it affects muscles that control eye movement, and it can cause carpal tunnel syndrome, in which compressed nerves in the wrist produce pain or weakness in the hand and forearm.

Autonomic neuropathy. The autonomic nervous system governs the body functions that you don't normally have to think about much, such as heartbeat, digestion, sweating and bladder control – but that become more of a concern if nerves are damaged. If you have any of the symptoms listed below, you need to talk to your doctor. Among the problems that can result from autonomic neuropathy are:

✱ Cardiovascular glitches, such as irregular heartbeat and a condition called orthostatic hypotension, in which your blood pressure fails to quickly adjust when you stand up, making you feel faint or dizzy. Deadened nerves can also fail to pick up pain from a heart attack.

Tests of nerves

While it's up to you to sound the neuropathy alarm, if you suspect you have nerve damage, your doctor can confirm and finetune the diagnosis with subtle tests. One way is to hold a tuning fork against body parts, such as your foot, to find out whether you can detect its vibration. Similarly, your doctor may touch you with a hairlike fine wire to gauge your response to delicate stimuli or apply heat or cold to make sure you could tell if you were being harmed by, say, scalding bathwater. If any of these tests indicate that you have nerve damage, your doctor will probably send you to a neurologist for further investigation and specialist advice.

✸ A condition known as gastroparesis, in which muscles of the gastrointestinal tract become slow and inefficient. Sluggish digestion not only causes problems like nausea, vomiting, bloating, diarrhoea, constipation and loss of appetite, but it makes blood-glucose patterns more difficult to predict and balance with insulin.

✸ Poor bladder function, in which nerves may have trouble telling when the bladder is full and don't empty the bladder completely when you void. One result is higher risk of urinary tract infections, which in turn can accelerate kidney damage.

✸ Sexual dysfunction, where men find it difficult to get or maintain an erection and women have vaginal dryness or tepid sexual response. Usually, sex drive is unaffected in both sexes.

✸ Dulled response to nervous symptoms of hypoglycaemia, such as shakiness, sweating and anxiety and a dangerous condition known as hypoglycaemic unawareness.

✸ Profuse sweating and poor regulation of body temperature.

Keeping the verve in nerves

In the case of nerve damage, closely controlling blood glucose – your top priority – can reduce your risks by as much as 60 per cent. Once neuropathy develops, treatments vary depending on how the nerve damage is affecting your body. Among the steps you can take to minimise damage and discomfort:

✔ **Get in touch with your feelings.** As with most diabetes complications, the sooner you pick up on nerve damage, the more you can do to keep it from escalating. Don't dismiss sensations or difficulties that disappear. In many cases, symptoms come and go or swing from mild to severe. Tell your doctor immediately if you experience:

● Tingling, numbness, burning or prickly pain in your arms, legs, hands or feet. Stay alert – the sensations can be very subtle at first. Try to be especially aware of unusual sensations in the feet, which are often affected first, or at night, when symptoms are usually worse

● Sensitivity to touch – even the light brushing of your sheets against you when you're in bed

● Leg cramps that may come and go, especially at night

- Difficulty sensing the position of your feet or toes, or a sense that you can't keep your balance
- Calluses or sores on your feet
- Wasting of the muscles in the feet or hands
- Weakness and difficulties walking
- Dizziness or faintness, particularly after standing or sitting up
- Digestive problems such as diarrhoea, constipation, indigestion, nausea and vomiting
- Problems with urination
- Erectile dysfunction in men or vaginal dryness in women.

✅ **Adjust your healthy eating plan.** Check with your dietitian to see if changes in the foods you eat regularly may help keep some symptoms of neuropathy in check. For example, if you're suffering from gastroparesis, you may want to try eating smaller and more frequent meals.

✅ **Boost your Bs.** In some cases, neuropathy is fostered by a deficiency in the vitamins B6 and B12, both of which are involved in the function of the nervous system. You can get vitamin B6 from avocados, bananas, poultry, pork, potatoes and fish like tuna, while B12 is found in animal foods, including meat, chicken, fish, seafood, eggs and dairy foods, including milk and yogurt. Do not take nutritional supplements without first discussing it with your doctor, diabetes educator or dietitian. Metformin can reduce the absorption of vitamin B12, so if you are taking this medication, it is important to monitor your B12 levels regularly.

✅ **Supplement your nerve health.** See page 199 to learn about alpha-lipoic acid, an anti-oxidant supplement that can help protect the nerves and ease the pain of neuropathy.

✅ **Reach for relief.** Try to temper the pain of polyneuropathy with over-the-counter pain relievers – especially aspirin, since it also carries the bonus of cardiovascular benefits. (If you're already taking small doses of aspirin daily, ask your doctor about adjusting the amount.) You may also find relief from topical creams containing capsaicin, a compound found in hot chillies that alleviates pain by interfering with signals that nerve cells send to the brain. When using these creams, be very careful to keep them away from the eyes and other sensitive parts of the body.

✅ **Ask about medication.** Medications are available to help control many of the specific conditions that can result from neuropathy. Sildenafil (Viagra) for sexual dysfunction is just one example. There are also medications that help you empty your bladder, ward off episodes of low blood pressure and treat gastroparesis. You might also benefit from taking a tricyclic antidepressant – not because you've got the blues but because they've also been found to take the edge off neuropathy pain. Give these medications time to work, as it often takes several weeks for them to become effective. Your doctor might also recommend an anticonvulsant drug, which can reduce the pain caused by nerve damage.

✅ **Don't smoke and limit alcohol.** Smoking damages blood vessels and the combination of nerve and blood vessel damage is the major cause of serious foot complications in people with diabetes.

Sidestepping foot problems

Your feet can take more than the usual beating when you have diabetes. Poor circulation from damaged blood vessels slows the healing process and makes your feet more prone to infection, while nerve damage can dull sensation and leave you oblivious to injuries that can quickly get out of control. This could result in some very serious complications that may need surgical intervention to resolve.

In the grand scheme of things, foot hassles may seem somewhat mundane. However, avoiding such hassles by looking after your feet is of utmost importance. If ignored and left untreated for long, what may seem like minor irritations can eventually put you at risk of actually losing a foot – or at worst a leg – as well as tissue death, known as gangrene.

Check your feet carefully every day and don't ignore broken skin, corns, calluses, bunions, ingrown toenails and other seemingly minor irritations. The way to avoid serious problems is to talk to your doctor or podiatrist right away. Of the thousands of amputations performed every year in Australia on people with diabetes, most could have been prevented.

It all begins with some form of injury that abrades or breaks the skin, the protective barrier that keeps germs out of your body. Perhaps your shoes aren't a good fit or you stepped on a stone. Once the damaged area becomes infected, healing may prove difficult, especially if you keep walking on it or aren't aware that it's there, and an open sore, or ulcer, can quickly develop. This is a reason to call your doctor or podiatrist. Infection from uncontrolled ulcers can burrow deeper into your skin and eventually reach the bone, putting the entire limb at risk. When you've had diabetes for a long time, feet may also become vulnerable to a condition called Charcot's foot, in which numbness and poor reflexes from neuropathy cause missteps that destroy joints in the foot.

Fortunately, paying special attention to your feet can go a long way towards keeping them healthy. Here are some of the most important steps you can take.

✅ **Always wear shoes.** Your shoes provide protection from blows, scrapes and sharp objects. You'll significantly improve this protection if you avoid going barefoot (especially at the beach, where sand can cause abrasions and debris can puncture the skin) or wearing open shoes, such as thongs or sandals. If you have foot problems, including reduced sensation, it's also a good idea to wear shoes indoors to avoid the risk of injury.

✅ **Do a daily check.** Give your feet a check once a day, perhaps at bedtime, going over them with both your eyes and your hands. Let your doctor know if you find evidence of

Take-charge tips

Finding shoes that fit is important for anybody, but doubly so for people with diabetes. Your podiatrist can help if you have trouble finding the right footwear, but you should be able to score comfortable shoes off the rack if you heed these tips:

Follow three fit factors. Don't settle for just any shoe, unless it meets all three criteria for a good fit:

- The tip of the shoe should extend about the width of your thumb beyond your longest toe.

- The ball of your foot should fit comfortably – without cramping the toes – into the widest part of the shoe.

- The heel should fit snugly without slipping when you walk.

- ○ **Measure every time.** Don't just tell the salesperson your size – get a new measurement. Changes in weight, blood circulation and foot structure can make your foot a different size or shape to what it was.

- ○ **Try on both shoes.** One of your feet is probably slightly larger than the other, so make sure shoes fit both feet. If necessary, buy for your larger foot and see your podiatrist about padding the other shoe.

- ○ **Don't assume it will stretch.** Shoes may mould better to your feet the longer you wear them, but don't let a salesperson tell you the basic fit will improve with time. The shoe should fit – now.

- ○ **Buy late in the day.** Feet swell by as much as 5 per cent over the course of the day, so shopping in the afternoon will ensure that feet aren't cramped when you put new shoes on in the morning.

- ○ **Ask about returns.** If you've lost sensation in your feet, you can't trust how shoes feel in the shop. Bring them home and wear them around the house for half an hour, then check your feet. If you see areas of redness, which indicate pressure from a poor fit, take the shoes back and swap them.

any problems. Besides blisters, cuts, bruises, cracking, peeling or other obvious signs of damage, look for areas that are shaded differently (either paler or redder), which could indicate persistent pressure from shoes. Feel for areas of coldness, which could be a sign of poor circulation, or warmness, which might be evidence of an infection, along with redness or swelling. If you have trouble seeing the bottoms of your feet, place a mirror on the floor and look at the reflection. If you have poor vision, ask a family member or friend to inspect your feet for you.

✓ **Wash and dry.** Keep your feet clean by washing them every day with lukewarm water and soap. (Avoid hot water, which, if you have neuropathy, may scald you without your knowing it.) Avoid soaking your feet, which will soften skin and make it more vulnerable to infection. Dry feet by blotting (not rubbing), making sure you dry between the toes to discourage fungal infections. Use a moisturising cream to prevent dryness and cracking, but don't put it between your toes, where it may encourage skin to wear away.

✓ **Clip with care.** Keep your toenails neatly trimmed, cutting them straight across to prevent ingrown nails and filing rough edges to avoid damaging adjacent toes. Some podiatrists advise against using nail clippers for fear that you'll accidentally cut the skin. If you're concerned, consider using a file or an emery board (go no shorter than the ends of your toes) or having someone help.

✓ **Get a clean start.** Begin each day by putting on a fresh pair of socks made of a breathable material like cotton, cotton blend or wool, which keeps moisture away from skin and helps keep your feet dry. Make sure socks fit well without bunching up, and don't wear socks with seams that will rub your feet, potentially causing pressure sores. If your feet tend to sweat a lot, change your socks throughout the day as needed.

✓ **Wear good shoes.** Footwear should provide both comfort and protection. Leather uppers are best because they conform to the shape of your foot and breathe so that feet perspire less. Opt for low heels for stability and soles made of crepe or foam rubber for cushioning. Have at least two pairs of shoes that you wear regularly so you can alternate from one day to the next, giving shoes time to air out between each wearing. New shoes should never be worn for more than a few hours at a time. Before putting on shoes, shake them out and feel inside to make sure there's no debris that could cause pressure or irritation.

✓ **Touch base with your doctor.** A foot examination needs to be done by your doctor, a podiatrist or a diabetes educator trained in foot assessment, at least every 6 months – more often if you have signs of neuropathy or poor circulation or you've already had foot ulcers, in which case you must see a podiatrist regularly. (Bring your most-worn pair of shoes to the appointment so your podiatrist can check wear patterns.) But don't wait for your 6-monthly check-up if you notice any changes in your feet. Not every minor cut demands medical attention, but call your podiatrist or doctor if you develop an infection or sore, your foot is punctured by a sharp object, a toe becomes red and tender, or you notice any change in sensation, such as numbness, pain or tingling. Do not use acid treatments or over-the-counter wart or corn removers, and never try to perform do-it-yourself 'bathroom surgery' to treat problems like warts, corns, calluses or ingrown toenails.

Dodging dental disease

People with diabetes are two to three times more likely to be affected by tooth decay and gum infections. The main reason is that high blood-glucose levels encourage the activity of bacteria in the mouth contributing to decay and the development of plaque. Diabetes can also reduce the body's resistance to infections, which can increase blood-glucose levels further.

Warning signs to watch for:

- bleeding gums when you brush or floss your teeth
- red, swollen, or sore gums
- receding gums
- pus between the teeth and gums
- bad breath
- loose or separating teeth
- change in your bite or jaw alignment
- changes in the fit of your dentures.

If you experience any of these problems, see your dentist urgently.

What can I do?

- Keep your blood-glucose levels well controlled to discourage bacteria and infections
- Brush your teeth at least twice per day using a soft, rounded bristled toothbrush and use dental floss daily
- Watch for early signs of gum disease such as redness or bleeding when you brush or floss
- Visit your dentist at least every 6 months
- Don't smoke

- Avoid soft drinks, including the diet variety. If you can't resist, use a straw
- Avoid frequent snacking – leave at least 2 hours between eating or drinking so that saliva can neutralise acids in the mouth. If you do snack, choose fruit, yogurt, cheese and raw vegetables
- Drink plenty of water, particularly after eating
- Chew sugar-free gum after meals to increase saliva production, which protects against tooth decay.

The stages of gum disease

Plaque and tartar build-up. When we eat, remnants of food together with saliva and bacteria cause the development of plaque. If not removed properly, through regular brushing and flossing, this plaque hardens into tartar which builds up around the gumline, making it harder to brush and clean between the teeth.

Gingivitis. The gums become red, swollen and tender and are likely to bleed during brushing and flossing. It can be improved by regular cleaning with your dentist and taking more care with your brushing and flossing at home.

Periodontitis. If gingivitis isn't treated early, it can progress to a stage where the gums pull away from your teeth, causing a gap, which can become infected. Without treatment, the infection destroys the bone around your teeth and you could require gum surgery or even lose your teeth.

complementary therapies

You're following an eating plan, watching your weight, getting regular physical activity and possibly taking medication or insulin for your diabetes. Can anything else help? Certain herbs and supplements show promise for bringing down blood glucose and protecting the eyes, nerves, kidneys and heart when used in conjunction with conventional diabetes management practices. And other complementary therapies may reduce stress. Should you try them? You are strongly advised to first consult your doctor, dietition or diabetes educator. And remember: these therapies must only be used in addition to – never instead of – your usual diabetes treatment.

The wonders of modern medicine have given us insulin and oral medications to help manage blood glucose and statins to lower the risk of heart-related complications. But what about the world of not-so-modern medicine? For thousands of years healers from different cultures relied on natural therapies, many of them herb-based, to treat conditions like diabetes. Can any of them help you? While diabetes organisations in Australia approach complementary therapies with caution, Diabetes New Zealand does not recommend their use.

More and more people – and even some doctors – are starting to ask that question as interest in so-called alternative medicine continues to grow. According to one US study, visits to registered medical practitioners remained stable through the late 1990s, but visits to alternative therapists jumped by 47 per cent. Perhaps more surprising, surveys also find that as many as 60 per cent of physicians have recommended complementary therapies to patients – a reflection of the fact that more than 75 medical schools in the United States now provide training in various types of alternative medicine. However, while this may lend an air of credibility and, in some cases, scientific validation to the case for alternative medicine in the United States, Australians and New Zealanders remain openly cautious about the true value of these sorts of complementary therapies.

What is alternative medicine?

In many ways, what you define as 'alternative' depends on your culture. Many alternative therapies come from Eastern regions, such as Asia and India, where healing traditions tend to be less scientific than they are in the West. But not all Western countries view medicine the same way, either. Germany, for example, has a long history of incorporating herbal therapies into conventional medicine and conducting research into their benefits. However, in Australia and New Zealand, herbal supplements, while growing in popularity, still play less of a role in mainstream medicine.

'Alternative' medicine often suggests a form of treatment that is taken instead of conventional medical treatment, which could potentially be very dangerous. 'Complementary', however, emphasises the fact that alternative therapies may sometimes be useful as an adjunct to traditional medical care but should never be seen as a substitute – as many alternative practitioners will be the first to tell you. In fact, it is very important that you ask your doctor about any supplement or alternative treatment you want to try, and inform other members of your diabetes team what you're using. Many complementary treatments, especially herbs, can interfere with other medications and may affect the way your doctor has advised you to treat your diabetes.

How to judge complementary therapies

One way to summarise the difference between complementary and conventional medicine is that the former is more art and the latter is more science. That balance is beginning to shift as more research is done into the potential benefits of complementary therapies. But one of the main drawbacks is that, in many cases, the scientific evidence that a therapy works is sketchy, and safety risks are often not well understood.

That doesn't necessarily mean that complementary medicine is automatically worthless or dangerous. But it does give you reason to approach it with an open mind – including a healthy openness to scepticism. Marketing and promotional material (along with much of the information published in books or on websites promoting complementary medicine) makes supplements and other products sound good. But it's important to be wary of the ways manufacturers typically get their point across:

? DID you KNOW...

The word drug comes from the French term drogue, meaning 'herb' – an indication that herbal remedies are not as far removed from conventional medicines as you might think. In addition to aspirin, many mainstream drugs have been developed from substances found in plants, including metformin, morphine and quinine.

Unquestioning faith. Sometimes labels and advertising will state what a product is used for as if there is no doubt that it works.

Vague research. In other cases, 'research' or 'studies' are cited with no further details about who conducted it.

Testimonials. A favourite 'proof' that a therapy works is to quote somebody (preferably a celebrity) who says it was good for him or her. But from a scientific perspective, anecdotes are the least convincing form of evidence.

History. The fact that a therapy has been used for hundreds or even thousands of years is often held out as evidence of effectiveness, but tradition is not necessarily proof.

The standards for studies

Why is the research so sparse on complementary remedies? Partly, it's a matter of money. No one can patent a natural product such as a herb, and pharmaceutical companies, which fund much of the research into conventional medicines, generally aren't willing to sink development dollars into products on which they have no exclusive claim.

So how can you tell if a complementary treatment will work for you? The only real answer – as is true for many drugs as well – is to try it and see, if your doctor approves. But before you discuss it with your doctor, gather plenty of information about the therapy and consider the research that's been done on it.

When evaluating research, you can get a sense of its value by looking at the criteria that researchers themselves use. In the world of medical science, the best studies are those that are:

Big. Your diabetes isn't the same as the next person's, so if you and someone else both take the same supplement, you can expect slightly different results. Even the best conventional medications don't work for some people. In other cases, a person's health may improve for reasons that have nothing to do with the treatment being tested. Getting reliable findings therefore depends to some degree on conducting tests that involve as many people as possible. Most studies of complementary therapies, however, are disappointingly small.

Human. Scientists often start with lab tests to determine a substance's chemical properties and effects. These experiments are a good start, but they can't reliably predict what will happen in the human body. Animal tests are more informative, and the most informative are those tests done on people.

Controlled. The least reliable experiments are those in which people are simply given the therapy and asked if it makes them feel better. In many cases, people will say yes even when the treatment is known to have no medical benefit – a phenomenon known as the placebo effect. Better experiments are controlled, meaning that one group of people gets the real treatment while a second group gets a fake one so that results can be compared and the possible impact of the placebo effect can be factored in.

Double-blind. To further guard against the placebo effect, it's best that study subjects don't know which treatment they're getting. To make absolutely sure that subjects are kept in the dark – that they won't get an inkling from the researchers, through body language or other subtle clues, of whether they're getting the real medicine or not – the people administering the treatments shouldn't know who's getting what, either.

Peer-reviewed. The most reliable studies are those that not only meet all the above criteria but also have been assessed as valid by other experts in the field before being published in what's known as a peer-reviewed journal.

The natural medicine cabinet

Some of the most popular complementary therapies for assisting diabetes management are herbal and plant-based supplements that you can find at health-food shops and many pharmacies and supermarkets. Do they work? For the most part, the jury is still out, but research so far suggests that a few may be of some value.

Whether to use complementary remedies is a personal decision you'll need to make in consultation with your doctor. Certainly, you need to approach them with caution. Don't simply assume that 'herbal' means 'safe', because, in most cases, thorough research on long-term effects has not been done. The fact is, many medicinal herbs do have effects on the body – which is reason for both hope and concern. The information presented below is not an endorsement of these therapies, but it can start you thinking about whether certain supplements may be useful to you.

Aiming for glucose control

The major goal of herbal therapies for diabetes is the same as for medication and insulin: to bring down high blood glucose. Here's where it's important to emphasise that these therapies are complementary: even if they work, you should never take them as a substitute for your insulin or regular medication, though they might be useful in lowering the doses you require.

It's extremely important that you monitor your blood glucose closely if you take these remedies, for two reasons. First, you won't know how effective they are unless you measure their impact on your glucose. Second, if they're able to bring blood glucose down, you need to be on the alert for an increased possibility of hypoglycaemia. Among the herbs that show the most promise for lowering blood glucose are:

Gymnema. Known botanically as *Gymnema sylvestre*, this plant is native to Africa and India, where its Hindi name translates as 'sugar destroyer'. The name aptly describes what it does to the sense of taste. Placed on the tongue, it impairs the ability to distinguish sweetness and bitterness – perhaps one reason it's been used to treat diabetes in India for more than 2000 years.

Although most herbalists generally regard gymnema as the most powerful herb for blood-glucose control, it hasn't been studied in experiments that are both controlled and double-blind. Nonetheless, the US research that has been done suggests that the herb has promise. In one of the best controlled (but not blind) studies, insulin requirements were cut in half for 27 people with type 1 diabetes who took a 400 mg extract of gymnema for 6 to 30 months, while the insulin needs of the control group didn't change.

It's thought that gymnema might work by boosting the activity of enzymes that help cells use glucose. Be aware that safety studies haven't been performed (and be especially cautious if you're pregnant or breastfeeding or have liver or kidney disease), but the herb is not known to cause serious side effects.

WHAT the STUDIES show

A 2002 US study of 145 people who had recently been hospitalised for heart attack or angina found that 74 per cent had used some form of complementary or alternative medicine in the previous 6 months – typically, herbal or nutritional supplements. About a third were taking supplements that could thin their blood or interact with heart medications they were taking. Most patients told their doctors what they'd been taking – but 25 per cent did not.

Fenugreek. Better known today as a spice hailing from the Mediterranean and Near East than as a medicine, fenugreek has nevertheless been put to a variety of uses over the centuries. For example, records dating back to 1500 BCE indicate that it was used to induce childbirth in ancient Egypt. In Europe, the German Commission E, which regulates herbal medicine, has approved it for use in an inflammation-fighting poultice.

Numerous animal trials and a few small studies conducted with a total of about 100 people in the US have suggested that fenugreek seeds can lower blood glucose. In one of the largest (though not double-blind) studies, 60 people with type 2 diabetes who took 25 g of fenugreek daily showed significant improvement in their overall blood-glucose control, post-eating glucose levels, urine glucose and cholesterol levels.

The reason for these benefits may not be all that mysterious. Fenugreek is a legume – a relative of chickpeas, lentils, peanuts and green peas – and is rich in fibre, which naturally slows digestion and the absorption of glucose. But laboratory research also indicates that fenugreek contains an amino acid shown to boost the release of insulin that might be useful if you have type 2 diabetes.

Don't take fenugreek supplements if you're pregnant, breastfeeding or if you have liver or kidney disease, and don't ingest it within 2 hours of taking an oral diabetes medication because it may interfere with the body's absorption of the drug. Also be cautious if you're taking blood thinners, with which fenugreek may interact.

Cinnamon. One of the oldest and most popular spices, cinnamon is usually added to provide taste and aroma to meals, but has also been used for centuries in Chinese medicine. Animal studies have shown that it can improve blood-glucose levels and insulin action, and a number of human studies have now shown benefits for blood-glucose control. Cinnamon is a rich source of anti-oxidants called polyphenolics and it is thought that these may be responsible for its benefits.

A meta-analysis of eight randomised controlled trials published in the *Journal of Medicinal Food* in 2011 found that cinnamon intake, either as whole cinnamon or cinnamon extract, significantly reduced fasting blood-glucose levels – by around 0.5 mmol/L compared to a control group. The studies ranged from 4 to 16 weeks and used varying amounts of cinnamon ranging from 250 mg to 6 g, with most using between 500 mg and 1 g per day. The authors point out that the reduction in fasting glucose (around 5.8 per cent) is similar to that seen with the diabetes medication metformin, which has been found to reduce FBG by around 4.5 per cent.

While its long-term use as a spice suggests that it is safe, there have been some concerns about consuming high doses of cinnamon. The authors suggest that consuming a water extract of cinnamon may be preferable to whole cinnamon, which has been linked to a possible increase in cancer risk in high doses. Large quantities of cinnamon also have the potential to interact with warfarin, so anyone taking this medication should check with their doctor before taking cinnamon.

Bitter melon. Also known as bitter gourd, balsam pear, karella or (scientifically) *Momordica charantia*, bitter melon is a dietary staple in Southeast Asia and India. Actually a vegetable, it has long been a folk remedy for diabetes in the East, and a number of studies in people (none of them double-blind) suggest it may indeed have some benefits. In one uncontrolled study of 18 people who had recently been diagnosed with type 2 diabetes, 73 per cent of those who drank about half a cup of bitter-melon juice (which lives up to its unpalatable name) saw significant drops in blood-glucose levels. In another study, five people who took 15 g of bitter melon in powdered form (available in capsules) brought their blood glucose down by 25 per cent in 3 weeks.

Substances in bitter melon are thought to block glucose absorption in the intestine.

In addition to having a terrible taste, bitter melon can cause side effects like gastrointestinal distress and headaches, and it should not be taken if you're pregnant or breastfeeding.

Ginseng. In Chinese, *gin* means 'man' and *seng* means 'essence' – perhaps not only because the ginseng root's shape sometimes resembles a human figure but also because, supposedly, the root can treat just about everything. In fact, ginseng's genus name, Panax, comes from two Greek words for 'cure' and 'all'. Ginseng is said to have whole-body effects that make it broadly useful for building resistance to disease, recovering from illness, combating the physical effects of stress and even promoting longer life (not to mention boosting your sex drive).

Can you take seriously something that sounds too good to be true? Some of the research into ginseng's effects on diabetes, while far from conclusive, is unusually strong and has appeared in respected peer-reviewed journals. In one 2002 study from the University of Illinois in the US, in the journal *Diabetes*, overweight mice with type 2 diabetes that were injected with an extract of Asian ginseng (one of two types of ginseng) normalised their blood glucose, dropped 10 per cent of their body weight and lowered their cholesterol by about a third.

Two years earlier, a Canadian study from the University of Toronto, in the *Annals of Internal Medicine*, found that 10 people who took 3 g of American ginseng (the other type) 40 minutes before eating reduced their post-meal glucose levels by about 20 per cent compared with a control group. An earlier published US study found that taking ginseng lowered HbA1c numbers in people with type 2 diabetes.

It's not clear how ginseng works, but slowing carbohydrate absorption, boosting glucose uptake and improving insulin secretion have all been suggested. So has the idea that ginseng, which can cause excitability, simply makes people more active. Other possible side effects include headaches, increased blood pressure and insomnia. Ginseng can interfere with certain heart medications and the blood thinner warfarin. When buying ginseng, steer clear of Siberian ginseng, which is completely unrelated to the 'true' ginsengs and is possibly inferior. Also be warned that ginseng is expensive to cultivate, so it's often adulterated with other substances, such as caffeine.

Ginseng is traditionally consumed in teas. Look for tea bags containing the powdered root. Such teas are sometimes labelled 'red ginseng'. This ginseng has been steamed and dried, a process that turns it red. 'White' ginseng is simply the dried root.

Other potential blood-glucose levellers

It has been suggested that a number of other plant-based supplements have the ability to lower blood glucose, based on preliminary research that's even less conclusive than that for those supplements discussed above. This group includes:

Aloe vera. It's a plant most famous for the soothing qualities of the gel extracted from its leaves, but taking it internally may lower blood glucose, according to a handful of trials performed mostly in Britain. In one study, five people with type 2 diabetes who took half a teaspoon of aloe vera every day for 4 to 14 weeks dropped their fasting blood-glucose results from an average of 15.2 mmol/L to 8.3 mmol/L.

Bilberry. Related to the blueberry and grown in Europe and Canada, bilberry is a folk remedy for diabetes, though no human studies have been done on its blood-glucose effects. In animals, it's been shown to lower blood glucose by 26 per cent and triglycerides by 39 per cent, potentially making it even more beneficial if you have heart disease. The safety of the extract hasn't been established (high doses may interact with blood thinners), but it's safe to eat it as a fruit.

Coriander. This popular herb is used in traditional Chinese medicine for a variety of purposes, but an animal study published in a British nutritional-science journal found that it lowered blood glucose when introduced into the food and drinking water of mice with diabetes.

Prickly pear. Also known as nopal, this cactus is a Mexican folk remedy for diabetes and has been studied in a number of small, uncontrolled trials. In two of them, people with type 2 diabetes who consumed 500 g of nopal (which is a very large amount!) saw their blood glucose drop significantly within a few hours. One suspected mode of action is prickly pear's high fibre content. Perhaps not surprisingly, possible side effects include gastrointestinal distress.

Pterocarpus marsupium. The bark of this tree from India contains a compound, called epicatechin, that some studies have found improves the function of insulin-producing beta cells in the pancreas. In one study from India of 97 people with type 2 diabetes, 69 per cent of those taking 2 to 4 g of the herb daily achieved good glucose control within 12 weeks.

Nerves: a touchy subject

There are also those natural remedies that don't lower blood glucose, but they may one day prove useful for reducing the impact of certain health complications that occur as a result of high blood glucose, such as neuropathy. That's not easy to prove, though, because nerve damage occurs slowly, over a very long period of time, while studies of natural remedies tend to be short-term. But at least two supplements seem to show some promise in negating neuropathy.

Alpha-lipoic acid. Sometimes called ALA for short, alpha-lipoic acid is a powerful antioxidant that works to protect cells against the damaging effects of molecules known as free radicals. These chemical scourges are thought to contribute to neuropathy brought on by diabetes, and numerous studies suggest that ALA can stave off damage to nerves caused by free radicals. ALA may also reduce harmful swelling of nerves by blocking an enzyme that causes a glucose by-product (called sorbitol) to build up inside nerve cells.

The body produces small amounts of ALA on its own, and you get a certain amount from foods such as meat and spinach. But neither of these sources provides enough to exert a therapeutic effect – especially since people with diabetes may be prone to low levels of ALA.

What are the effects of ALA? A number of high-quality studies around the world have addressed that question, and the answers, while not yet conclusive, are intriguing. For example, a Mayo Clinic study in the US has shown that after having just 3 months of ALA supplementation the ability of nerves to conduct signals in people with diabetes was significantly improved. And yet another university study of more than 300 people with diabetes in Germany found that people taking 600 mg of ALA for 3 weeks experienced less pain and other symptoms of polyneuropathy.

Yet results have been mixed in some of the largest trials, conducted in Germany in a series of studies called ALADIN – for Alpha-Lipoic Acid in Diabetic Neuropathy. In one double-blind trial involving 328 people with type 2 diabetes, those who received daily ALA injections for 3 weeks felt significantly less pain from neuropathy than those receiving a placebo. But a larger follow-up study found little difference in symptoms between people treated with ALA injections and tablets for 9 months and those not receiving the real medication.

However, looking beyond the issue of effectiveness is the question of safety. A meta-analysis of 15 randomised controlled trials published in the *European Journal of Endocrinology* in 2012 found that treatment with injection of ALA (at doses of 300–600 mg per day) for 2 to 4 weeks was safe and improved nerve conduction speed and other neuropathic symptoms. While the safety of ALA hasn't been formally established, the substance has been used to treat diabetes in Germany for more than 30 years without reports of serious side effects. Still, animal studies suggest that it is toxic to rats who are deficient in thiamin, so some natural therapists suggest that you take a supplement of this B vitamin when using ALA.

Gamma-linolenic acid. Though the name sounds somewhat similar to ALA, gamma linolenic acid (GLA) is an essential fatty acid whose most concentrated source in nature is found in the oil from a wildflower called evening primrose (so called because its yellow petals open at dusk). Normally, the body makes all the GLA it needs from other types of fat, but some research indicates this process may be impaired in people with diabetes, suggesting that supplementation may be a good idea. You need GLA because the body converts it to *prostaglandins* – hormone-like substances that regulate a variety of functions, including inflammation, dilation of blood vessels and hormone activity. Getting more gamma-linolenic acid is thought to help prevent neuropathy in part by boosting the flow of nutrients and oxygen to nerves.

At least one decent-size, controlled, double-blind, peer-reviewed study backs up the claim that evening primrose helps to prevent neuropathy. This investigation, which involved 111 people with neuropathy, found that those who took 480 mg of GLA daily scored significantly better on 13 out of 16 tests for nerve damage after a year than those people who received a placebo. Another double-blind study, though much smaller (22 people), produced similar results with a smaller dose of GLA, contained in about 4 g of evening primrose oil.

Because evening primrose oil has been studied as a complementary treatment for a variety of common problems (including eczema and rheumatoid arthritis) and is widely used throughout Europe, it has a fairly long safety record and is not known to cause serious side effects. However, small numbers of people who take evening primrose oil may experience headaches or gastrointestinal distress.

Natural eye protection

Can complementary therapies protect eyes from the weakening and bursting of blood vessels that occur with retinopathy? Certain supplements may be helpful, though the evidence for them is not as strong as for some of the therapies recommended for other aspects of diabetes.

L-carnitine. L-carnitine is a type of amino acid – small units of organic material that link together to form proteins. A form of L-carnitine called acetyl-L-carnitine, or ALC, is known to have a potent anti-oxidant effect and has been proposed as a treatment for both diabetic retinopathy and diabetic nerve disease. You can get L-carnitine from high-protein foods, such as beef and lamb, along with dairy products, but at least one European study suggests that some people with diabetes may be naturally deficient in the amino acid.

Is it possible that L-carnitine can prevent eye damage? Most of the evidence that hints at any sort of benefit comes from animal research. A combined analysis of two large studies in people with diabetic peripheral neuropathy (DPN) published in the *European Journal of Endocrinology* in 2012 found that those who took at least 2 g per day of acetyl-L-carnitine had a reduction in pain scores. One study showed an improvement in nerve conduction while the other didn't, and one showed signs of nerve regeneration. The researchers recommend it should be used early in the disease process for maximum benefit and that further research is needed to confirm the effectiveness of ACL for the prevention and treatment of DPN.

Bilberry. In addition to its reputed ability to lower blood glucose, bilberry (also known as blueberry) is used to treat a variety of eye problems, including diabetic retinopathy. Evidence that bilberry improves vision is partly anecdotal: for example, during World War II, Royal Air Force bomber pilots claimed they could see better on night raids after eating bilberry. But there's reason to believe its benefits might be real. Bilberry is rich in flavonoids – vitamin-like anti-oxidant plant substances, some of which are known to strengthen tiny blood vessels like those that nourish the retina. Bilberry is particularly packed with flavonoids known as antho-cyanosides, which have been shown both to make blood vessels less leaky and fragile and to shore up connective tissue like that of the retina.

One small, controlled, double-blind study of 14 people with retinal damage from diabetes or high blood pressure found that bilberry produced significant improvements in blood vessels in the eye. But little other controlled research has been done to show how well bilberry works. Still, it may be worth discussing it with your doctor or dietitian. Bilberry supplements generally aren't known to have adverse effects, and the fruit is certainly safe – as are other foods containing anthocyanosides, such as blackberries and grapes.

Help for the heart and kidneys

Complications of diabetes are often interrelated, and that's certainly true of heart and kidney disease. For example, kidney disease can raise blood levels of cholesterol and triglycerides, which not only boosts your risk of cardiovascular disease but also further accelerates kidney damage. A number of supplements may run interference against this vicious cycle.

OPCs. If you pay attention to scientific names, you might guess that OPC supplements – short for oligomeric proanthocyanidin complexes (also sometimes referred to as PCOs) – share common ground with the flavonoids in bilberry. The two, in fact, are closely related and seem to have similar effects. OPCs, found primarily in grapeseed extract, are powerful anti-oxidants and appear to strengthen blood-vessel walls, making them less leaky – important for protecting the delicate capillaries that filter wastes in the kidneys.

Little controlled research has been done to show how well OPCs might protect the kidneys. In one study from France (where grapeseed extract was first popularised), people with diabetes or high blood pressure who took 150 mg of OPCs daily were able to decrease the leakiness and fragility of blood vessels in the kidneys. However, these results are highly preliminary. Still, tests have been done on OPC safety, and it's come up clean, aside from occasional allergic reactions and mild gastro-intestinal problems. However, high doses may interfere with blood thinners, such as warfarin or aspirin.

Garlic. The ancient Greeks said that this pungent herb could clear the arteries – and modern research suggests that that may be only the beginning. Dozens of studies since the 1980s have looked at garlic's effects on a variety of cardiovascular risks, and, while not always consistent, results have generally been positive. Fortunately for you and the person standing next to you, garlic in the powdered, capsule form used in many studies won't give you garlic breath.

Many of these studies, when taken together, suggest that garlic can lower cholesterol by as much as 9 to 12 per cent, bring down blood pressure by 5 to 10 per cent, prevent blood from clotting around artery obstructions, make blood vessels more pliable and also lower your overall risk of heart attack. The research isn't perfect, though. For example, in one particular study, where garlic was shown to be just as effective as a prescription cholesterol-lowering medication, the participants all made changes to their healthy eating plans that could well have affected the results of the study. Still, the balance of evidence suggests that garlic has real benefits for the heart and blood vessels.

However, it's possible that garlic may also thin the blood, so check with your doctor before taking garlic supplements if you're also taking aspirin or other blood-thinning medications or other supplements with blood-thinning effects, such as ginkgo or high doses of vitamin E.

L-carnitine. In addition to its possible benefits for the eyes, this amino acid has been shown in controlled studies to reduce death rates in people who have had a heart attack, relieve symptoms of intermittent claudication in the legs and improve heart function in people with

Buyer beware

Even if studies show that a herb or a natural remedy works, there's no guarantee the one you buy will. Although supplements aren't considered medicines, they are therapeutic goods and are therefore subject to government regulation. Complementary medicines available for supply in Australia are included on the Australian Register of Therapeutic Goods Association (ARTG) as 'listed' (low risk) or 'registered' (higher risk) medicines. This is shown on the product label by the designation 'AUST L' or 'AUST R' respectively, followed by a unique number. Still, quality control is largely at the whim of manufacturers. Among the potential problems:

Shoddy production. With no one looking over their shoulders, there is no guarantee that manufacturers will actually fill bottles with what the label says is inside.

Natural variation. Even if the manufacturer does care about quality, plants of the same species that are raised in different places or under different growing conditions can vary significantly in their chemical make-up.

Lack of knowledge. In many cases, nobody really knows which part of a plant produces the desired therapeutic effect (the root versus the leaves, for example). So the manufacturer may responsibly provide the herb that you want – just not the part that gives the desired results.

Responsible manufacturers understand these problems and do their best to ensure quality. To identify quality products, check the label for:

- the botanical name if the product is plant-based

- the recommended dose in milligrams

- a batch or lot number and expiry date

- the manufacturer's name and address

- a statement that the product contains a standardised extract, which ensures a certain dose of the active ingredient.

angina. In one study, for example, people who took 4 g of L-carnitine a day after experiencing a heart attack had a death rate of 1.2 per cent over the course of a year, while those who took a placebo had a death rate of 12.5 per cent. The people taking the L-carnitine also had better blood pressure, lipid profiles and heart rates. Paradoxically, the best dietary sources of L-carnitine – namely beef, lamb and dairy products – are not necessarily the most heart-healthy foods if they are the full-fat varieties.

Gamma-linolenic acid. Though primarily used to treat diabetic neuropathy, GLA (typically from evening primrose oil) may help the heart as well. In one 5-year study of 102 people who had just been diagnosed with diabetes, those whose diets were enriched with linolenic acid (a precursor to GLA) developed fewer cardiovascular problems and suffered less heart damage compared to a control group.

The nutritional pharmacy

Certain vitamins may help manage blood glucose and reduce the risk of complications. They're best when they come from foods – but should you get more of them from supplements? Discuss these two with your doctor, diabetes educator or dietitian.

✸ **Chromium.** Your daily requirement for chromium, a still-mysterious trace mineral, is estimated at a meagre 50 to 200 mcg. Some studies find that taking supplements in amounts upwards of 500 mcg brings down blood glucose (though other studies find no benefit). It's thought that chromium might help cells use insulin. The amounts used in studies are higher than the generally estimated 'safe and adequate' limit of 200 mcg. Should you take it? As there is no evidence of chromium deficiency in Australia, it's best to discuss it with your doctor or dietitian.

✸ **Magnesium.** This mineral lends a hand to many chemical processes in the body, and it may help cells use insulin. Deficiencies (common in people with diabetes) may promote eye damage. The usual daily value is 400 mg, but some research finds that taking as much as 2 g a day helps people with type 2 diabetes use insulin more effectively. Doses that high often produce diarrhoea. Avoid high doses if you have kidney disease, or are pregnant or breastfeeding. You will obtain more magnesium by eating more green, leafy vegetables and whole grains.

Exploring other therapies

Taking a supplement feels like taking conventional medication because they both come in tablet and capsule form. But other types of complementary therapies seem like a different animal altogether. For instance, there are mind–body approaches, techniques linked with Eastern ideas about energy flow and yet other unconventional or scientifically unproven ideas.

Do these therapies work? Each needs to be judged on its own merit, but it seems clear from research that more is involved with achieving healing and health than causing chemical changes with medications or fixing the body with surgery. Even conventional medicine – by controlling for a placebo effect, in which thinking you'll get better can seem to make it happen – tacitly acknowledges that the mind and body are closely entwined. Theories holding that stress and other mental states can affect the immune system, once largely dismissed, are now more widely accepted as studies continue to reveal connections between the nervous and the immune systems.

That doesn't mean that every therapy without a plausible explanation is valid and waiting for science to catch up. But some complementary therapies do seem to offer promise. Although they may require an investment in time or money, they probably pose few risks.

Biofeedback: the mind–body loop

Doctors long assumed that automatic functions such as breathing, heartbeat and body-temperature regulation were beyond our control. In fact, that's one reason the nervous system was classified as having two distinct parts – the voluntary one, in which conscious thoughts make your fingers wiggle, for example, and the autonomic one, in which the body, on its own, for instance, makes your heart pump faster when you're in danger or stressed. The two systems were once thought to be independent of each other and, in fact, not even on speaking terms.

But, biofeedback – a process of gaining insight into physiological functions by using instruments that measure them – has shown that these systems, like the superpowers during the Cold War, have hidden communication links that allow the two to influence each other. With biofeedback, you're hooked up to a computerised machine that monitors body functions, such as sweating or brain activity. With training, you can learn to recognise your body's responses to stress and other states and exert conscious control over them.

? DID you KNOW…

There are several forms of biofeedback, which measures different changes in the body. One type monitors blood flow in the extremities, such as the hands and feet, by measuring skin temperature. Another type gauges anxiety by measuring how much you sweat. A third type tracks muscle activity by sensing electrical activity from the firing of nerves in muscle fibres. A fourth type detects stress and other mental states by measuring brain waves.

Research in the US has found biofeedback to be helpful for more than 100 different conditions, and numerous studies suggest that it may help manage diabetes and its complications. For example, one study published in a US journal found that people using biofeedback were able to boost skin temperature in their toes by increasing blood flow by 22 per cent. Other studies in people with diabetes have shown that biofeedback can help reduce stress and lower blood pressure, and (perhaps as a result) may be able to help stabilise blood glucose.

To take advantage of biofeedback, you'll need to learn control techniques from a trained practitioner (discuss it with your doctor), but once you've mastered them, you can practise biofeedback at home.

Is the force with you?

According to traditional Chinese medicine, good health depends on a balance of yin and yang – the positive and negative aspects of the universal life force known as chi, which flows through 14 meridians in the body. Is there anything to it? Some research suggests that traditional acupoints along the meridians differ slightly from the surrounding skin in electrical and magnetic properties while also containing dense concentrations of blood vessels and nerves. Lab tests on animals suggest that acupuncture releases endorphins and other chemical messengers that may help relieve pain.

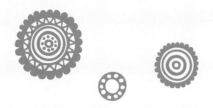

Acupuncture: therapy with a point

According to traditional Chinese medicine, the real reason you develop diseases like diabetes is that you suffer imbalances in the flow of life energy, or chi, through your body. Chi is thought to run through an invisible system of meridians, or energy pathways, that can be influenced by the insertion of extremely thin needles at specific sites known as acupoints.

In the West, acupuncture has been dismissed by many as quackery, at least in part because the meridian system doesn't correspond to any known part of the anatomy. But acupuncture has gained a certain amount of credence in Western medicine – it's not unusual to find practitioners who have medical degrees – because studies suggest that it may actually ease certain conditions, particularly nausea and pain. (The treatment itself can feel irritating but generally doesn't hurt.)

Much of the research into acupuncture's effects on diabetes comes from China, where it is more accepted, which some doctors view as cause for scepticism. Still, in one review of several Chinese studies published by a researcher at a university in Beijing, acupuncture appeared to cut blood-glucose levels by about half, on average. It was also seen to improve symptoms of neuropathy and heart disease. In the West, an English study found that 67 per cent of people with type 2 diabetes with chronic pain from neuropathy were able to get significant relief through acupuncture.

If you're considering trying acupuncture, talk to your doctor first, before finding a licensed practitioner, and expect to need as many as 25 treatments over a period of 2 to 3 months.

Magnets: an attractive option?

The idea that magnets can influence health isn't new. It was popular in the early twentieth century, but magnet therapies were discredited because of a lack of evidence that they worked. Recently, though, the idea has again begun gathering adherents. Treatments range from holding magnets next to afflicted areas of the body to lying on magnetic mattresses.

In the case of diabetes, magnets aren't thought to stabilise blood glucose, but there's some evidence that they may be useful in relieving pain from neuropathy, especially in extremities like the feet. In one pilot study in which 14 people with peripheral neuropathy wore magnetic innersoles in their shoes for 4 months, 75 per cent of those with diabetes (and 64 per cent of the group as a whole) improved – and some said their pain disappeared altogether. Other studies have produced similar results, though these findings are still preliminary.

Theories that magnets might help promote health aren't as wacky as they might seem. Tiny amounts of magnetic energy are involved in a vast range of biochemical processes in the body, from cell division and energy exchange right down to the subtle forces that hold the body's atoms together. It's thought that magnets may have therapeutic effects by drawing blood (which contains iron-rich haemoglobin) into areas that need more oxygen and nutrients, affecting the flow of ions that help blood-vessel walls relax, or stimulating the nervous system.

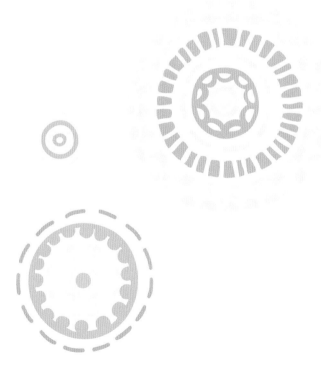

living well *with* diabetes

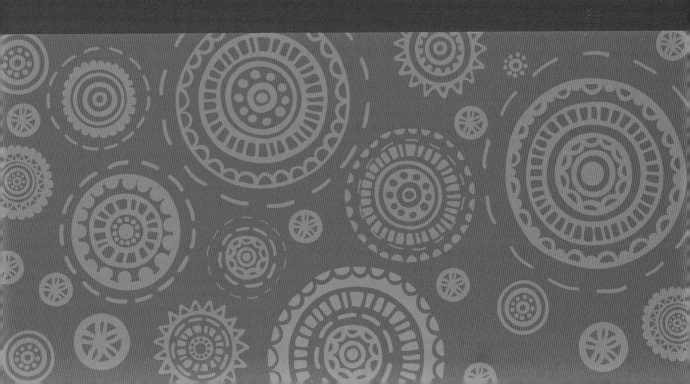

Diabetes isn't just a physical disorder; like any chronic condition it's also an ongoing emotional challenge. At various points, you're likely to face anger, frustration and possibly feelings of depression, and just plain being burned out from dealing with it. Learning how to cope is a must. You'll also need some know-how for handling diabetes when you're temporarily unwell or when you're travelling. The bottom line is that diabetes doesn't need to get you down – or slow you down. It's a matter of finding out all you can about living well with diabetes.

Diabetes is a chronic condition – something you have to live with for the rest of your life. It requires daily attention, which can seem a burden at times. But a key fact to remember is that, while you shouldn't deny the challenges of diabetes, there's no reason that every aspect of an enjoyable life can't be just as rewarding for you as for anybody else.

Quality of life is an important element in diabetes care: it's the point of everything you do to manage your condition – from eating healthily, walking regularly and taking daily insulin injections or medication. The better care you take, the less likely you are to experience the complications that account for most of the suffering that goes with diabetes. When it comes to blood glucose, better control means a better life.

This isn't just an attempt cheer you up. In an attempt to shed light on how to live well with diabetes, researchers have studied quality-of-life issues in people with diabetes. One US study compared quality of life in people with diabetes who had good blood-glucose control with peers who didn't. Those with good control had milder symptoms, felt better and were more likely to feel mentally sharp than the other group. As a result, they tended to be more productive and less restricted in every aspect of life.

But living well with diabetes goes beyond blood-glucose control. It also means managing your emotions (a significant part of dealing with diabetes) and contending with a raft of practical issues from day to day.

The feelings factor

'How are you feeling?' There are two ways to interpret that question. One is how you're feeling physically, which people tend to think of first. The other – equally as important – is how you're feeling emotionally. Indeed, a growing body of international research shows that mental and physical health are tightly entwined. If you're feeling emotionally unbalanced, then your health may follow.

Studies find, for example, that people who suffer such negative emotions as anger, depression and anxiety tend to have higher rates of heart disease and weaker immune-system response than people with a more positive outlook – important considerations for people with diabetes. That doesn't mean you need to worry about ruining your health if you're already feeling bad. But paying careful attention to your emotional wellbeing can help you to start improving it.

Why diabetes can be a downer

Anybody with diabetes will probably agree that there's truth to the notion that having a chronic disease makes your life more difficult than that of someone who does not (or, at least, difficult in different ways). Still, it's interesting to note that, according to one recent study of people with chronic conditions (including diabetes, liver infection and gastrointestinal disease), those with diabetes tended to do better on the quality-of-life front. This study found that the daily grind of dealing with diabetes – including tasks like testing and taking tablets or insulin – doesn't faze people as much as might be expected. The real battle, it turns out, is with emotional, psychological and social issues. It's easy to see why this potentially life-threatening disease can take a toll:

It never goes away. Diabetes is for life. Even though it's possible to delay or ward off the most debilitating consequences, the knowledge that you're engaged in a never-ending battle can make you feel weary and defeated.

It's often hidden. Diabetes is considered a silent, invisible disease in two different respects. First, even while it's progressing you may not feel any symptoms, which can foster a deceptive sense that you don't really have a

> **? DID you KNOW...**
>
> A connection between diabetes and emotions was noticed at least as far back as the seventeenth century, when British physician Thomas Willis theorised that an emotional state he called 'profound sorrow' caused diabetes. For more than two centuries, the idea persisted that diabetes might have psychological origins. Today's view is that while negative emotions may make diabetes more difficult to deal with or accelerate the disease process, they're far more likely to be a consequence of the illness than a cause.

disease. As a result, you may find it tempting to stray from your eating plan, regular physical activity or treatment. (Or you may have the impression that no matter what you do, diabetes is secretly eating away at your health.) The other hidden aspect of diabetes is that it's not obvious to others. On the surface, everything about you may seem 'normal', while underneath, you realise that you're different from those around you in a fundamental way. This can make you feel socially awkward, especially in settings where food is being served.

It's inconsistent. It would be easier if diabetes followed a predictable course that was the same for everyone, but it doesn't. For one thing, your diabetes is different from the next person's (based on your diabetes type, blood-glucose levels, pancreatic function, insulin resistance and other factors). But your own case of diabetes may also be subject to seemingly erratic changes. For example, blood glucose can move up and down in response to a wide

variety of influences, from illness to physical activity (not to mention medication and insulin treatments), and it can be difficult to predict when glucose might drop too low and cause a hypoglycaemic episode or spike up too high.

Coping with your emotions

Life's already an emotional rollercoaster without the added burden of diabetes, so you don't always need to hold your disease responsible for your ups and downs. In fact, doing so may make you feel more helpless and out of control (and prevent you from solving problems not related to diabetes). But it's useful to recognise when diabetes does fan the flames of feeling – and address the emotions head-on.

The first step is to recognise that mood swings are a natural phenomenon with diabetes – even apart from the emotional challenges of managing the disease. Variations in your blood-glucose levels can affect your mood directly. Low glucose levels can make you nervous, irritable and anxious, while high blood glucose can make you feel fatigued and down in the dumps. That means the steps you take to control your blood glucose can have an emotional payoff as well. Still, you can expect to contend with negative feelings that have nothing to do with blood glucose but everything to do with having diabetes.

Diagnosing depression

Doctors distinguish between run-of-the-mill lows that come and go in response to events in your life and the clinging cloudiness of clinical depression, which can hang around for weeks without letting up. If you're clinically depressed, medication may help. You may be clinically depressed if five or more of the following are true of you for at least 2 weeks straight:

○ You feel sad, empty, anxious or irritable just about all the time.

○ You take little interest or pleasure in most, if not all, of your daily activities.

○ You lack energy.

○ Your normal appetite changes or you've lost or gained a significant amount of weight.

○ You feel agitated or sluggish in your responses.

○ You feel worthless or guilty.

○ You have trouble sleeping – or you sleep more than usual.

○ You have difficulty concentrating or making simple decisions.

○ You often find yourself thinking about dying or suicide.

Defeating depression

Everybody feels low at least some of the time, and common sense suggests that having a chronic disease is ample reason to feel down. In fact, people with diabetes may be as much as four times more likely than the rest of the population to feel depressed, and they may also suffer from depression longer. All of which suggests that depression is normal if you have diabetes. But you don't have to accept low moods as inevitable or beyond your control.

✔ **Be alert to symptoms.** Read over the criteria for clinical depression (see 'Diagnosing depression', above) and consult a doctor if you think that you may qualify. Your problem may have a physiological cause that can be remedied

by, say, adjusting your diabetes medication or taking you off certain tablets that can have depressant side effects (including some blood-pressure medications and antihistamines). Otherwise, your doctor or psychiatrist can prescribe antidepressant medications that fine-tune levels of certain chemicals in the brain. SSRIs (selective serotonin reuptake inhibitors) are likely candidates because they're effective and generally have fewer side effects than other antidepressants, though they can cause such side effects as nervousness, insomnia, lack of appetite and dulled sexual response.

✔ **Talk it out.** Sharing your feelings is one of the most effective ways of taking an emotional burden off your shoulders – which is why counselling is a mainstay of treatment for depression. Start off by asking a friend or loved one if you can talk to them about what you're going through. And assure them that you're not expecting them to solve your problems, but that lending an ear would really help you to try to manage your own feelings.

✅ **Socialise more.** Just being with other people in a social setting or a group like a community club, volunteer organisation, or religious congregation can take your mind off your troubles, brighten your mood and make you feel less alone.

✅ **Stick with the program.** Don't let your low mood derail your self-care program, especially when it comes to regular physical activity. In fact, physical activity has been shown to lift mild or moderate depression.

✅ **Don't drink.** Because it's a depressant, alcohol won't drown your sorrows, it will only aggravate them. Drinking in excess, of course, will also add empty kilojoules to your eating plan and possibly erode your self-discipline.

Attacking anger

Most people go through a predictable cycle of emotions after they're first diagnosed with diabetes, typically starting with a this-can't-be-true sense of denial that eventually gives way to anger when you realise you're in it for the long haul. You may feel that your body has betrayed you, that your life has been turned upside down or that you don't deserve something like this and it just isn't fair.

Stop anger in its tracks

According to many behavioural-medicine experts, you can soothe your pent-up anger by asking yourself four key questions about what's provoking you:

○ Is this important?

○ Is my reaction appropriate?

○ Can I change the situation?

○ If I can, is it worth taking action?

If you answer 'no' to any of these questions, the only rational choice is to calm down. While anger isn't always rational, forcing yourself into an objective frame of mind can often be calming in itself.

These are normal responses that may make you irritable for weeks and even months at the outset. As you gradually accept your diabetes and settle into a self-care routine, your anger may cool down. But it's also possible that anger will persist, especially if you find yourself frustrated by your diabetes. For example, your best efforts at glucose control may not be producing the results you want. You may resent the intrusion diabetes has made on your daily routine or feel irritated by having to change your eating or activity patterns.

Frustration is a part of dealing with diabetes, but unchecked anger isn't healthy for your relationships, your mental health or your body.

As with depression, anger is linked with higher rates of heart disease. It can seem a difficult emotion to control, but if you're alert to it and prepared to contend with occasional flare-ups, you can get the upper hand. Here's how.

✓ **Take responsibility.** Making progress towards peace means working towards an attitude of acceptance – not only of the diabetes itself but of the emotional toll it takes as well. Diabetes can be frustrating, and it can make you angry. Those are realities, and it's okay to recognise them as such. This allows you to take a step back and see a bigger picture in which your emotions aren't overwhelming and out of control but rather predictable responses for which you can begin to take responsibility. Part of this responsibility involves understanding where your anger is coming from, and not unfairly blaming other people or circumstances. If you stay calmer, those around you will as well, and you'll most probably find less fuel to fire your outbursts.

✓ **Look for patterns.** Try to predict when you're most likely to experience feelings of annoyance, frustration or rage. Is it always having to check your blood-glucose levels? Or getting high readings when you're trying to do your best? Do certain topics of conversation make you annoyed? If you don't know when you tend to get angry, try writing down what's happening every time you do get angry to see if patterns start to reveal themselves. In some cases, simply knowing your triggers can give you a greater sense of control. And, of course, it can help you to avoid them.

✓ **Ignore the bait.** An exercise that some experts suggest is to think of yourself as a fish being baited by a hook. On the hook is a trigger for your anger. Do you take the bait or recognise it for what it is and simply pass it by? Consciously choosing not to bite lets you take control of your anger by refusing to let another person or situation determine your feelings.

✓ **Change your mental channel.** Sometimes, even when you approach anger rationally, you still feel peeved. In those cases, try shifting your thoughts. If you're fuming while stuck in traffic, turn on the radio or listen to a book on tape or CD. Mentally replay last night's football game or TV crime drama. Repeat a quiet phrase such as 'Calm down' or a favourite prayer, if that would better suit you.

Seeking an anxiety antidote

If you're feeling depressed, it's quite likely that you're a bit anxious as well – the two emotions often occur together. But even if you're not feeling down, having diabetes can give you plenty of cause for worry. For starters, there's the fear of complications that may impair your quality of life in the future. Even if you're really committed to monitoring and managing your diabetes, the unseen and unfelt nature of the disease can foster a nagging sense of dread.

Worrying about your diabetes is normal and, to some extent, even healthy because it helps motivate you to follow your treatment plan. But anxiety can sometimes acquire a life of its own and can become counterproductive and unhealthy. If your fears are more intense than they need be, crop up frequently or persist even when circumstances no longer justify them, they can distract you from the better things in life, undermine your ability to manage your disease and paralyse more positive thinking. To release yourself from the grip of fear:

✅ **Talk to your doctor.** Remember that nervousness and such symptoms as rapid heartbeat are signs of hypoglycaemia as well as anxiety, so your first step is to test your blood glucose to see if you are having a hypo or if you are just anxious. If you are having a hypo, treat it immediately (see page 73 for how to treat a hypo). Secondly, have your doctor evaluate your recent blood-glucose history. In some cases, a bout of anxiety might simply require an adjustment in your insulin or medication. If that's not the problem, your doctor or specialist can refer you to a mental-health professional, who may advise you to take the appropriate medication to treat your anxiety.

✅ **Talk back to yourself.** Anxiety can blind you to positive emotions and cause you to focus only on negatives and potential catastrophes. You might fear that a slight slip from your blood-glucose goals is the first step down the road to vision loss or that if you take time to be active regularly, you'll never get all your work done and you'll be fired. Pay attention to automatic thoughts, which set the tone for your mental state. If they tend to be negative, try to be as objective as possible and ask yourself if evidence supports your thinking or whether you might be wrong. Look back to challenges you successfully met in the past for proof that things can also work out for the better.

✅ **Keep a bedside notepad.** Worries have a way of intruding on your thoughts in the middle of the night. If anxiety keeps you up, keep a notepad and pen by your bed so that you can jot down what's bothering you. Try writing concrete steps you can take to resolve your concerns; this provides a reassuring sense that you've tackled the problem. Getting better sleep will make you feel more refreshed and energetic in the morning, and this can help you keep your anxieties in perspective.

Putting stress in its place

Too much stress isn't good for anyone, but it may be especially bad for people with diabetes. It can prevent you from effectively managing your condition by thwarting your intentions to eat healthily, keep up with your physical activity program, and remember to do regular blood-glucose tests. Worse still, there's considerable evidence that stress makes blood glucose rise.

One way to explain this effect is that hormones released when you're tense or extremely pressured – particularly cortisol and epinephrine – pump glucose into blood from storage sites in the liver so the body has more energy available to meet a challenge. So-called stress hormones can have other harmful effects as well. One recent study finds that stress inhibits the ability of blood vessels to expand, which might make it a factor in heart attacks.

The best way to deal with stress is simply to avoid whatever it is that's making you tense.

But since that's not always possible, you can benefit from taking other steps:

✓ **Invest in relationships.** Numerous studies find that surrounding yourself with family and friends buffers the strain of stress better than just about anything else. Social support leaves you feeling less isolated while bolstering your sense of control, which alone can make life seem less daunting. When speaking with loved ones (especially a partner), avoid put-downs and negative language; studies have found that sniping can produce a marked increase in stress hormones.

✓ **Join a program.** Ask your doctor or diabetes educator if they could recommend a good stress-management program to suit you. One research study, published in 2002, found that people with diabetes who participated in such management programs could significantly improve their HbA1c results – enough to hit blood-glucose targets shown to reduce the risk of various diabetes complications.

✓ **Follow your faith.** Religious belief can help put the trials and tribulations of life in a reassuringly larger perspective or – if faith doesn't come easily to you – provide an opportunity to receive social support through communal worship, along with a sanctuary from life's storms.

✓ **Express yourself.** People who make a point of writing down their thoughts in a journal tend to feel less stress and may even be better able to resist illness than those who

Does stress cause diabetes?

A study published in Diabetes Care in 2010 found that, in comparison with those who didn't report any extremely stressful life events, those who reported work- or finance-related stressful events were significantly more likely to have the metabolic syndrome. The more stressful events a person experienced in any of the areas assessed, the greater the risk. The researchers also found that the accumulation of stressful life events was associated with individual components of the metabolic syndrome, including insulin resistance, obesity and high triglycerides (blood fats). The metabolic syndrome, also known as syndrome X or the insulin-resistance syndrome, is a collection of symptoms (including raised blood-glucose levels, blood fats, blood pressure and carrying weight around the middle) that occur together and can increase the risk of type 2 diabetes, heart disease and stroke.

don't. And don't feel self-conscious about the way you write or what you write as it's not intended for other people to read. Just be sure to write down honest feelings about what's bothering you. In one study, those who kept a journal had measurable improvements in immune function while those who repressed their thoughts saw declines.

Battling 'diabetes burnout'

Though dealing with diabetes 24 hours a day can seem overwhelming at first, many people willingly adjust to a new lifestyle of dedicated self-care. But over time, a creeping sense of fatigue and frustration can set in – what some experts call 'diabetes burnout'. When you're burned out, you may not feel outright depressed, just sick and tired of the never-ending daily grind. As a result, you may find that your all-important motivation begins to wane.

Even though burnout won't directly cause physical changes in the body, feeling frustrated – often because you may sense that you're not making progress against your disease – can have an impact on your health. You may start to slack off your healthy eating plan, physical activity, medication or regular testing.

Talking with your doctor, psychologist or a counsellor is your first step if diabetes care is wearing you down. Your doctor may be able to make adjustments in your treatment – fewer injections using different combinations of insulin, for example – to ease your burden. A psychologist or counsellor may be able to suggest new ways of thinking that can boost your sense of purpose. But then you'll need to take steps to help you fortify your resolve.

✅ **Check your goals.** At some point earlier in your treatment, you and your diabetes team established objectives for your self-care: blood-glucose targets, healthy eating plan, physical activity goals. These were probably based on what you thought possible then, but it may be time to review your list of objectives. Pretend you're starting over. Knowing now what you didn't know then, do you feel your goals are reasonable? Feeling successful in meeting your objectives is a key to staying motivated.

✅ **Evaluate your progress.** Maybe you haven't made as much progress as you would like. But be objective about what you have accomplished. How has your blood-glucose control improved? How about your weight or your overall fitness? Have you managed to be disciplined about testing and taking medication? You may find that you've done better than you give yourself credit for. On the other hand, your frustration may be a good sign; it means you actually are motivated to do better.

✅ **Identify problem areas.** If you're like most people, you've probably been more effective with some elements of your self-care than with others. But don't let your lack of progress in one area colour the entire picture. Instead, try to isolate the aspects of your care with which you have the most trouble. Is it a challenge to control your appetite? Are you forgetting to take your medication or insulin? Is finding time for physical activity a constant battle?

✅ **Seek solutions.** Once you've identified problem areas, you can start finding solutions. Why do you feel a particular challenge is such a struggle? What could change to make it more manageable? For example, if your eating is the issue, ask your dietitian if there are changes to your meal plan that may make it more appealing to you and your personal preferences. If you really don't like your activity program, try to find something that blends fitness and fun, to keep you motivated.

✅ **Enlist support.** Remember, you're not in this alone. Talk to other people with diabetes for perspective, ideas and encouragement.

Four top stress-relief strategies

To tame tension, it helps to tackle both its physical and its psychological dimensions. Here are some of the most important steps you can take, according to experts in stress-management:

1 Fill the balloon

Deep breathing has been shown to rapidly calm the body's physical response to stress. Done properly, three breaths can lower your heart rate and blood pressure. It's a very powerful tool, but people generally don't understand how to do it. Most people tend to take shallow breaths that make the chest expand, with the diaphragm pushing upward. Deeper, stress-relieving breaths, however, should make the diaphragm move downward, not upward, expanding your belly. Imagine a balloon under your belly button that you're trying to fill. As you breathe in, imagine the balloon expanding, then slowly let the air out.

2 Put the present in your thoughts

Most stress comes from worrying about the past or the future. You'll feel less stress if you can stay focused on the here and now, where there's a finite number of things you have to deal with. Start by simply acknowledging – and accepting – what you're feeling right now, without thinking about why or what to do about it. We tend to think in run-on sentences. Just think, 'I'm frustrated' and end the sentence there. If your mind strays to the future, consciously bring it back to the moment at hand. Deep breathing can help you stay centred on the here and now.

3 Be grateful for what you have

Whenever it seems appropriate make a point of being grateful. This can encourage an awareness of what's good about the present moment, and how things we take for granted (regular meals, a place to live, a hot shower every morning) are worthy of our gratitude.

4 Be kind to yourself

Most of us judge ourselves harshly, straining for perfection and beating ourselves up for mistakes. Consciously say to yourself, 'I don't have to be perfect'. Feeling more forgiving of yourself will not only relieve tension, it'll also improve the way you treat others, which leads to better relationships and further stress reduction over the long term.

Join a diabetes support group (ask your doctor or diabetes educator for a recommendation), or find an Internet chat group that you're comfortable with. Enlist friends to join you in your physical activity program or to keep them posted on your progress. Knowing that someone else is interested in you can help spur you on. Many companies have walking clubs that encourage staff to step out of their offices during lunchtime. If you work in an office, check with the social club or human resources department about what's on offer – or set up a walking group yourself and start recruiting your colleagues to join you.

Contact your diabetes association for more information about local support groups in your area or visit Diabetes Counselling Online (www. diabetescounselling.com.au).

✅ **Keep your eyes on the prize.** Try to stay focused on the quality of life you gain by controlling your diabetes rather than on the negatives – namely, the complications – that you avoid. It's a subtle distinction, but cringing in fear of consequences is generally a less effective motivator than striving for more joy, freedom and flexibility in your life.

How to think about diabetes

When you have diabetes, your attitudes are tugged in two seemingly opposite directions. On the one hand, you need to make maintaining good blood-glucose control a top priority. On the other hand, you want to be able to live as normal a life as possible and not to feel constantly restricted by the disease. So, the questions are, 'Should diabetes always be in the top of your mind, or should you try not to dwell on it?'

These questions represent a spectrum with two unhealthy extremes on either end. One is denial (especially common in the early days after diagnosis), in which you fail to realise or accept all the changes necessary to take charge of diabetes and ensure quality of life over the long haul. The other is obsession, in which you desperately strive for perfection in every aspect of your treatment to the extent that you think about little else.

Try to incorporate a little of both extremes into your attitude about diabetes. A bit of denial allows you to set aside gloomy thoughts of complications so that you can concentrate on enjoying your life today. And a certain amount of obsession encourages you to be diligent about your care. But taken too far, both outlooks can threaten your health – denial because it leads to poor glucose control and obsession because your inevitable failure to achieve perfect control leads to disappointment and discouragement. Finding the right balance depends in part on the way you approach life as a whole.

✅ **Seek serenity.** The familiar adage that we need to have the courage to change the things we can, the serenity to accept the things we can't and the wisdom to know the difference applies particularly well to diabetes. It's important to take responsibility for your

> **? DID you KNOW...**
>
> A recent study of people with type 1 diabetes finds that the more positive a person's attitude towards having diabetes, the better their physical and mental health are likely to be. Researchers concluded that how a person thinks about their diabetes has a significant impact on such outcomes as related heath complications.

disease and do everything in your power to manage it, but also to let go of the idea that you'll ever exert total control over diabetes – or any other aspect of your life.

✓ **Embrace ambiguity.** If you wrestle with questions of whether you consider yourself sick versus well, or in control versus at the mercy of your disease, step back and ask why it's necessary to have all the answers. As is true for most aspects of life, the path of wisdom may be to simply accept the situation's inherent ambiguities.

✓ **Know yourself.** The real issue in how you think about diabetes may be how you think about yourself. Do you see yourself as a person with a disease or someone who's loving, creative, resourceful and appreciated by family, friends and community? The less you define yourself by your diabetes, the easier it will be to see the measures you take to manage your diabetes as stepping stones to fulfilling your other important roles in life.

Sex and diabetes

Despite vast improvements in knowledge, many myths continue to exist in the community about diabetes and sex. The good news is that there's no reason you can't have a full and satisfying sex life if you have diabetes. But you need to understand how your disease can affect different aspects of your sexuality and sexual function.

First, bear in mind that sexual intimacy can be physically vigorous, burning kilojoules. That means that, like physical activity, it may put you at risk of hypoglycaemia if you are taking insulin or certain diabetes tablets. To keep your blood glucose stable, it's wise to take glucose readings before and after intercourse to get an idea of how your body responds. It's not always possible to plan ahead, but if you can, try having a sugary drink or a small snack beforehand or immediately afterwards (you may find it useful to keep some quick-acting carbohydrate on your bedside table).

For women

It is not clear exactly how much diabetes impacts on sexuality in women. However, it is known that women with type 1 diabetes are more likely to have certain problems associated with sex-related functions. Among them:

Blood-glucose fluctuations. Though not a universal experience, many women notice their blood glucose rises a few days before their monthly period begins. Researchers suspect

If you're pregnant and have diabetes

Without planning, having a baby when you have diabetes increases the risks both for your child and for you, but plenty of women with diabetes have healthy pregnancies and healthy babies.

Before conceiving, get a thorough evaluation for complications of diabetes, such as retinopathy, kidney damage, nerve damage and high blood pressure – all of which can be made worse by pregnancy. To guard against complications and protect the health of your baby, you should be prepared to control your blood glucose even more tightly than before, not only during your pregnancy but for 3 months before you conceive. While women with diabetes have babies with birth defects in only 2 to 3 per cent of cases, those numbers more than triple if blood-glucose levels are not tightly controlled.

Tight control not only reduces the risk of birth defects but keeps the baby from growing too large, which raises the risk of delivery problems. If you have type 1 diabetes, you'll probably need more insulin injections and may be advised to switch to a pump. If you have type 2, and take diabetes tablets, you may need to start taking insulin. Looking after your diabetes and working closely with your diabetes team throughout your pregnancy will maximise your chances of having a healthy baby and minimise the complications.

(though not all agree) that fluctuations in female sex hormones, such as oestrogen and progesterone, temporarily make cells more resistant to insulin. If you suspect this is a problem for you:

✳ For several months, keep a record of when your period begins, then compare it to your daily blood-glucose records. If you find a distinct correlation between your glucose levels and your menstrual cycle, talk to your doctor about adjusting your insulin or doses of medication at that time.

✳ Consider an alternative cause. Some doctors think the real reason blood glucose rises before your period is that the cravings and irritability of premenstrual syndrome make you eat more – or more erratically – thereby causing unusual peaks and valleys in blood-glucose levels. Try eating at regular intervals to keep blood glucose stable, and avoid having alcohol and caffeine, which can affect your mood.

✳ If you take oral contraceptives, ask your doctor which pill is best for you. Monophasic oral contraceptives, which contain fixed amounts of oestrogen and progestin, appear to keep blood-glucose levels more stable than triphasic oral contraceptives and progesterone-only contraceptives. If the contraceptive you're taking has adverse side effects, notify your doctor immediately and discuss other contraceptive options.

Vaginal dryness. Women with diabetes sometimes find they lack natural lubrication during sexual arousal, though this problem isn't limited to people with high blood glucose. To deal with it, try using water-based lubricants, available at any pharmacy. Check with your doctor if the problem continues: you may have low oestrogen levels that can be boosted with topical oestrogen cream or hormone replacement therapy (HRT). Weigh the HRT option carefully, though. It may solve the lubrication problem, but it may raise the risk of other health problems.

Infections. Excess glucose in the blood encourages the growth of fungal organisms and bacteria, making women with diabetes more prone to yeast infections and vaginitis. If you have vaginal discharge or itching, see your doctor for treatment.

For men

Sex can sometimes seem more straightforward for men, but the male sexual response is also a complex melding of mind and body involving numerous systems that can be affected by diabetes.

The major difficulty men may face is erectile dysfunction (also called impotence), the inability to achieve or maintain an erection – a problem that often occurs with age and is hardly limited to men with diabetes. In many cases, the cause is purely physical. When you have diabetes, poor circulation can prevent blood from properly engorging chambers in the penis, and nerve damage can interfere with signals involved with sexual response. (Fortunately, the nerves that enable orgasm are seldom impaired.) But

depression and anxiety can cause erectile dysfunction as well, and sexual difficulties may involve a combination of factors. Try these steps:

✅ **Narrow it down.** Talk to your doctor about possible causes so you know how to treat the problem. It may be a simple matter of adjusting one of your medications. Many medications, including some for high blood pressure, can interfere with sexual function. However, if erectile dysfunction seems to happen on and off, strikes suddenly or occurs in some circumstances but not others, there may be a psychological component. If you gradually and consistently lose function over time, there's probably a physical cause. Make an appointment for you and your partner to discuss options with your doctor.

✅ **Oral medication.** Sildenafil (Viagra) and vardenafil (Levitra) are taken about an hour before sex. Viagra can last for up to 6 to 8 hours and Levitra up to 48 hours. Tadalafil (Cialis) is taken between 30 minutes and 12 hours before sex and works for up to 24 hours. Your doctor will advise whether any of these medications are right for you.

✅ **Injected medication.** Another option is alprostadil (Caverject). Like oral medications, it relaxes smooth-muscle tissue in the penis to boost blood flow, but it's injected into the penis or inserted into the urethra in pellet form. Alprostadil can also have untoward side effects – your erection may not subside as normal after sex and, if injected, can cause bruising at the injection site, resulting in pain or discomfort.

Planning for sick days

Being sick takes an extra toll if you have diabetes because it can throw off your blood glucose and put you at risk for significant short-term complications. The best way to deal with sickness is to know what to do in advance. Speak with your doctor, diabetes educator and dietitian to work out a strategy you can quickly put into action the next time a cold, the flu or some other illness strikes.

Illness is a form of stress that – like emotional stress – rouses the body's defences. One effect is that the liver steps up glucose production to provide more energy. At the same time, stress hormones are released that make cells more insulin resistant. The net result is that blood glucose can rise dramatically when you're unwell. Among the serious problems that can result are:

- ✸ **Ketoacidosis.** If available insulin isn't enough to move glucose into cells (mostly a problem with type 1 diabetes), and your blood-glucose levels rise above 20 mmol/L, the body will start tapping its fat stores, releasing toxic ketones and putting you at risk of a coma if left untreated.

- ✸ **Hyperosmolar Hyperglycaemic State (HHS).** When blood glucose in people with type 2 diabetes gets too high, the body tries to get rid of glucose through the urine, which can produce severe dehydration that can also lead to coma if left untreated.

To keep your blood glucose in check when you're unwell and help yourself feel better faster, follow these steps:

- ✅ **Step up your monitoring.** It's more important than ever to keep careful track of your blood-glucose levels, so you'll need to test yourself more often than you usually do – every 2 hours at first. If your blood glucose goes higher than 15 mmol/L, and you have type 1 diabetes, test your urine for ketones (or your blood if your meter tests blood ketones). If ketone results are positive – or if your blood glucose consistently hovers above 15 mmol/L – call your doctor.

- ✅ **Eat as well as you can.** Illness can ruin your appetite (especially if you have trouble keeping food down), but you need to continue to provide your body with the energy it needs. Work with your dietitian to develop a sick-day menu that fits in with your eating plan – perhaps one featuring foods that offer good nutrition but are easy on the stomach, and eat small amounts frequently throughout the day.

- ✅ **Get plenty of fluids.** This familiar advice is doubly critical when you have diabetes because water is drawn into excess glucose and excreted in the urine, which can cause dehydration. Drinking a half to three-quarters of a cup of sugar-free fluids every hour is essential. This helps to keep your temperature down and prevent dehydration. If you can't eat, you will also need small amounts of any drink containing sugar (about three-quarters of a cup each time), such as fruit juice or soft drink.

✓ **Never stop your medication.** When you're sick, unless your doctor instructs you otherwise, you must continue to take your oral medication or give yourself insulin injections even if you're not eating when you're sick. In fact, your doctor may want you to take more insulin when you're unwell and will advise you of the exact amounts depending on your blood-glucose readings.

✓ **Watch the over-the-counter remedies.** Some common over-the-counter medicines, such as cough syrup and nasal decongestants, can raise blood glucose. Check with your doctor before taking any over-the-counter medication, herbal remedy or dietary supplement when you're unwell.

✓ **Keep alert to danger.** Keep testing for ketones and know the signs of ketoacidosis (which include stomach pain, vomiting, chest pain, difficulty breathing, feelings of weakness, sleepiness, fruity-smelling breath, blurry vision) and of dehydration (extreme thirst, dry mouth, cracked lips, sunken eyes, mental confusion, dry skin). Seek urgent medical assistance if you have ketones or any of the symptoms listed above.

Driving and diabetes

Your general health is a significant contributor to road safety. As diabetes has the potential to impact on one's ability to drive, people with diabetes are required to meet certain medical standards.

Australian driving guidelines

Australian medical standards released by Austroads in March 2012 'Assessing Fitness to Drive 2012' are intended to improve safety for all road users. They are in place to provide guidance to doctors and driver licensing authorities on how to assess the fitness to drive of private and commercial drivers of heavy and light vehicles and motorbikes.

How diabetes might affect your ability to drive

Diabetes may affect your ability to drive through:

- A hypoglycaemic event or hypo (where your blood-glucose levels fall below 4 mmol/L) which, left untreated, may lead to unconsciousness.

- Persistently high blood-glucose levels leading to diabetes complications such as vision loss and heart disease. Nerve damage, especially in the feet, causing loss of sensation can also pose safety issues.

What's changed in Australia?

A significant change in the guidelines is that 'satisfactory control' is now defined as an HbA1c level of less than 9 per cent (or 75 mmol/mol). The HbA1c is a measure of your blood-glucose level average over the preceding 3 months. It is not your daily blood-glucose level.

The general target for most people with diabetes is an HbA1c of less than 7 per cent. By aiming for an HbA1c of less than 7 per cent, you are less likely to develop long-term complications.

An HbA1c greater than 9 per cent generally shows that blood-glucose levels have been high most of the time. It can also mean blood-glucose levels have swung between highs and lows over the previous 3 months, which means the person is at an increased risk of hypoglycaemia. Those with an HbA1c greater than 9 per cent are at increased risk of complications that can affect their fitness to drive, such as vision impairment, heart disease and nerve damage, especially in the feet.

If you have an HbA1c above 9 per cent, it does not automatically mean you will lose your licence. Assessing Fitness to Drive is a guide only and allows doctors to make their own judgement about the 'satisfactory control' of their patients' diabetes on a case by case basis.

In New Zealand there are generally no driving restrictions for people with well-controlled diabetes. However, your medical practitioner will seek to ensure that you are adhering to your medication regime and maintaining a reasonable level of glycaemic control while minimising the number of hypoglycaemic episodes.

People with diabetes should always be aware of the risks of hypoglycaemia and be regularly monitored, with particular attention to the emergence of diabetic complications that can affect fitness to drive. A referral to a specialist may be necessary if concerns are raised.

When to tell

Diabetes managed with diet and exercise.
If your diabetes is managed with diet and exercise, you do not need to advise your driving authority that you have diabetes, whether you hold a private or commercial driver licence.

Diabetes managed with glucose-lowering medications other than insulin

- Private licence holders treated with glucose-lowering medications other than insulin may generally drive without restrictions. However, you need to tell your driving authority you have diabetes and also have your fitness to drive reviewed by a GP every 5 years.
- Commercial licence holders on metformin alone require an annual review by a GP.
- Commercial licence holders treated with medications other than metformin require an annual review by a diabetes specialist (endocrinologist).

Diabetes managed with insulin.
If you manage your diabetes with insulin, you must tell your local DLA.

- Holders of a private conditional licence require a 2-yearly review by a GP.
- Those with a commercial licence require a yearly review by a diabetes specialist.

Driver responsibility checklist

- Take medication as prescribed
- Check blood-glucose levels before driving and ensure reading is above 5 mmol/L
- Carry a blood-glucose meter and do not delay or miss a meal or snack
- Carry fast-acting carbohydrates
- Check BGLs every 2 hours during driving
- Treat mild hypo symptoms
- Attend medical reviews as advised by diabetes care team
- Feel awake and alert at all times
- Carry identification that says I have diabetes
- Advise my DLA that I have diabetes.

When you've had a severe hypo

If you have recently had a severe hypo (where you were unable to treat yourself), stay off the roads for a period of time. It often takes many weeks for blood-glucose levels to stabilise and the warning symptoms of hypos to return.

If you're unsure whether to report a severe hypo to your local driving authority, get advice from your diabetes team. They can work with you and your driving authority to manage your condition if required.

In New Zealand a person who experiences a severe hypoglycaemic episode while driving, irrespective of whether a crash occurred, should be advised to stop driving. At least a month is recommended, during which time remedial action needs to be undertaken. Specialist review will almost certainly be required.

It's important to remember that if you report your condition to your driving authority, it doesn't necessarily mean you will lose your licence. It just means that you might have to see your doctor more often and there may be some restrictions placed on your driving. However, remember that this is done for your safety and that of other road users.

Of course, it goes without saying that alcohol and driving are not recommended, not even in small quantities.

Travelling with diabetes

Most of us love to pack our bags and hit the trail (road, rail or air) with family and friends. Fortunately, there's no reason why diabetes should hold you back from travelling, as long as you take some reasonable precautions to make sure that while you're away, your blood glucose is under control.

Your mantra is 'Plan ahead'. Your doctor may want to give you a thorough examination before you depart, depending on how long you'll be gone, so it's important to discuss your plans. For smooth sailing, heed the following advice.

✓ **Keep diabetes supplies close at hand.** If you are travelling by plane, pack your medications, insulin, needles, test strips, lancets, ketone strips and other supplies in your carry-on bag with extra insulin. If you're travelling with a companion, pack half of everything in their hand luggage in case yours gets lost or stolen during the journey.

✓ **Pack a snack.** Carry a snack such as a piece of fruit, a muesli bar, trail mix, a sandwich or crackers in case your blood-glucose levels start to drop when you don't have immediate access to other food. If you are at risk of hypoglycaemia, always carry some fast-acting carbohydrate, such as glucose tablets or jelly beans. If you eat your snacks throughout the journey, make sure you replenish your supplies at every available opportunity.

✓ **Anticipate airport security.** With the increased security at airports these days, expect your supplies to get a thorough once-over. Current Australian air regulations require all diabetes supplies, including syringes, pen needles and insulin-delivery systems, to be carried on board in your hand luggage. In Australia, your NDSS card is accepted as proof that you need to carry diabetes equipment. You should also carry scripts for all your medications, clearly labelled with your name by the pharmacy. To get through customs you will also need several copies of a letter from your doctor outlining your condition, your medication and the equipment you use. These guidelines are subject to change, and individual airlines may have different rules, so be sure to call ahead for current policies before you leave.

✅ **Mind your meals.** If you're flying, you may choose to advise the airline in advance that you have diabetes, which will in turn be passed on to the cabin crew. You may wish to pre-order meals that are low in saturated fat and high in fibre when you make your bookings. When you're en route, wait until your meal is in sight before you take your pre-meal insulin in case the service is unexpectedly slowed or cancelled. When travelling by car, try to stick to your regular mealtime schedule to keep your blood glucose stable. If that's not possible, carry snacks along with you and monitor your blood-glucose levels regularly (every 2 hours or so). Don't drive unless your blood-glucose level is over 5 mmol/L. Be alert to symptoms of low blood glucose, such as nervousness, sweating and crankiness. If you feel a hypoglycaemic episode coming on, pull over immediately and eat something. Wait until your blood glucose has returned to normal before continuing on.

Take-charge tips

Planning a trip can be a challenge, but it's an even bigger challenge when you have diabetes. Follow this basic advice.

○ When it comes to supplies, such as medication, insulin, test strips and lancets, the rule of thumb is pack twice as much as you think you'll need. It's easier to carry extra than to get more on the road.

○ Wear medical identification that alerts people that you have diabetes.

○ Arrange travel insurance for your health and your belongings and make sure your health cover applies to both pre-existing conditions and the places you will visit.

○ In case you need to restock while you're away, have your doctor give you prescriptions for refills. Each script must include your name, the name and type of medication and your doctor's details. Get a letter from your doctor outlining your condition and medication in case you need to see a doctor while you're away.

○ Also ask your doctor to prescribe a glucagon kit, which contains an emergency dose of a hormone that someone else can give you by injection if you have a severe hypoglycaemic attack.

✅ **Get in the zone.** Travelling across different time zones can throw your normal insulin and meal schedule completely out of kilter, but you can compensate for the disruption if you're careful. When adding hours to your day by travelling west, you may need to take more insulin. When losing hours by travelling east, you may need less. Check with your doctor for specific recommendations. As for timing your injections and meals, wear two watches or use your smartphone. Keep one set on your home time and the other adjusted to your travel time. When you reach your destination, adjust the second watch to local time.

✅ **Organise for overseas.** If you're travelling outside the country, be aware that insulin you find abroad may be sold in different strengths than the insulin standardised in Australia and New Zealand. Your best bet is to stick to your own supplies by taking much more insulin with you than you'll need for the entire trip. Insulin is stable at room temperature (under 30°C), but extreme heat or cold will destroy its effectiveness. When travelling by car, always store your insulin supply in the boot, which is the coolest place. You may also consider whether you need a small insulated bag if you're travelling through extreme temperatures; discuss this with your diabetes educator. Also remember to take a liberal supply of syringes or pen needles and lancets with you, too. It's not going to be much help to you if you have your self-testing kit and insulin supply without the other necessary equipment that goes with them.

Exercising on the road

It's tough to stay physically active when travelling – but not impossible. Try to keep your body in gear by planning ahead and snatching opportunities as they arise:

- During long flights, walk the aisle as often as you can to help your circulation. Support stockings or socks can help to prevent swelling and may reduce the risk of clotting in the veins of your legs. However, it's a good idea to check with your doctor before you go as to whether this is suitable for you.

- Pack comfortable clothes for regular walks when you arrive at your destination, including sensible shoes.

- Don't forget your swimsuit in case the opportunity arises to do a few laps at your hotel pool, or nearby, on arrival.

- If you're away on business, wear dressy walking shoes rather than more formal dress shoes to encourage walking during breaks or before and after meetings.

- Use airport delays time for around-the-terminal walking sessions. When you're making connections, steer clear of the moving footpaths (conveyor belts) and walk the distance under your own power.

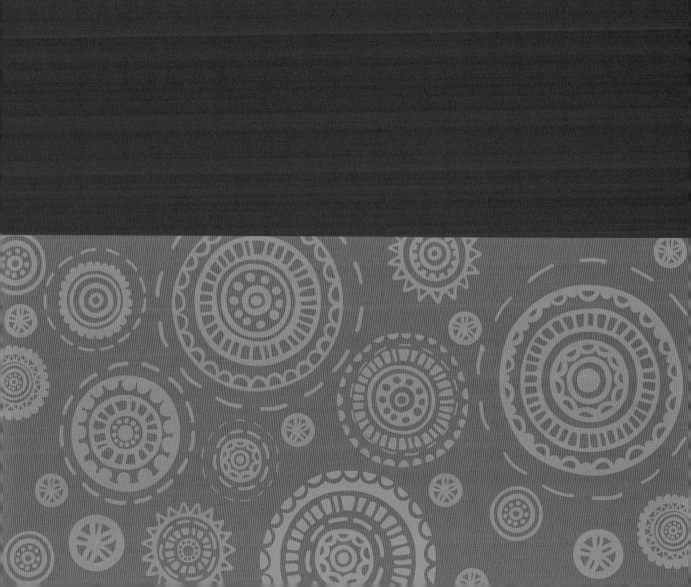

breakthroughs *of the* future

A cure for diabetes is still out of reach – but not by much if progress continues at its current pace. Research is yielding fresh insights into the disease and what causes it, and new medications and techniques to treat it are in the works. Recent advances may offer a realistic way in the future of improving diabetes control and delivering insulin. These include an artificial pancreas and transplanting islet cells into the pancreas to eliminate the need to inject insulin altogether.

I magine not having any treatments for diabetes: no insulin, no tablets to control blood glucose, no medical procedures for complications in the eyes or kidneys – and little hope for a long or healthy life. That was the situation during the first part of the twentieth century, but this book has shown how diabetes care has made great strides in a relatively short time. And today the pace of innovation is gathering speed.

As the prevalence of diabetes has grown, understanding how the disease works and finding effective new treatments has taken on even greater urgency. As a result, researchers are continually making advances that make the future of diabetes care look brighter than ever before. While much about managing diabetes will remain in the hands of those who have it (particularly in relation to lifestyle issues), we can be confident of a greatly improved outcome for those people as years go by. To some extent, the future is already here. Consider some of the important advances that have taken place within just the past 5 years or so:

✸ New types of insulin provide even more options for keeping blood glucose stable throughout the day and after meals. These include the new insulins Glargine (Lantus) and Levemir (Determir), which stay evenly active for up to a period of 24 hours, and rapid-acting Lispro and Insulin Aspart, which start to work within 5 minutes of taking them.

✷ New glucose-monitoring methods that allow you to test your blood glucose without pricking your finger. Known as continuous glucose-monitoring systems (CGMS), these are worn like an insulin pump and give a glucose reading every 1 to 5 minutes.

Building on the present

Few medical advances come out of the blue. Instead, they're built on previous groundbreaking work. That means researchers aren't resting on their laurels when it comes to improvements they've made but are forging ahead with new insights and developments. Some of what we can look forward to seeing in coming years:

Continuous glucose-monitoring systems (CGMS). A continuous glucose monitor (CGM) is a device that measures glucose levels continuously throughout the day and night, every 1 to 5 minutes. This gives the wearer access to between 288 and 1440 glucose readings every 24 hours, providing a much better picture of overall glucose control compared to traditional blood-glucose monitoring, which is really just a single point in time.

Continuous glucose monitors consist of three main parts: a sensor, a transmitter and a monitor.

⬦ The sensor is a small disposable glucose-sensing device that is inserted just under the skin (usually on the stomach), in a similar way to inserting an insulin pump catheter. The sensor measures the glucose level in the interstitial fluid between the cells, similar to measuring glucose levels in the blood. A new sensor needs to be inserted every 6 to 7 days, depending on the device. The CGMS may also be combined with a pump where the pump becomes the receiver rather than a separate device. In this case, you just need to buy the transmitter and sensors.

✷ The transmitter is attached to the sensor and sends glucose readings to the wireless receiver.

⬦ The receiver is a handheld device, similar in size to a traditional blood-glucose meter, which displays glucose readings. This can be worn on a belt or waistband, like a pager or insulin pump, and gives a glucose reading every 1 to 5 minutes, depending on the device.

CGMS provides a number of benefits over regular monitoring, including being able to show trends in your glucose levels from minute to minute, including overnight; being able to set alarms if your glucose level falls too low or goes too high and allowing you to finetune your insulin, food intake and exercise to obtain optimal glucose control.

Despite these benefits, there are a number of barriers to using CGMS, including availability and cost. At this time only two types of CGMS are available in Australia, and private health funds in Australia do not cover the actual devices or the sensors, making them unaffordable for most. CGMS is also not as accurate as regular blood testing, particularly when glucose levels are changing rapidly, such as after a meal or during intense exercise. Since they also need to be calibrated regularly with a regular blood-glucose test, they are not an alternative to your regular testing.

Current CGM Systems. There are currently three CGM systems that have FDA (US Food and Drug Administration) approval and are available in Australia.

- The Guardian REAL-Time Continuous Glucose Monitoring System (Medtronic Minimed) gives a reading every 5 minutes.
- The MiniMed Paradigm® REAL-Time System and Paradigm Veo System devices work alongside the Minimed Paradigm insulin pumps, with the pump acting as the receiver. It gives readings every 5 minutes. For more details visit www.medtronic-diabetes.com.au
- The Dexcom G4 ® Platinum is approved for use in adults with type 1 or type 2 diabetes and recently approved for children over 2 years of age. Dexcom gives a reading every 5 minutes with the sensor lasting for 7 days. It may be used as an independent unit for people on multiple injections or in conjunction with the Animas Vibe insulin pump. For more details visit www.dexcom.com and www.amsl.com.au

New standards for care. Whatever advances in medications or treatments for complications may be in the works, the most important way to deal with diabetes will still be to control blood glucose as tightly as possible. As studies continue to shed light on how high blood glucose poses risks for diabetes, heart disease and complications, the medical community is moving to make standards of care more stringent. It's not just a matter of semantics: lowering your HbA1c a small amount with healthy eating and physical activity can potentially make even the most exciting new medications and medical therapies unnecessary.

The future of insulin delivery

If you take insulin, finding any way besides injection to get it into your body is probably on your wish list – and scientists are working hard to make just that happen. That may sound like a tall order, considering that injections have been the only delivery system available in the more than 90 years that insulin has been used. Still, while challenges remain, novel alternatives may be just around the corner.

Numerous methods (including eye drops, rectal suppositories and wax pellets placed under the skin) have been tried unsuccessfully throughout the years, but researchers haven't yet run out of ideas.

Inhaled insulin. Inhaled insulin delivery systems provide rapid-acting insulin as a dry powder that is inhaled through the mouth into the lungs (similar to asthma inhalers), where it passes into the bloodstream. These devices have been developed and found to work successfully, but due to a lack of significant benefit and interest, manufacturers are no longer pursuing the development of inhaled insulin.

Oral insulin. Researchers have been stymied for years in their attempts to develop insulin you can swallow because the hormone is naturally broken down during digestion before it reaches the bloodstream. However, a number of approaches in development may overcome this barrier. One method being explored in both the United States and Europe is to encase tablets in a resin or plastic coating that breaks down only after the medication reaches the bloodstream. Another tactic is to avoid the gastrointestinal tract altogether by using a spray or patch that allows insulin to be absorbed through the cheek.

Using molecular messengers. On the distant horizon of the coming decades is the prospect of loading insulin into designer molecules called nanoshells – tiny hollow spheres made of silica and coated with gold. On their injection into the body, a hand-held infra-red laser would be used to heat the nanoshells, causing them to release small amounts of insulin. Theoretically,

each nanoshell injection could provide needle-free insulin for months at a time.

Insulin patches. These are placed on the skin to give a continuous low dose of insulin. Before meals, the user pulls off a tab on the patch to release extra insulin. The main challenges with patches are the ability to get the insulin through the skin and to deliver accurate doses.

The disease frontier

Researchers still have much to learn about diabetes and how to prevent it. In type 2 diabetes, for example, it isn't clear how the body becomes insulin resistant or why obesity poses such great risks. In type 1 diabetes, which can be only partly attributed to genes, the disease's environmental triggers are still largely mysterious.

Here are some of the ways researchers are trying to get at the roots of diabetes and thus shed light on its prevention and treatment.

Looking ahead. During the next decade, Australian and overseas scientists will continue to explore new treatments to improve diabetes control, a cure for type 1 and type 2 diabetes and valuable new tools that include non-invasive methods of monitoring blood glucose.

Boosting insulin power. No matter how closely you control blood glucose with insulin, it's difficult to get perfect results. Among the challenges are that blood glucose can

A diabetes forecast

One encouraging finding from the US Diabetes Prevention Trial–Type 1 that is also applicable to people with diabetes in Australia and New Zealand is that the presence of certain types of antibodies known as human leukocyte antigens, or HLAs, is closely associated with development of type 1 diabetes. While most HLAs protect the body, others seem to target islet cell products in the pancreas, such as insulin. By looking at specific antigens, we can now tell with greater precision whether someone is likely to get type 1 diabetes within the 3-year period following the test.

still swing too high after meals and too low when you're not eating – and when control is good, you tend to gain weight. Enter amylin, a hormone that's released by beta cells in the pancreas at the same time that insulin is secreted. People with type 1 and type 2 who require insulin are deficient in amylin. This has led researchers to try to stabilise blood glucose with a synthetic amylin replacement called pramlintide. It appears to work by suppressing secretion of another hormone (glucagon) that raises blood glucose and brakes digestion by slowing the movement of food from the stomach to the small intestine. Clinical trials from the United States have been encouraging. In a recent year-long study of some 538 people with type 2 diabetes, those who got pramlintide injections with their meals dropped their

HbA1c scores without changing their insulin dosage or experiencing hypoglycaemia – and they also lost weight into the bargain.

Preventing type 1. The Intranasal Insulin Trial (INIT II) began in Australia in 2006 with the aim of developing a vaccine for type 1 diabetes. The study is testing whether intranasal administration of insulin to children and young adults with a family history and positive antibodies for the disease will delay or prevent the onset of type 1 diabetes. Previous research has suggested that giving intranasal insulin can induce protective immunity, thus acting as a vaccine against type 1 diabetes. The trial is building on the results of the INIT I trial, which demonstrated an acceptable safety profile and an immune effect in children and young adults at risk of type 1 diabetes who were given intranasal insulin. The INIT II trial is designed to test the effectiveness of this potential vaccine and to assist in finding a suitable dose range in a larger population. The trial is taking place at a number of centres across Australia and New Zealand with first-degree relatives (mother or father, brother or sister, son or daughter) and second-degree relatives (grandmother or grandfather, aunt or uncle, niece or nephew, half-sister or half-brother) of people with type 1 diabetes.

Unlocking secrets with medications. Many medications are developed in 'backward' fashion – that is, scientists don't always understand why they work, just that they do. But a medication's effectiveness may provide clues about the mechanisms of the disease itself. In the case of type 2 diabetes, scientists are scrutinising thiazolidinediones, also called glitazones – drugs that help lower blood glucose by making cells more sensitive to insulin. Insulin resistance is a key trait of type 2 diabetes. Glitazones are interesting because they don't just have beneficial effects in one type of cell but work across the board in fat, liver and muscle cells – all places affected by diabetes. Through studies that aim to understand how the glitazones achieve their effects, researchers may be able to develop even better medications in the future.

Searching for triggers. If the origins of type 1 diabetes are only about half genetic, environmental factors must play a role, too. But which factors? One unsubstantiated theory is that exposure to cow's milk early in life may make children more susceptible to diabetes, possibly because of protein similarities between milk and pancreatic beta cells. An international study based in Europe called TRIGR (Trial to Reduce Diabetes in the Genetically At-Risk) is testing this idea by following diabetes rates in children who are breastfed for the first 6 months of life versus those who are exposed at an earlier age to cow's milk. Preliminary results suggest that the risks are significantly lower for those who drink less cow's milk. Similarly, the TEDDY (The Environmental Determinants of Diabetes in the Young) study and DAISY (Diabetes Autoimmunity Study in the Young) are following newborns at risk of type 1 diabetes (due to having a first-degree relative with type 1) and those from the general population up to 15 years of age

to try to identify factors that may trigger or protect against the development of type 1 diabetes, including dietary factors, infections, vaccinations and psycho-social stressors. The final results of both studies will not be available until around 2017.

Fingering faulty genes. Research is moving forward to find the genes responsible for causing diabetes, regulating functions like insulin production or contributing to complications. For example, an international team of researchers called the Type 1 Diabetes Genetics Consortium is collecting genetic data on families around the world and analysing it for clues about which genes might contribute to type 1. Meanwhile, another US study is looking to find genes that play a role in diabetic nephropathy, or kidney damage, which appears to run in families.

Understanding the genetics of diabetes could have almost limitless practical payoffs in new medications and therapies. For instance, researchers at the Joslin Diabetes Center, in Boston, USA, recently announced that they had isolated and cloned the third of three genes thought to be responsible for regulating insulin production by beta cells in the pancreas. They now believe they can use these genes to make cells other than beta cells manufacture insulin. Such genetically modified cells may possibly then be implanted in people as beta-cell substitutes.

Pursuing peptides. Protein fragments called peptides help regulate a number of processes in the body that may contribute to type 1 diabetes, and scientists are working to develop peptide-based therapies to treat the disease. One drug seeks to fend off assaults on the pancreas by triggering the release of cytokines, hormones that regulate immune-system cells and appear to stop the progression of newly diagnosed type 1. In animal studies and preliminary trials in people, this new drug appeared to preserve insulin function without affecting the immune system's ability to protect the body from infection.

Preventing diabetes onset. Australian researchers have recently shown that the cells of our immune system can be manipulated to prevent type 1 diabetes. Our immune cells, or white blood cells, include B cells and T cells. B cells make antibodies and present 'antigens' to T cells, allowing them to recognise and kill invaders. Previous research has shown that groups of B cells migrate to the pancreas, and tell T cells to kill the cells that produce insulin. The study in mice that develop type 1 diabetes found that using a special molecule called BCMA, which blocks a hormone responsible for controlling the survival of B cells, a special type of T cell (called a regulatory T cell) increased and prevented the autoimmune attack on the insulin-producing cells in the pancreas. After this treatment, none of the mice developed type 1 diabetes – a significant finding, as other B cell depletion methods have only delayed or reduced the incidence. BCMA is already being used in clinical trials for other autoimmune diseases, such as Sjogren's Syndrome and Lupus, providing hope that it will soon be trialled in humans with type 1 diabetes.

However, all of the research activities listed here are still in the experimental phase of development and not for use at this time.

Working on weight loss

Keeping your weight down is a critical factor in controlling type 2 diabetes, but much about how the body regulates appetite, metabolism, fat accumulation and other factors isn't well understood. As rates of obesity in Australia and New Zealand continue to climb along with rates of diabetes, public-education campaigns have been launched to bring attention to the dangers of obesity in both adults and children. In the meantime, researchers are devising new ways to help you manage your weight.

The main principles of weight loss remain the same: to lose excess kilos you need to burn more kilojoules than you take in. But many people find this difficult because the body seems programmed to keep weight consistent. Much of the research into obesity seeks to understand just how the body's internal controls work. Here are some recent insights.

Finding 'fat' genes. What you do (or don't do) has a lot to do with how much you weigh, but it's also clear that body weight runs in families. By some estimates, as much as 40 to 70 per cent of such traits as body mass and fat formation in the gut are determined by your genes. Now that the human genome has been mapped, scientists are trying to zero in on the genes – and there are likely to be many – that contribute to weight control. One exciting development was the discovery of a genetic defect that curbed production of the appetite-regulating hormone called leptin. Now researchers are looking at clusters of genes on two different chromosomes that may predispose people to abdominal fat and insulin resistance. The hope is to determine how the relevant genes interact with each other and eventually be able to custom-design drugs that can address the flaws that contribute to obesity in an individual's genetic make-up.

Leveraging leptin. Genetic defects may not be the most important influence on leptin. In fact, most obese people have ample amounts of the hormone but don't seem to benefit from its ability to signal when appetite is satisfied. Researchers aren't sure why, but they may now have another piece of the puzzle. In an exciting development, US scientists have identified a protein that appears to help regulate signals that allow leptin to work. The protein has two important effects: it makes laboratory mice stay slim, even when they are fed a high-fat diet, and it boosts insulin sensitivity. This makes the protein, called PTP1B (protein tyrosine phosphatase 1B), a potentially powerful agent against both obesity and type 2 diabetes. This research has not yet gone beyond animal testing, but it provides an intriguing basis for further study.

Suppressing the appetite. Everyone dreams of a safe tablet that would act as a switch to turn off appetite. But it's unlikely that a single chemical agent will do the trick because the urge to eat is regulated by a complex biochemical process with many players. Still, researchers are working to identify the players in the hope of tackling a few of them to give people trying to lose weight an edge.

One candidate described recently in a British science journal is a molecule called OEA (oleyleth-anolamide). Levels of OEA in the intestine increase when you eat. Scientists believe the compound helps trigger feelings of fullness that make you stop eating. In studies at the University of California in the US, rats that were given OEA reduced their food intake and their weight. A chemically similar drug developed by a French company is now being tested in people.

Another prospect is a compound called C75, which appears to curb appetite by affecting several brain chemicals at once. Obese lab rats injected with C75 ate less even after fasting, according to one study. What's more, the compound seems to increase metabolism to make animals burn more energy, which means it may boost weight loss by both cutting and burning kilojoules.

Obesity and the brain. If you remember the high-fashion emaciated look of a few years ago known as 'heroin chic', then you have a picture of what narcotics do besides blow your mind: they curb the appetite and make you lose weight. Wasting your mind and body is hardly a path to good health, but the link between weight loss and pleasure-producing chemicals in the brain hasn't been lost on scientists. Of particular interest is dopamine, a neurotransmitter produced when you satisfy urges such as sex and eating. Brain researchers at Brookhaven National Laboratory in the US have found that obese people have fewer sites, or receptors, on cells for dopamine to dock with than people of normal weight. The scientists speculate that overeating may be caused by a greater need for stimulation to produce satisfaction. The implication of this is that other activities that boost dopamine in the brain – such as physical activity – can help to take the edge off cravings.

Other studies by the same researchers indicate another difference in obese people: areas of the brain that process sensual signals received from the mouth, lips and tongue about food are more active than they are in normal-weight people. This raises the possibility that drugs that make food less palatable may help people lose weight despite sensory hot spots in the brain.

Controlling complications

If you follow all the advice you find in this book, your prospects for avoiding future complications may well be bright even without any more medical advances. In fact, the most important developments in preventing damage from diabetes continue to focus on understanding how tight control of blood glucose can reduce your risks. But researchers are also looking into ways to minimise the impact of diabetes on your health even if blood glucose does get out of hand.

Such advances are potentially significant because many people with diabetes – especially type 2, which usually develops without symptoms over a long period of time – already have complications by the time they're diagnosed.

Eye protection

Vision loss, which can lead to blindness, is perhaps one of the complications of diabetes that people fear the most. Good blood-glucose control will significantly reduce your risk of eye problems – by as much as 76 per cent. And medical advances should improve those odds even further. Among the possibilities being explored to put a damper on diabetic eye damage are:

Macular oedema is a form of diabetic eye disease that occurs when damaged blood vessels in the eye begin to leak fluid near the center of the retina, known as the macula. If left untreated, it can lead to vision loss. Diabetic macular oedema is usually treated with laser therapy, but a recent study has found that combining laser treatment with an injection of a drug called ranibizumab (Lucentis) into the eye resulted in significantly greater improvements in vision than laser treatment alone. Ranibizumab works by blocking a chemical signal that stimulates blood vessel growth, which can prevent blood vessels from leaking fluid and causing macular oedema.

Help from ACE inhibitors. Already used to bring down high blood pressure, ACE (angiotensin-converting enzyme) inhibitors have shown potential for improving insulin sensitivity and preserving kidney function. Now research suggests that ACE inhibitors may improve circulation to the eyes. If taken before blood vessels proliferate from retinopathy, the drugs may help reduce the risk of proliferation and haemorrhaging in the future.

A nervy proposition. One of the ways high blood-glucose levels can lead to complications is that blood glucose converts to a substance called sorbitol, a modified form of glucose that's especially prone to building up in tissue. In the eyes, sorbitol contributes to clouding of vision, while in the nerves it traps water in cells, which can impair function by making nerves swell. Scientists have found that an enzyme called aldose reductase speeds the conversion of blood glucose to sorbitol, and pharmaceutical companies are working to develop drugs that block the enzyme's effects. So far, aldose reductase inhibitors have not impressed many clinicians, but research continues in the belief that more effective drugs are still to be found.

Head-to-toe help

From the heart to the kidneys to the feet, here are the most promising advances currently in the works for treating or preventing other complications of diabetes.

Double-duty drugs. Like ACE inhibitors, another class of drugs that may have unforeseen benefits are thiazolidinediones, also called glitazones. In addition to making cells more sensitive to insulin and preventing

> ## WHAT the STUDIES show
>
> Diabetes and heart disease are so closely linked that high blood levels of insulin are used as a marker for cardiovascular risk. Now a US study finds that a molecule called proinsulin, a precursor of insulin, predicts heart disease risk even better than insulin. When researchers examined 1456 people, they found that elevated proinsulin levels roughly doubled heart disease risk, even in people without diabetes.

damage to the kidneys and eyes due to high blood pressure, some studies have indicated that glitazones may help relax the endothelium, a layer of cells lining the blood vessels and cavities of the heart. If the effect is demonstrated in further studies, glitazones may prove to be useful in fighting cardiovascular complications while they lower blood glucose.

Grappling with growth hormone. Studies suggest that naturally occurring growth hormone may help trigger the onset of kidney damage from diabetes. In one study, for example, lab mice with diabetes whose cells were genetically programmed not to respond to growth hormone didn't develop kidney disease, while other diabetic mice did. Now researchers are working to develop a class of drugs that – when the likelihood of serious disease warrants it – can block growth hormone's action by claiming a 'parking space' on cells normally reserved for the hormone. There's also evidence that so-called growth hormone antagonists may help prevent diabetic eye disease.

Stopping the stiffening. Another process that contributes to damage from complications is a stiffening of tissues due to advanced glycosylation end products, or AGEs – structures that form when sugars bind with the amino acids of proteins in a process sometimes likened to the toughening of browned meat. AGEs appear to contribute to virtually every major complication of diabetes, including retinopathy, nerve damage, high blood pressure, foot ulcers and cardiovascular disease. Impeding their action has long been a research priority. While some chemical agents have shown promise, few have been found to be both effective and safe. But work on AGE inhibitors continues. Scientists are also looking at drugs that may be able to break up the links between proteins created by AGEs after they have formed.

Biological skin substitutes. Though other complications might sound more dire, poorly healing foot ulcers are the most common reason people with diabetes enter hospitals. One way to treat them has been skin-graft operations, which require anaesthesia and can be hampered by infection and scarring. But an emerging type of therapy can circumvent these concerns by using what's known as biological skin substitutes, or living skin equivalents. Sometimes called 'living bandages', they're biotechnology products that contain the ingredients of skin (such as collagen and other proteins) and fuse with your own tissue to significantly speed healing.

Replacing the pancreas

Whether you have type 1 or type 2 diabetes, part of your problem is that your pancreas isn't working as it should. In type 1 diabetes, the pancreas makes no insulin. In type 2 diabetes, the condition of your pancreas – particularly the beta cells that make insulin – may deteriorate as the disease progresses. Which begs the question: Why not replace the old, broken parts with new, functioning ones?

Pancreas transplants are nothing new, but they're not a widely prescribed treatment, either. The major barrier is that the body rejects foreign tissues, which means patients must take drugs that suppress the immune system, potentially causing serious complications. There's also the limited availability of donor organs. For these reasons, pancreas transplants are currently offered only to people with type 1 diabetes who have severe complications and need lifesaving transplantation of another organ – most commonly the kidney.

Islet cell transplants

There may be no reason to get rid of the entire pancreas – which produces digestive enzymes and hormones besides insulin – if it's only the beleaguered beta cells that are in trouble. That's the idea behind islet cell transplants, in which surgeons replace clumps, or islets, of cells – including beta cells – that are clustered throughout the pancreas.

The procedure was pioneered in animals as far back as the 1970s and has since been made possible in people. In fact, hundreds of people have received islet cell transplants around the world. Initially the success rate was poor, as the immunosuppressant drugs given to prevent rejection were toxic to the beta cells. But major advances in the past few years have made this a viable option for some people with type 1 diabetes. This is the result of the work of Canadian researchers who developed what is known as the 'Edmonton Protocol' using a combination of immunosuppressant drugs that prevent rejection while also stopping the immune system attacks that cause type 1 diabetes in the first place.

Islet cell transplants using the Edmonton Protocol are now being done in Australia through the Australian Islet Transplantation Program (ITP). Islet cells, taken from donor pancreases, are given as a transfusion under local anaesthetic using ultrasound to guide the needle. Most people have a significant reduction in their insulin needs following the first infusion, but generally need a second or third infusion to be free of injected insulin. However, just as with a whole pancreas transplant, they need to take immunosuppressant drugs indefinitely to prevent rejection, and this

The supply-side challenge

Even if techniques for islet cell transplants are refined, a significant barrier to making the procedure a mainstream treatment is the lack of donor pancreases from which cells can be extracted.

To resolve this dilemma, researchers are looking for ways to produce islet cells without having to rely on donors. Studies are now looking at how islet cells multiply, in the hope that ways can be found to make them grow faster – work already being pioneered in animals. Researchers are also looking into the possibility of using cells from such animals as pigs, in humans.

The most significant (and controversial) area of research involves the use of embryonic stem cells – cells that have the capacity to become virtually any type of cell in the body. Lab studies have shown that stem cells can be genetically manipulated to produce insulin, suggesting that they might make a viable source for transplants. Other options might be to use adult stem cells extracted from bone marrow or blood, which may hold promise for producing insulin, or to convert liver cells into insulin-making cells. Animal research has also suggested that stem cells can be developed from unfertilised eggs instead of embryos; if it can be done in humans, this would skirt the ethical issues surrounding the use of embryonic tissue.

makes the procedure suitable only for those with severe hypoglycaemic unawareness or complications that significantly affect their quality of life.

However, despite the optimism, islet cell transplants are still far from perfect. Some of the transplants have been found to fail with time, and the long-term side effects of the new immunosuppressant drugs are not well understood. But as studies continue, researchers are hopeful that powerful new approaches to restoring pancreatic function will eventually become more widely available.

An artificial pancreas

Even with all the progress being made on the transplant front, some researchers believe a different approach is even closer to becoming a reality – developing a mechanical system that mimics the insulin-controlling functions of the pancreas. Such a system requires two basic parts: an internal monitor to keep track of blood-glucose levels and a dispensing device to automatically respond to glucose changes by releasing just the right amount of insulin to keep blood glucose stable.

The basic elements of such a system – an insulin pump and a continuous glucose meter – have already been invented. These are available for use but not yet in a closed-loop system (where the CGMS 'talks' to the pump and tells it how much insulin to give based on glucose readings). An artificial pancreas will integrate the two technologies, with the sensor being able to communicate with the pump to provide the right amount of insulin at the right time.

The results of a trial of such an automated system show that children wearing the pump and sensor combination spent significantly more time with blood-glucose levels in the normal range, and were less likely to experience hypoglycaemia. Researchers are now working at perfecting this technology, which will include testing it in real-life situations, with the hope of making it commercially available in the near future.

CAREFUL CONSIDERATIONS

Ever since she was diagnosed with type 1 diabetes at age 11, Kerry Brunson resigned herself to daily insulin injections and blood-glucose tests for the rest of her life. By her late 30s, that view hadn't changed, but her condition had.

'As I got older, I had less awareness of when my blood glucose was getting too low', she says. 'My family could sense it more than I could. My children would say, "Mum, are you okay? You need something to eat." My kids and my husband would follow me around making sure I was all right.' There were times her husband would find her convulsing in her sleep from low blood glucose, but the final straw was when she had two seizures while alone with her kids.

She sat down to watch TV, fell unconscious and went into convulsions. The children had to phone emergency and watch their mother being taken away in an ambulance while neighbours stayed with them until her husband, Ed, came home. 'I have no recollection of what happened', says Kerry, 'but it was really upsetting for the kids. It scared me, too: what if the kids were with me and I lost control behind the wheel?' Something had to change. On the advice of her diabetes educator, she tried an insulin pump. Since then Kerry hasn't looked back. 'My lifestyle is so much freer, I have more flexibility in timing meals and the best thing of all – no more of those terrifying hypos.'

> *'…I feel so much more confident and positive about my life…'*

Kerry says that for the first time in years, she can eat when she (and the rest of the family) want to, she has better control over her blood glucose with improved HbA1c tests and, because of all of this, she feels a lot better about herself.

'The insecurity is gone', says Kerry. 'I feel so much more confident and positive about my life.' Even though her blood-glucose tests were reasonable when she was injecting, she couldn't seem to avoid those hypoglycaemic episodes that created stress for everyone day after day. 'For the first time since I was diagnosed, I really feel in control of things', she says.

For people who are prepared to pay for the pump, plus the ongoing costs of the infusion set and related items, perform at least five to six blood-glucose tests a day and have a mechanical device attached to their body on a permanent basis, the insulin pump can be life changing – just as it has been for Kerry. However, it is clearly not for everyone and its use needs to be discussed thoroughly with your doctor or diabetes educator. In New Zealand, some pumps are available free, but the ongoing costs are not funded. In Australia, most private health funds will cover the initial cost of a pump, and consumables are subsidised on the NDSS.

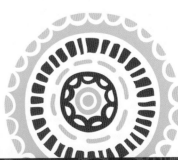

recipes

Breakfast

Carrot, apricot and pecan muffins

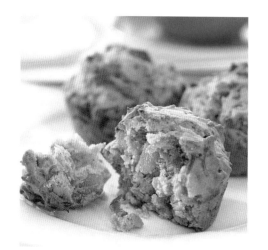

Make a batch of these healthy muffins to keep in the freezer. Take a muffin out the night before – by the time breakfast comes, it will be thawed.

Preparation: 20 minutes • Cooking: 35 minutes • Serves 6 (makes 12)

½ cup (60 g) pecans
1¾ cups (250 g) plain flour
1¾ tsp baking powder
1 tsp ground cinnamon
pinch of salt
½ cup (130 g) unsweetened
  puréed cooked apple
¼ cup (55 g) white sugar
¼ cup (60 g) firmly packed
  soft brown sugar

2 tbsp canola oil
1 medium egg
1 medium eggwhite
4 large carrots (about 300 g),
  grated
⅓ cup (45 g) dried apricot
  halves, coarsely chopped

1 Preheat the oven to 190°C. Lightly coat a 12-hole American-style muffin tray with cooking spray; each hole should be about 6 cm diameter. Or, line each muffin hole with a paper liner.

2 Toast the pecans on a small baking tray for 5 minutes, or until lightly fragrant. When they are cool enough to handle, chop them coarsely.

3 Sift the flour, baking powder, cinnamon and a pinch of salt into a bowl. Combine the apple, both sugars, the oil, whole egg and eggwhite in a separate bowl, then stir in the pecans, grated carrot and apricots.

4 Make a well in the centre of the flour. Stir in the carrot mixture until just moistened. Spoon into the prepared muffin holes and bake for 30 minutes, or until a skewer inserted in the centre of a muffin comes out just clean. Cool for 10 minutes in the tray, then transfer to a wire rack to cool completely.

NUTRITION PER SERVING 1644 kJ, 8 g protein, 15 g fat (1 g saturated fat), 58 g carbohydrate (27 g sugars), 5 g fibre, 209 mg sodium. GI: medium

Cheese and onion rarebit

There are many versions of Welsh rarebit (or rabbit). The one here is richly flavoured with cheese and thickened with breadcrumbs to add texture, and is spooned over thinly sliced red onions before being grilled until golden and bubbling. A spinach, apple and celery salad is the perfect partner.

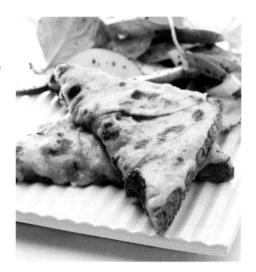

Preparation: 15 minutes • Cooking: 10 minutes • Serves 4

100 ml low-fat milk
½ tsp mustard powder
1 cup (120 g) firmly packed grated fat-reduced tasty cheese
½ cup (30 g) fresh salt-reduced, wholemeal breadcrumbs
4 thick slices multigrain bread
1 small red onion, thinly sliced

FOR THE SALAD
1 tbsp walnut oil
2 tsp red wine vinegar
2 tsp poppy seeds
¼ tsp freshly ground black pepper
200 g baby spinach leaves
2 red apples, quartered, cored and sliced
2 celery stalks, sliced

1 Preheat the grill to high. Put the milk, mustard powder and cheese in a small heavy-based saucepan and stir over a low heat until the cheese has melted and the mixture is smooth. Remove from the heat and stir in the breadcrumbs. Cool for 3–4 minutes, stirring occasionally, until thickened to a spreading consistency.

2 Meanwhile, arrange the slices of bread on the grill tray and toast on both sides under the grill.

3 While the bread is toasting, make the salad. Put the oil, red wine vinegar and poppy seeds in a salad bowl and season to taste with pepper. Whisk to mix. Add the spinach, apples and celery, but do not toss the salad.

4 Top the toast with the slices of red onion, then spoon the cheese mixture over the top, spreading it out to cover the toast completely. Return to the grill and cook for 2–3 minutes, or until the cheese mixture is golden brown and bubbling. Toss the salad and serve with the rarebits.

NUTRITION PER SERVING 1178 kJ, 18 g protein, 10 g fat (2 g saturated fat), 29 g carbohydrate (16 g sugars), 8 g fibre, 376 mg sodium. GI: low

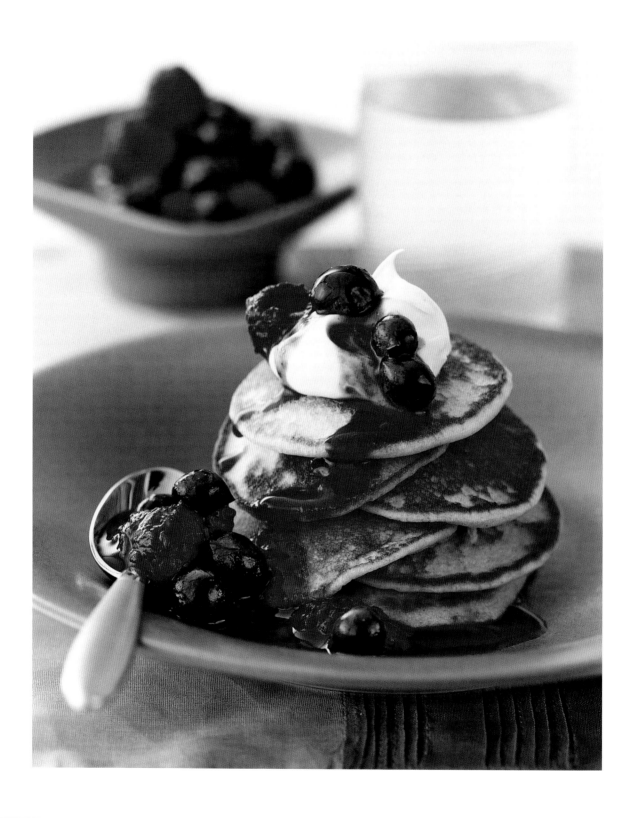

Pikelets with berries and yogurt

Pikelets are easy and fun to make and are perfect for breakfast, afternoon tea or even a simple dessert. Served with yogurt and sweet, succulent berries, they are irresistible.

Preparation: 10 minutes • Cooking: 25 minutes • Serves 4 (makes about 24)

1 cup (140 g) self-raising
   flour
2 tsp caster sugar
1 medium egg, beaten
1 tbsp olive oil spread
150 ml low-fat milk
1 tbsp canola oil

1⅓ cup (200 g) blueberries
1 tsp honey
1¾ cup (220 g) frozen
   raspberries, thawed, any
   juices reserved
¾ cup (195 g) plain low-fat
   yogurt

1 Sift the flour into a bowl and stir in the sugar. Make a well in the centre, then add the egg, melted spread and a little of the milk. Gradually stir the flour into the liquids and pour in the remaining milk a little at a time, to make a fairly thick, smooth batter.

2 Heat a large shallow ovenproof dish in a low oven, then turn off the heat and line the dish with a tea towel (this is for keeping the pikelets warm).

3 Heat a large heavy-based frying pan over a medium heat and grease it with 1 tsp of the oil. Using a tablespoon, pour the batter from the pointed end (rather than the side of the spoon) to make neat, round pikelets. Depending on the size of the pan, you should be able to cook 4–6 pikelets at once, but make sure you leave enough space round them so you can turn them easily. Cook for about 2 minutes, or until almost set and bubbles are breaking on the surface; the pikelets should be golden brown underneath.

4 Using a palette knife or spatula, turn the pikelets over and cook for a further 1–2 minutes, or until golden brown on the other side. Transfer to the prepared dish, wrap in the tea towel and keep warm while you cook the remaining pikelets. Grease the pan lightly with 1 tsp oil before cooking each batch.

5 Place the blueberries in a bowl and stir in the honey. Add the raspberries and lightly crush the fruit, leaving some berries whole. Serve the pikelets warm with the honeyed berries and yogurt.

NUTRITION PER SERVING 1262 kJ, 11 g protein, 9 g fat (2 g saturated fat), 43 g carbohydrate (18 g sugars), 5 g fibre, 335 mg sodium. GI: medium

Snacks/Appetisers

Goat's cheese toasts

These easy-to-make savoury bites are made by topping toasted slices of crusty French bread with slices of roma tomato and tangy goat's cheese, then sprinkled with pine nuts and fresh herbs. Choose your favourite type of goat's cheese: delicate or strong in flavour; soft or firm in texture.

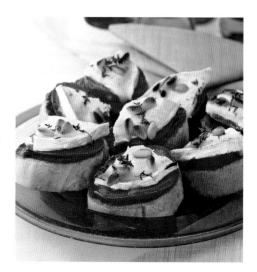

Preparation: 15 minutes • Cooking: 10 minutes • Makes 16

1 French bread stick, cut into 2.5 cm slices
1/3 cup (80 ml) tomato purée (passata)
2 tbsp sun-dried tomato paste
4 roma tomatoes
110 g goat's cheese
1 tbsp extra virgin olive oil
2 tbsp pine nuts
few sprigs of fresh thyme or oregano

1 Preheat the grill to moderate. Place the bread slices on the grill tray and lightly toast on both sides.

2 Mix together the tomato purée and tomato paste and spread a little of the mixture over each toast, covering the surface completely.

3 Slice the tomatoes lengthwise, discarding a slim slice from the curved edges, to give 4 flat slices from each tomato. Lay a slice of tomato on top of each toast.

4 Place 1 small slice of firm goat's cheese or about 1 tsp soft goat's cheese on top of each tomato slice, then drizzle with a little of the oil. Scatter a few pine nuts and herb sprigs over the top.

5 Grill for 4–5 minutes, or until the cheese is beginning to melt and the pine nuts are golden. Serve the toasts hot.

NUTRITION PER TOAST 367 kJ, 3 g protein, 5 g fat (2 g saturated fat), 8 g carbohydrate (2 g sugars), 1 g fibre, 124 mg sodium. GI: high

Caramelised onion tartlets

Croustades – made from thin slices of bread pressed into patty tins, brushed with olive oil spread and baked until crisp – are a great alternative to pastry for savoury tartlets. Both the croustades and filling can be prepared ahead, then warmed and assembled for serving.

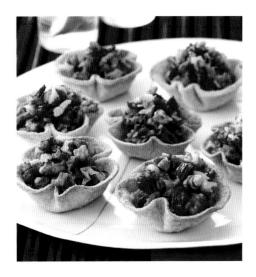

Preparation: 20 minutes • Cooking: 35 minutes • Makes 12

12 thin slices white bread
1 tbsp olive oil spread
1 tbsp extra virgin olive oil
2 large onions, thinly sliced
¼ cup (35 g) sun-dried tomatoes packed in oil, drained and roughly chopped

2 tsp finely chopped fresh thyme
¼ cup (30 g) walnut pieces

1 Preheat the oven to 230°C. Lightly spray a 12-hole deep patty pan or muffin tin with cooking spray. Using a 7.5 cm pastry cutter, cut a disc from each slice of bread. Flatten each bread disc with a rolling pin, then press into the oiled patty tins to line them evenly, curving the edge of the bread slightly to make large scalloped edges.

2 Brush the bread cases with the melted olive oil spread and bake for 8–10 minutes, or until crisp and golden. Set aside in a warm place until ready to fill.

3 Heat the oil in a large heavy-based frying pan with a well-fitting lid. Add the onions and stir well. Cover with the lid and cook over a low heat for 20 minutes, or until the onions are very soft.

4 Remove the lid, turn up the heat and cook rapidly, stirring, until the onions turn a dark golden brown. Remove from the heat and stir in the sun-dried tomatoes and thyme.

5 Divide the onion filling among the croustades, then scatter the walnut pieces over the top. Serve hot.

NUTRITION PER SERVING 471 kJ, 3 g protein, 5 g fat (1 g saturated fat), 14 g carbohydrate (3 g sugars), 2 g fibre, 136 mg sodium. GI: high

Gingered crab filo parcels

These Chinese-style, triangular parcels of crisp, light filo pastry enclose a ginger-flavoured filling of crabmeat, water chestnuts and corn. They look and taste wonderful and are really easy to make. Prepare them ahead for a party, then bake just before serving with a sweet chilli dipping sauce.

Preparation: 50 minutes • Cooking: 15 minutes • Makes 18

1 can white crabmeat (about 170 g), drained
1 can sliced water chestnuts (about 230 g), drained
  and coarsely chopped
1 can (310 g) corn kernels, drained
4 spring onions, chopped, green parts reserved
1 tbsp finely chopped fresh ginger
1 fresh red chilli, deseeded and finely chopped
2 tbsp Chinese rice wine or dry sherry

¼ tsp salt
¼ tsp freshly ground black pepper
2 tbsp canola oil
2 tbsp sesame oil
6 sheets filo pastry (about 45 x 30 cm each)
1 tbsp sesame seeds
sweet chilli sauce to serve

1 Preheat the oven to 200°C. Combine the crabmeat, water chestnuts, corn, spring onions, ginger, chilli and Chinese rice wine in a bowl and season with salt and pepper to taste. Mix together the canola and sesame oils in a cup.

2 Stack the filo sheets on top of one another and roll up the sheets loosely, rolling from a short side. Using a sharp knife, cut the roll across evenly into three pieces. Cover two of these shorter rolls with plastic wrap to prevent them from drying out. Unravel the third roll, remove one of the strips and set the rest aside, covered.

3 Lay the strip of filo flat on the work surface, with a short end nearest to you, and brush with a little of the oil mixture. Place a heaped teaspoon of the crab mixture near the bottom, towards the right-hand corner of the short end, and fold the pastry diagonally over it. Continue folding

diagonally, over and over, until you reach the end of the strip, making a neat triangular parcel. Place on a baking tray, seam-side down.

4 Repeat with remaining strips of filo, uncovering them only when needed, until all of the crab mixture is used.

5 Lightly brush the tops of the parcels with any remaining oil mixture and sprinkle with the sesame seeds. Bake for 12–13 minutes or until crisp and golden.

6 Transfer the parcels to a wire rack and cool slightly. Meanwhile, shred the green tops of the spring onions for garnishing, to form 'brushes'. Serve the parcels warm, on a tray garnished with the spring onion brushes and a small dish of sweet chilli sauce.

NUTRITION PER SERVING 314 kJ, 2 g protein, 5 g fat (1 g saturated fat), 6 g carbohydrate (1 g sugars), 1 g fibre, 150 mg sodium. GI: none

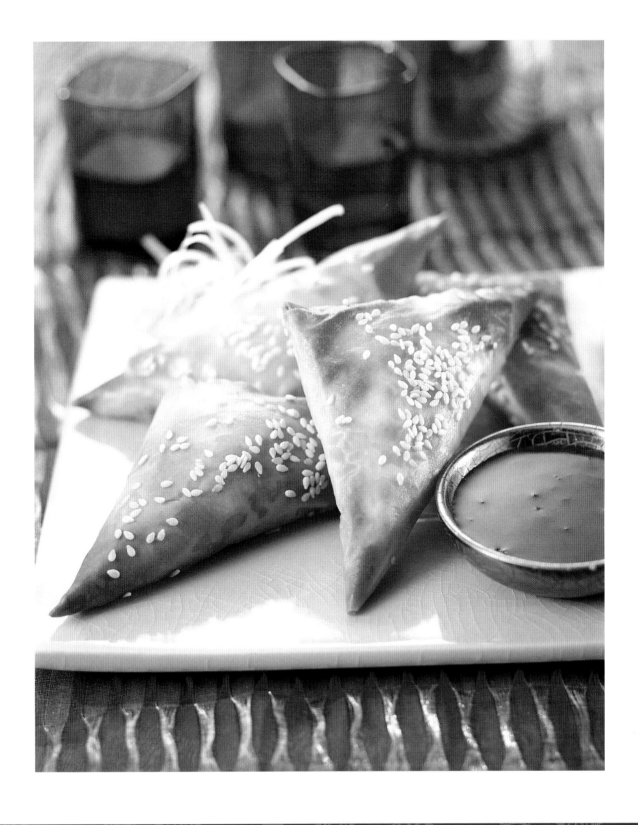

Lunch

Open-faced chicken sandwiches

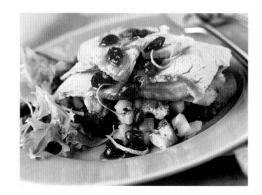

This chicken sandwich is made from tender slices of roasted chicken, smothered with a cranberry dressing and topped with a light herbed 'stuffing'.

Preparation: 30 minutes • Cooking: 20 minutes • Serves 4

6 slices white bread, about 150 g
300 g fresh-roasted chicken breast slices, warmed

FOR THE STUFFING
1 onion, chopped
2 green apples, peeled and chopped
2 celery stalks, chopped
¾ cup (180 ml) salt-reduced chicken stock
1½ tsp finely chopped fresh thyme or 1 tsp dried
¼ tsp dried mixed herbs

FOR THE DRESSING
½ cup (70 g) sweetened dried cranberries
40 ml salt-reduced chicken stock
1½ tbsp balsamic vinegar
1 tbsp honey
1 tbsp extra virgin olive oil
2 tsp grated orange zest

1 Preheat the grill to moderate. Toast four slices of bread on one side until golden, about 2 minutes. Tear the remaining bread into 1 cm pieces.

2 To make the stuffing, lightly coat an ovenproof frying pan with cooking spray and set over a medium–high heat. Sauté the onion, apple and celery for about 5 minutes, or until soft. Add the chicken stock, thyme, dried mixed herbs and bread pieces. Cook, stirring, until heated through, about 4 minutes. Transfer the pan to under the grill and grill for about 3 minutes, or until the top is browned. Stir the browned parts under and grill for a further 3 minutes.

3 For the dressing, combine the cranberries, stock, vinegar, honey, oil and zest in a saucepan over a medium–high heat. Bring to a simmer and cook, stirring, for 1 minute; remove from the heat.

4 For each sandwich, place a piece of toast on a plate, toasted-side down. Spoon some stuffing on top and cover with chicken slices. Drizzle with the warm dressing.

NUTRITION PER SERVING 1744 kJ, 28 g protein, 9 g fat (2 g saturated fat), 56 g carbohydrate (33 g sugars), 5 g fibre, 444 mg sodium. GI: medium

Egg and anchovy pan bagna

Pan bagna is a Mediterranean layered sandwich, often prepared in a hollowed-out round, rustic loaf. Here, eggs, anchovies, capers, basil and tomatoes – all ingredients from a classic salade niçoise – are layered in a long French loaf, then left so that the flavours can meld and soak into the bread. It's a great picnic lunch.

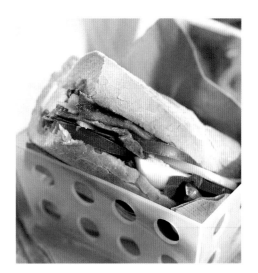

Preparation: 15 minutes • Cooking: 10 minutes, plus 1 hour chilling • Serves 4

4 medium eggs
1 tbsp extra virgin olive oil
1 garlic clove, crushed
1 large wholemeal French
  bread stick, about 250 g
4 ripe tomatoes, sliced
1 red or yellow capsicum, or a
  mixture of both, deseeded
  and very thinly sliced

½ red onion, very thinly
  sliced
100 g baby spinach leaves
6 anchovy fillets, halved
  lengthwise
1 tbsp capers, drained
1 handful of fresh basil
freshly ground black pepper

1 Place the eggs in a saucepan with enough cold water to cover them. Bring to the boil, then lower the heat slightly so that the water is boiling gently and cook the eggs for 8 minutes. Drain and rinse the eggs under cold running water to cool them quickly. Peel and slice.

2 Stir the oil and garlic together in a small bowl. Cut the bread open along its length, keeping it still attached along one side, like a hinge. With the loaf opened out flat, brush the garlic-flavoured oil all over the cut sides.

3 Layer the egg slices, tomatoes, capsicum, onion, spinach leaves and anchovies in the bread stick, scattering the capers and basil leaves among the layers. Make sure that each ingredient is evenly distributed along the loaf. Season with pepper, then close up the loaf and wrap in plastic wrap.

4 Leave to cool at room temperature for about 1 hour (or up to 3 hours in the refrigerator). Cut into 4 equal pieces before serving.

NUTRITION PER SERVING 1173 kJ, 16 g protein, 12 g fat (3 g saturated fat), 28 g carbohydrate (5 g sugars), 6 g fibre, 442 mg sodium. GI: high

Citrus and spinach salad

In this colourful salad, spinach is enhanced by sweet melon and citrus, and prosciutto adds a savoury touch. You can prepare the dressing in advance, but assemble the salad at the last moment to preserve as much vitamin C as possible. Serve with wholemeal bread.

Preparation: 15 minutes • Serves 4

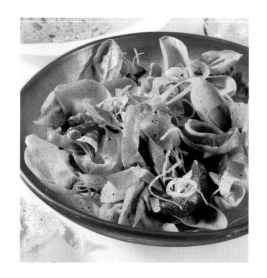

1 ruby or pink grapefruit
2 large oranges
250 g baby spinach leaves
250 g rockmelon flesh, cut
   into bite-sized cubes
1 capsicum, thinly sliced
2 spring onions, white parts
   only, very thinly sliced
50 g thinly sliced prosciutto,
   excess fat removed, cut
   into shreds

FOR THE DRESSING
1 tbsp balsamic vinegar
2 tbsp extra virgin olive oil
1 tbsp cream
½ tsp honey
freshly ground black pepper
4 slices wholemeal bread

1 To make the dressing, put the vinegar, oil, cream and honey in a small screw-top jar. Cover and shake until well blended. Set aside until needed.

2 Working over a bowl to catch the juice, peel the grapefruit, removing all the bitter white pith, then cut it into segments between the membranes. If large, cut the segments into bite-sized pieces. Set the grapefruit segments aside on a plate.

3 Using a citrus zester, take fine shreds of zest from the orange and set aside. Working over the bowl containing the grapefruit juice, peel the orange, removing all the pith, then cut the fruit into segments between the membranes, then

cut the segments into bite-sized pieces, if you like. Add to the grapefruit pieces and set aside.

4 Add 1 tbsp of the combined grapefruit and orange juices to the salad dressing and shake again to blend. Taste and add more citrus juice, if you like. Add pepper to taste.

5 Place the spinach in a large serving bowl. Add the orange and grapefruit segments, the melon, capsicum and spring onions and toss together. Shake the dressing, pour it over the salad and toss. Scatter the prosciutto and orange zest over the top and serve, with a slice of wholemeal bread per person.

NUTRITION PER SERVING 1262 kJ, 12 g protein, 16 g fat (4 g saturated fat), 27 g carbohydrate (18 g sugars), 8 g fibre, 436 mg sodium. GI: low

Melon, fetta and orange salad

Here, the classic starter of melon and prosciutto is transformed into a tempting salad with the addition of fetta, cherry tomatoes, cucumber and oranges. This serves four people for lunch, with warm ciabatta bread to mop up the juices, or six people as a starter.

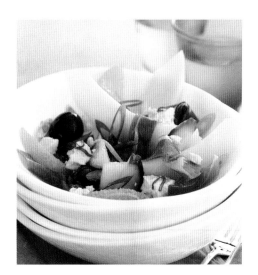

Preparation: 25 minutes • Serves 4

2 large oranges
1 small honeydew melon, peeled, deseeded and sliced
150 g cherry tomatoes, halved
⅓ cup (50 g) black olives
½ Lebanese cucumber, thinly sliced
4 spring onions, thinly sliced
4 slices of prosciutto, about 50 g in total, trimmed of all fat and cut into strips

⅓ cup (50 g) roughly crumbled salt-reduced fetta

FOR THE DRESSING
½ tsp orange zest strips
⅓ cup (80 ml) freshly squeezed orange juice
2½ tbsp extra virgin olive oil
1 tsp sesame oil
6 fresh basil leaves, shredded
freshly ground black pepper to taste

1 Make the dressing first. Mix the orange zest and juice with the olive oil, sesame oil and basil in a large salad bowl. Season with pepper to taste.

2 Cut the peel and pith away from the oranges with a sharp knife. Holding them over the salad bowl to catch the juice, cut between the membrane to release the orange segments. Add the segments to the bowl.

3 Add the melon, tomatoes, olives, cucumber, spring onions and prosciutto. Toss until the ingredients are well blended and coated in dressing. Scatter the fetta over the top and serve.

NUTRITION PER SERVING 1447 kJ, 10 g protein, 21 g fat (6 g saturated fat), 29 g carbohydrate (28 g sugars), 6 g fibre, 446 mg sodium. GI: medium

Dinner

Beef waldorf

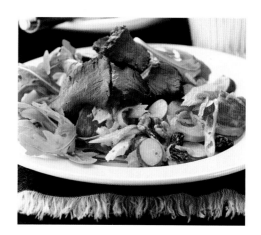

Raw fruit and vegetables are among the richest sources of essential vitamins and minerals. This tasty main-dish salad offers plenty of these vital nutrients and it's made extra delicious with a creamy mustard dressing. Serve with lots of crusty fresh bread for a satisfying and healthy meal.

Preparation: 20 minutes ● Cooking: 10 minutes, plus cooling ● Serves 4

2 fillet steaks (about 140 g each), trimmed of fat
¼ tsp extra virgin olive oil
salt and freshly ground black pepper
250 g radishes, thinly sliced
3 carrots, grated
1 medium yellow capsicum, deseeded and sliced
3 large celery stalks, sliced on the diagonal
3 spring onions, sliced on the diagonal
⅓ cup (35 g) walnuts

⅓ cup (55 g) raisins or sultanas
2 small green apples
2 tsp lemon juice
100 g rocket or watercress leaves

FOR THE DRESSING
2 tbsp wholegrain mustard
¼ cup (65 g) plain low-fat yogurt
2 tbsp 97% fat-free mayonnaise

1 Brush the steaks with oil and season with salt and pepper. Heat a ridged cast-iron grill pan or non-stick frying pan over a medium–high heat until hot. Add the steaks and cook for 3 minutes on each side for medium–rare or 4 minutes on each side for medium for 2 cm steaks; adjust slightly for more or less than this thickness. Remove the steaks from the pan and let cool for 15 minutes.

2 To make the dressing, put the mustard, yogurt and mayonnaise in a bowl and stir until combined.

3 Put the radishes, carrots, yellow capsicum, celery, spring onions, walnuts and raisins in a large bowl. Quarter and core the apples, then cut them into 2 cm cubes and toss in the lemon juice. Add to the bowl with half the dressing and turn to coat well. Season with salt and pepper.

4 To serve, pile the rocket on four plates and spoon the apple and vegetable salad alongside. Cut the steak into thin slices and arrange on top. Spoon the remaining dressing over the top.

NUTRITION PER SERVING 1214 kJ, 20 g protein, 11 g fat (2 g saturated fat), 27 g carbohydrate (25 g sugars), 6 g fibre, 405 mg sodium. GI: low

Spiced lamb with burghul

You may be familiar with burghul from the popular salad tabouleh. Here, it is cooked with spices, dried fruit and tender lamb cutlets to make a delicious Middle Eastern-style dish.

Preparation: 15 minutes • Cooking: 35 minutes • Serves 4

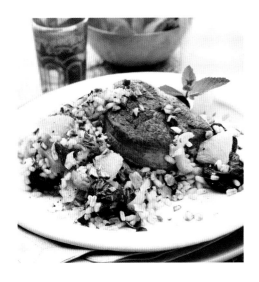

1 tbsp olive oil
4 lamb chops (about 400 g in total), trimmed of all excess fat
1 onion, chopped
2 tsp finely chopped fresh ginger
2 tsp cumin seeds
1 cup (180 g) coarse burghul
2 cups (500 ml) salt-reduced chicken or vegetable stock
juice of 1 orange
1 tsp honey

seeds from 6 green cardamom pods
1 cinnamon stick
½ cup (90 g) pitted prunes
⅓ cup (45 g) dried apricot halves, cut into slivers
2 tbsp chopped fresh mint
freshly ground black pepper
1 orange, segmented and segments halved
¼ cup (30 g) unsalted pistachio nuts, chopped
sprigs of fresh mint to garnish

1 Heat a large, deep, non-stick frying pan over a medium heat. Add the oil, and then the lamb cutlets and cook for 2 minutes on each side, or until nicely browned. Transfer to a plate.

2 Add the onion to the juices left in the pan (there shouldn't be any need to add any oil) and cook gently for 5 minutes, or until softened. Stir in the ginger and cumin seeds and cook gently for 1 minute.

3 Stir in the burghul, then add the stock, orange juice, honey, cardamom seeds and cinnamon stick. Bring to the boil. Reduce the heat and return the lamb to the pan, together with the prunes, apricots, mint and pepper to taste. Cover and simmer gently for 15–20 minutes or until the burghul is tender and all the liquid has been absorbed.

4 Stir in the orange segments and scatter the chopped pistachio nuts over the top. Serve garnished with sprigs of mint.

NUTRITION PER SERVING 2127 kJ, 31 g protein, 17 g fat (5 g saturated fat), 54 g carbohydrate (21 g sugars), 11 g fibre, 423 mg sodium. GI: low

Summer salmon and asparagus

Fresh young vegetables and succulent salmon make this an excellent speedy dish to prepare for special occasions, especially when asparagus is in season. Serve with boiled new potatoes for a memorable meal.

Preparation: 10 minutes • Cooking: 20 minutes • Serves 4

4 skinless salmon fillets (about 150 g each)
300 g baby leeks or chopped leeks
300 g tender asparagus spears
   (about 1½ bunches)
200 g sugar snap peas
⅓ cup (80 ml) dry white wine

200 ml salt-reduced fish or vegetable
   stock
1½ tbsp olive oil spread
salt and freshly ground black pepper
snipped fresh chives to garnish
600 g new potatoes

1 Run your fingertips over each salmon fillet to check for any stray bones, pulling out any that remain between the flakes of fish.

2 Arrange the leeks in a single layer in the bottom of a large shallow flameproof casserole dish with a tight-fitting lid. Lay the pieces of salmon on top. Surround the fish with the asparagus and sugar snap peas. Pour in the wine and stock, then dot the margarine over the fish. Season with salt and pepper.

3 Bring to the boil, then cover the casserole dish and reduce the heat so the liquid simmers gently. Cook the fish and vegetables for 12–14 minutes, or until the salmon is pale pink all the way through and the vegetables are tender.

4 Garnish with chives, then serve, accompanied with boiled new potatoes.

NUTRITION PER SERVING 1721 kJ, 38 g protein, 15 g fat (3 g saturated fat), 26 g carbohydrate (6 g sugars), 7 g fibre, 292 mg sodium. GI: medium

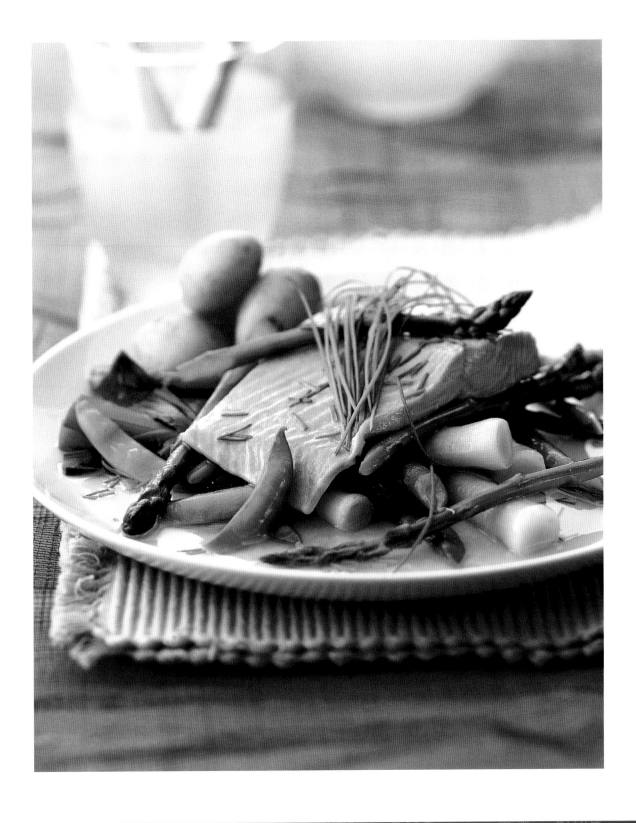

Marsala chicken with fennel

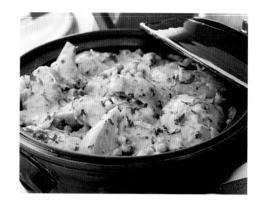

Cooking with a little wine – in this case the famous dessert wine from Sicily – gives great depth to a sauce: nearly all the alcohol and kilojoules burn away, leaving behind only flavour. This sauce is thickened with a mixture of egg and lemon juice, which is typically Mediterranean.

Preparation: 15 minutes ● Cooking: 45 minutes ● Serves 4

1 chicken (about 1.25 kg), jointed
6 tbsp plain flour
freshly ground black pepper
1 tbsp extra virgin olive oil
1 large leek, coarsely chopped
1 tbsp chopped fresh parsley
1 tsp fennel seeds
100 ml marsala

1½ cups (400 ml) salt-reduced chicken stock
2 fennel bulbs, trimmed and cut into chunks
2½ cups (400 g) shelled fresh or frozen peas
juice of 1 lemon
1 medium egg, lightly beaten
chopped fresh parsley to garnish
shreds of lemon zest to garnish

1 Remove the skin from the chicken joints, except for any small pieces, such as the wings. Season the flour with pepper and coat the joints.

2 Heat 2 tsp of the oil in a large frying pan and add the leek, parsley and fennel seeds. Cook over a medium heat until the leek is softened, stirring frequently. Remove from the pan with a slotted spoon and set aside.

3 Add the remaining oil to the pan and sauté the chicken for 6–7 minutes, or until golden. Remove the chicken from the pan and set aside. Pour in the marsala and let it bubble until it is reduced to about 2 tbsp of glaze. Pour in the stock, and return the leek mixture and dark meat chicken joints and wings to the pan (wait to add the breasts as they can overcook). Add the fennel

seeds. Cover and simmer over a low heat for about 10–15 minutes, then add the breasts and continue to cook, covered, for 15 minutes, or until all the chicken joints are tender. Add the peas for the last 5 minutes of cooking.

4 Using a slotted spoon, remove the chicken pieces and vegetables to a platter or serving bowl. Keep warm.

5 In a bowl, mix the lemon juice into the egg. Slowly add about ⅓ cup (80 ml) of the hot cooking liquid to the lemon and egg mixture, stirring well. Slowly stir this mixture back into the liquid in the pan. Return the chicken and vegetables to the pan and gently warm over a very low heat so the sauce doesn't curdle. Season to taste. Serve garnished with parsley and lemon zest.

NUTRITION PER SERVING 2107 kJ, 45 g protein, 21 g fat (6 g saturated fat), 26 g carbohydrate (10 g sugars), 8 g fibre, 444 mg sodium. GI: low

Roast vegetable and bean stew

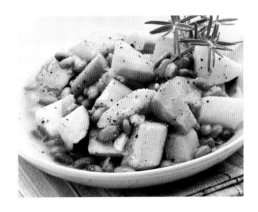

This easy, one-pot dish of root vegetables and red kidney beans makes a nourishing winter main course and it needs no accompaniments. It's particularly enjoyable with a glass of dry cider or apple juice.

Preparation: 20 minutes, plus overnight soaking
• Cooking: 3 hours • Serves 4

¾ cup (150 g) dried red kidney beans or pinto, soaked overnight in cold water
500 g pumpkin
300 g new potatoes, scrubbed and cut into 4 cm cubes
150 g carrots, cut into 4 cm cubes
150 g parsnips, cut into 4 cm cubes
2 large zucchini, cut into 4 cm cubes

2 tbsp extra virgin olive oil
1 garlic clove, finely chopped
salt and freshly ground black pepper
4 large sprigs of fresh rosemary, plus extra sprigs to garnish
1 cup (250 ml) dry alcoholic cider
1 cup (250 ml) salt-reduced hot vegetable stock

1 Drain and rinse the beans, then place them in a large saucepan and cover with plenty of cold water. Bring to the boil and simmer for about 2 hours, or until tender. Drain well.

2 Preheat the oven to 200°C. Remove the seeds and fibres from the pumpkin, then cut off the hard skin and cut the flesh into 4 cm cubes.

3 Put the pumpkin in a bowl and add the potatoes, carrots, parsnips and zucchini. Drizzle over the oil and toss to coat the vegetables evenly. Stir in the garlic and season with salt and pepper.

4 Lay the rosemary sprigs on the bottom of a large roasting tin and spread the vegetables on top in a single layer. Roast for about 30 minutes, turning once, until lightly browned.

5 Remove from the oven and stir in the drained beans, cider and stock. Cover the tin tightly with foil, then return to the oven and cook for a further 20–25 minutes, or until the vegetables are tender. Before serving, remove the rosemary stalks and garnish with fresh rosemary sprigs.

NUTRITION PER SERVING 1539 kJ, 15 g protein, 11 g fat (2 g saturated fat), 43 g carbohydrate (15 g sugars), 15 g fibre, 448 mg sodium. GI: low

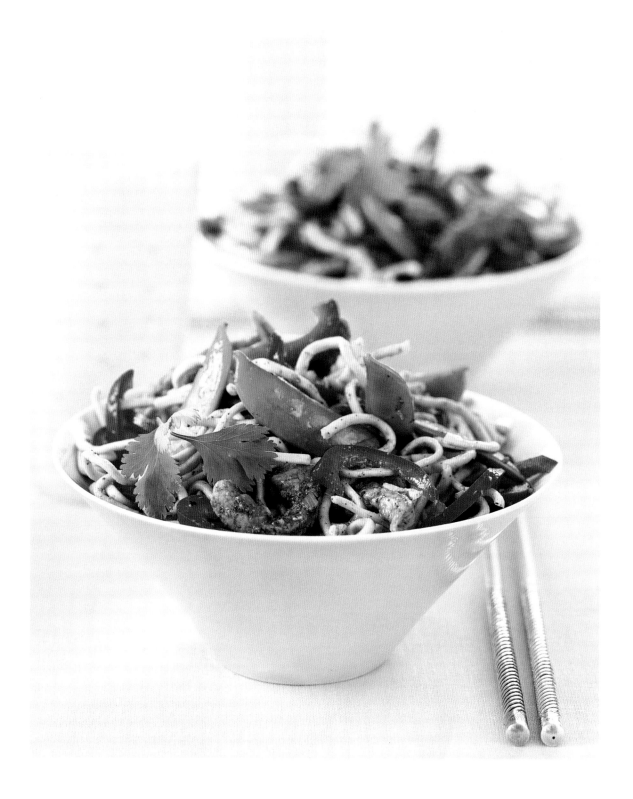

Five-spice pork

The simple Asian technique of stir-frying is perfect for preparing meals in a hurry. It is also a great healthy cooking method because it uses just a small amount of oil and cooks vegetables quickly so that most of their beneficial vitamins and minerals are preserved.

Preparation: 15 minutes • Cooking: 15 minutes • Serves 4

2 small pork fillets (about 200 g each), trimmed of all excess fat
250 g medium Chinese egg noodles
1 tbsp canola oil
1 large onion, finely chopped
1 large garlic clove, crushed
1 tbsp five-spice powder
500 g snow peas or sugar snap peas

2 medium red capsicums (or 1 red and 1 yellow or orange), deseeded and thinly sliced
½ cup (125 ml) salt-reduced hot vegetable stock
¼ tsp salt and pepper
fresh coriander leaves, to garnish

1 Cut each of the pork fillets across into 5 mm slices, then cut each slice into 5 mm strips. Cover and set aside.

2 Cook the noodles in a saucepan of boiling water for 4 minutes, or cook or soak them according to the packet instructions. Drain well and set aside.

3 While the noodles are cooking, heat a wok or a large heavy-based frying pan until hot. Add the oil and swirl to coat the wok, then add the onion and garlic and stir-fry for 1 minute. Add the five-spice powder and stir-fry for another minute.

4 Add the pork strips to the wok and stir-fry for 3 minutes. Add the snow peas or sugar snap peas and the capsicums and stir-fry for a further 2 minutes. Pour in the stock, stir well and bring to the boil.

5 Add the noodles to the wok and stir and toss for 2–3 minutes or until all the ingredients are well combined. Season to taste and serve immediately, sprinkled with coriander leaves.

NUTRITION PER SERVING 1821 kJ, 35 g protein, 8 g fat (1 g saturated fat), 54 g carbohydrate (6 g sugars), 5 g fibre, 345 mg sodium. GI: low

Desserts

Rhubarb and saffron crème brûlée

A tart compote of rhubarb makes a pleasing contrast to the rich custard here. This special-occasion treat is lightened by the fruit and its use of less egg yolk and cream (which is reduced-fat to boot), yet it still retains its rich indulgent nature.

Preparation: 25 minutes • Cooking: 40 minutes, plus cooling and at least 1 hour chilling • Makes 6

250 g rhubarb, chopped
juice of ½ orange
⅓ cup (75 g) caster sugar, or to taste
1 cup (250 ml) low-fat milk
2 pinches of saffron threads

3 medium egg yolks
1 whole medium egg
¼ cup (55 ml) light thickened cream
¼ cup (50 g) demerara sugar

1 Preheat the oven to 160°C. Put the rhubarb in a heavy-based saucepan with the orange juice and ¼ cup (55 g) of the caster sugar. Poach over a medium–low heat for 5–7 minutes, or until the fruit is tender and juicy, but still keeps its shape. Leave to cool.

2 To make the custard, heat the milk with the remaining caster sugar and the saffron in a heavy-based saucepan until bubbles appear around the edge. In a bowl, beat together the egg yolks, whole egg and thickened cream. Slowly add the hot sweetened saffron milk to the egg mixture, stirring to mix well.

3 Divide the rhubarb compote among six 150 ml ramekins. To ladle the custard mixture over the fruit, place the base of the ladle on top of the fruit and turn it slowly to gently ease in

the custard (if you pour the custard into the ramekins, it will mix with the rhubarb and will not form two separate layers).

4 Place the ramekins in a large roasting tin. Pour boiling water into the tin to come about two-thirds of the way up the sides of the ramekins. Bake for 25 minutes, or until set. Remove from the oven and leave to cool. Refrigerate for at least 1 hour or until quite cold.

5 Preheat the grill to high. Sprinkle 2 tsp of demerara sugar on top of each custard and smooth it with your finger to form an even layer. Grill close to the heat until the sugar melts and bubbles, keeping a close watch on it so that it doesn't burn. Remove from the heat and allow to cool for a few minutes, or until the sugar has hardened to a crust. Serve.

NUTRITION PER SERVING 706 kJ, 5 g protein, 5 g fat (2 g saturated fat), 24 g carbohydrate (24 g sugars), 1 g fibre, 52 mg sodium. GI: medium

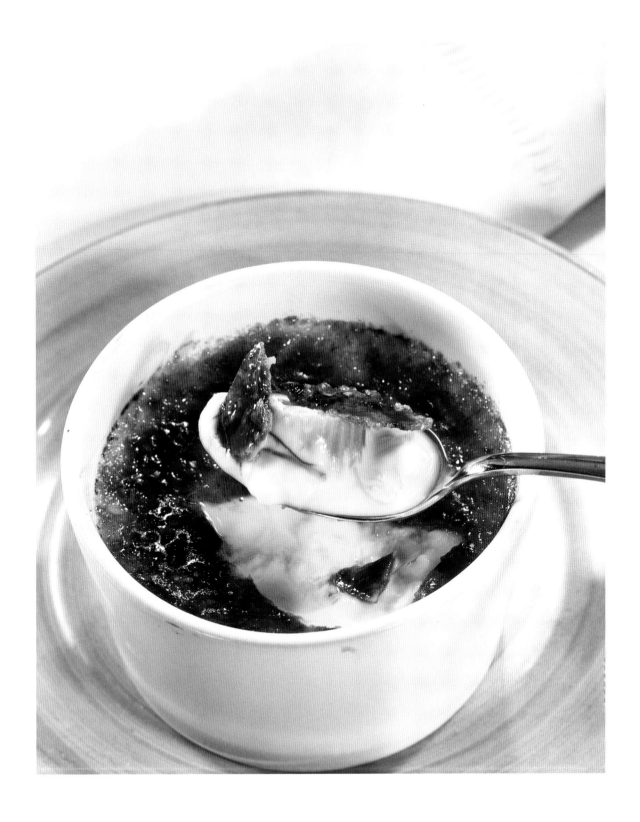

Mango mousse

Nothing signals summer's arrival more than the presence of juicy mangoes in the greengrocers. Prepare this light mango mousse to enjoy their vitamin-rich bounty.

Preparation: 20 minutes, plus at least 2 hours chilling
• **Serves 6**

3 mangoes (about 1 kg in total), peeled and sliced
¼ cup (60 ml) lime juice
½ tsp ground ginger
3 tsp powdered gelatine

1 cup (250 ml) water
2 tbsp sugar
½ cup (125 g) light sour cream

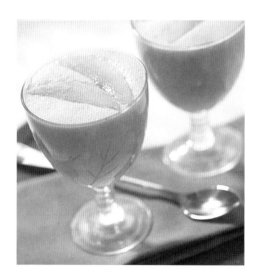

1 Reserve 12 small mango slices. Purée the remaining mango slices with the lime juice and ginger in a food processor.

2 Sprinkle the gelatine over ½ cup (125 ml) of the water in a small bowl. Let stand for 5 minutes, or until softened. Meanwhile, combine the sugar and remaining water in a small saucepan and bring to the boil. Stir the gelatine into the hot sugar mixture and cook, stirring, for 1 minute, or until the gelatine is dissolved.

3 Add the gelatine mixture to the mango purée and process until well combined. Add the sour cream and process briefly just to blend.

4 Spoon into dessert bowls or glasses, top with the reserved mango slices, cover and refrigerate for 2 hours, or until chilled and set.

NUTRITION PER SERVING 707 kJ, 4 g protein, 4 g fat (3 g saturated fat), 28 g carbohydrate (27 g sugars), 3 g fibre, 17 mg sodium. GI: medium

Baked almond-stuffed peaches

Baking fruit brings out its flavour wonderfully, and a stuffing is a simple way of making baked fruit special. Here peaches are filled with a mixture of dried apricots, almonds and amaretti biscuits. Many other fruits – nectarines, apples, pears or quinces – can be prepared in the same way.

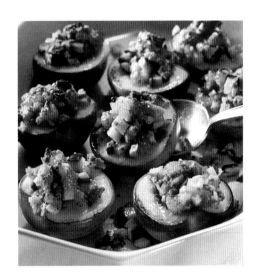

Preparation: 20 minutes • Cooking: 40 minutes • Serves 8

5 large ripe but firm peaches
10 dried apricot halves,
   finely chopped
6 amaretti biscuits,
   crumbled

2 tsp almond essence
1 tbsp brandy
1 eggwhite
⅓ cup (50 g) blanched
   almonds

1 Preheat the oven to 180°C. Cut the peaches in half and remove the stones. Arrange 8 of the halves, cut-side up, in a shallow baking dish. Set aside. Finely chop the remaining peach halves.

2 Combine the chopped peaches with the dried apricots, crumbled amaretti, almond essence, brandy and eggwhite. Stir until thoroughly combined.

3 Heat a small heavy-based frying pan and dry-fry the almonds, turning and tossing every so often, until they are lightly browned in spots. Remove and chop, in a food processor or by hand, to make a mixture of small chunks of nuts and ground nuts.

4 Add the chopped almonds to the fruit and amaretti mixture and mix well. Use the mixture to fill the hollows in the peach halves, heaping up the filling and pressing it gently together. Cover the baking dish with a tent of cooking foil.

5 Bake for 25–30 minutes, then remove the foil. Increase the oven temperature to 200°C and bake for a further 5 minutes, or until the nutty topping is lightly browned. The peaches are best served warm, but they can be chilled before serving, if you prefer.

NUTRITION PER SERVING 571 kJ, 4 g protein, 5 g fat (0.5 g saturated fat), 18 g carbohydrate (15 g sugars), 3 g fibre, 11 mg sodium. GI: low

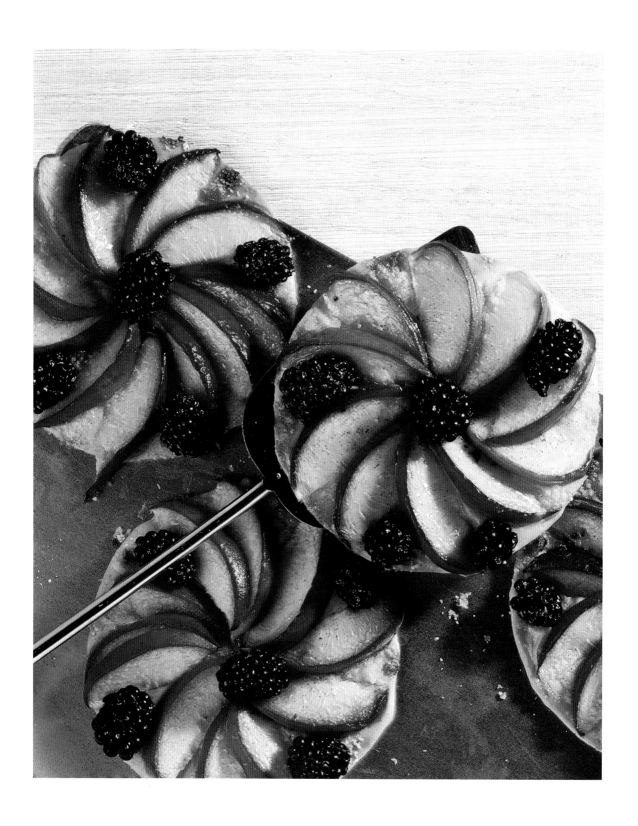

Peach and blackberry filo pizzas

These simple, attractive tarts have a crisp filo pastry base and a luscious fresh fruit topping. Filo pastry is made with very little fat, so is healthier than other types of pastry.

Preparation: 15 minutes • **Cooking: 15 minutes** • **Makes 4**

5 sheets filo pastry (about
   45 x 30 cm each), thawed if frozen
1 tbsp olive oil spread, melted
2 tsp ground almonds or hazelnuts

4 peaches
¾ cup (150 g) blackberries
1 tbsp vanilla sugar

1 Preheat the oven to 200°C. Place a sheet of filo on the work surface and brush very lightly all over with melted margarine. Top with another sheet and brush with margarine. Layer on the rest of the filo sheets, brushing with margarine each time and, finally, brush the top surface. Using a saucer measuring about 13 cm as a guide, cut out four discs from the layered filo. Transfer to a baking tray.

2 Sprinkle each disc with ½ tsp of the ground nuts, then set aside.

3 Cut the peaches in half, twist apart and remove the stones. Slice the peaches thinly. Place the slices on the filo pastry discs, fanning them out from the centre so they leave a little of the pastry edge uncovered all around. Divide the blackberries among the pizzas, then sprinkle each one with 1 tsp of the sugar.

4 Bake for 15 minutes, or until the pastry is golden brown and the peaches are very tender and lightly caramelised. Transfer to individual plates and serve within a few minutes or the pastry will become soft.

NUTRITION PER SERVING 746 kJ, 4 g protein, 4 g fat (1 g saturated fat), 30 g carbohydrate (21 g sugars), 6 g fibre, 146 mg sodium. GI: high

Resources directory

Diabetes

State and Territory Diabetes Organisations (Australia)
Contact your local state or
  territory office:
  Tel: 1300 136 588
ACT: www.diabetes-act.com.au
NSW: www.australiandiabetes
  council.com
NT: www.healthylivingnt.org.au
QLD: www.diabetesqueensland.
  org.au
SA: www.diabetessa.com.au
TAS: www.diabetestas.org.au
VIC: www.diabetesvic.org.au
WA: www.diabeteswa.com.au

Australian Diabetes Educators Association (ADEA)
Tel: (02) 6287 4822
www.adea.com.au

Diabetes New Zealand
Contact your area office, or the
  national office:
  Tel: 0800 369 636
www.diabetes.org.nz

Diabetes South Africa
Tel: (086) 111 3913
email: national@diabetessa.org.za
www.diabetessa.co.za

Diabetes Youth New Zealand
email: contact@diabetesyouth.
  org.nz
www.diabetesyouth.org.nz

Diabetic Society of Singapore
Tel: (65) 6842 6019
www.diabetes.org.sg

National Diabetes Institute (Malaysia)
Tel: (03) 7876 1676
www.diabetesmalaysia.com.my

Edgar National Centre for Diabetes and Obesity Research (New Zealand)
Tel: (03) 474 7775
www.otago.ac.nz/diabetes

Juvenile Diabetes Research Foundation (Australia)
Tel: (02) 9966 0400
www.jdrf.org.au

Medic Alert Foundation (Australia)
Tel: 1800 882 222
www.medicalert.com.au

Medic Alert Foundation (New Zealand)
Tel: 0800 840 111
www.medicalert.co.nz

National Diabetes Services Scheme (NDSS) (Australia)
Tel: 1300 136 588
www.ndss.com.au

New Zealand Society for the Study of Diabetes (NZSSD)
Tel: (03) 474 0999 extn 8510
www.nzssd.org.nz

Eyes

Glaucoma Australia
Tel: 1800 500 880; (02) 9906 6640
www.glaucoma.org.au

Optometrists Association Australia
Tel: (03) 9668 8500
www.optometrists.asn.au

Royal Australian and New Zealand College of Ophthalmologists
Tel: (02) 9690 1001
www.ranzco.edu

Royal New Zealand Foundation for the Blind
Tel: 0800 243 333; (09) 355 6900
www.rnzfb.org.nz

Vision Australia
Tel: 1300 847 466
www.visionaustralia.org.au

Feet

Australasian Podiatry Council
Tel: (03) 9416 3111
www.apodc.com.au

Podiatry New Zealand
Tel: 0800 769 393
www.podiatry.org.nz

Food and nutrition

Dietitians Association of Australia
Tel: 1800 812 942; (02) 6163 5200
www.daa.asn.au

Dietitians NZ
Tel: (04) 477 4701
www.dietitians.org.nz

Food Standards Australia and New Zealand (FSANZ)
Australia
Tel: (02) 6271 2222
www.foodstandards.gov.au
New Zealand
Tel: (04) 978 5630
www.foodstandards.govt.nz

Glycemic Index Foundation (Australia)
Tel: (02) 9020 6100
www.gisymbol.com

New Zealand Nutrition Foundation
Tel: (09) 489 3417
www.nutritionfoundation.org.nz

Nutrition Australia
Check the website for details of
    the office in your area.
www.nutritionaustralia.org

Heart

Heart Foundation (Australia)
Tel: 1300 362 787
www.heartfoundation.com.au

National Heart Foundation (New Zealand)
Tel: (09) 571 9191
www.nhf.org.nz

Indigenous health

Aboriginal Medical Service
Contact your local Aboriginal
    Medical Service or the
    Aboriginal Health team in
    your area.

Australian Indigenous HealthInfoNet
www.healthinfonet.ecu.edu.au

Mental health

Beyond Blue (Australia)
Tel: (03) 9810 6100
www.beyondblue.org.au

Diabetes Counselling Online
Tel: (08) 8365 4424
www.diabetescounselling.com.au

Lifeline (Australia)
Tel: 131 114
www.lifeline.org.au

Lifeline (New Zealand)
Tel: 0800 543 354
www.lifeline.co.nz

Physical activity

A Healthy and Active Australia (Department of Health and Ageing)
www.healthyactive.gov.au

Diabetes Exercise and Sport Association of New Zealand
www.desa.org.nz

Exercise and Sports Science Australia (ESSA)
Tel: 07 3862 4122
www.essa.org.au

Smoking

Quitline 137 848 (Australia), or
0800 778 778 (New Zealand)

Quit Now (Australia)
www.quitnow.gov.au

The Quit Group (New Zealand)
www.quit.org.nz

Other contacts

Amputees Federation of New Zealand
Tel: (03) 455 6347
www.amputee.co.nz

Health Navigator New Zealand
www.healthnavigator.org.nz

Kidney Health Australia
Tel: (03) 9674 4300
www.kidney.org.au

Kidney Health New Zealand
Tel: 0800 KIDNEY (0800 543 639)
www.kidneys.co.nz

National Amputee Associations and Support Groups (Australia)
Tel: 1800 810 969
www.amputeesnsw.org.au

National Stroke Foundation (Australia)
Tel: 1800 STROKE (787 653)
www.strokefoundation.com.au

Stroke Foundation of New Zealand
Tel: 0800 STROKE (787 653)
www.stroke.org.nz

Index

Page numbers in **bold** print refer to
main entries

A

abdominal fat, 42, **44**, 110, 111, 112, 217, 239
abdominal squeeze (exercise), **127, 129**
Aboriginal Medical Service, **275**
Aboriginal people, 16, 41, 44
acarbose, **149–50**
acceptance, 214, 215, 219
Accredited Exercise Physiologists, 26
Accredited Practising Dietitians, 85
Acesulphame K, 104
acetaminophen, 151
acetyl-L-carnitine, 201
acinar cells, 35
acinus, 35
activity plans, **116–18**
Actrapid, 154
acupuncture, **206**
adolescents, **15**
adrenaline, 33
adult-onset diabetes *see* type 2 diabetes
Advil, 179
aerobic activity, 22, **112–13**, 118, 141
age at onset, **36, 37**, 41, 42
age risk factor, 16
AGEs, 242
A Healthy and Active Australia, 275
air pollution, 40
airport security, **227–8**
ALADIN, 200
albumin, 77, 80, 177, 178
alcohol, 21, 22, 89, 186
    blood glucose &, 60, **74**, 101
    depression &, 214
    drawbacks of, 100, **101–2**
    driving &, 227
    medications &, 101, 145, 148, 150
    men &, 101
    premenstrual syndrome &, 222
    standard drinks of, **101**
    women &, 101
aldose reductase inhibitors, 241
Aleve, 179
Alitame, 104
allergic reactions, 148, 151, 154–5
almond-stuffed peaches, Baked (recipe),
    271
almonds, 92, 97
aloe vera, **198**

alpha-blockers, 151
alpha-glucosidase inhibitors, **149–50**
alpha-lipoic acid, 185, **199–200**
alprostadil, 223
alternative medicine *see* complementary
    therapies
alternative therapists, 192, 193
Alzheimer's disease, 112
ambiguity, **221**
American ginseng, 198
amino acids, 31, 196, 201, 202, 242
amputation, 173, 186
Amputees Federation of New Zealand,
    275
amylin, 236
aneurysms, 172, **174**
anger, 211, **214–15**
angina, 170, 196, 203
angiotensin-converting enzyme inhibitors,
    151, 171, **174–5**, 178, **240–1**
angiotensin II receptor blockers, 174
animal fats, 173, 175, 179
animal insulin, 154–5
animal tests, 194, 196, 197, 198, 200, 201,
    238, 239, 241, 243
Animas Vibe insulin pumps, 234
ankle swelling, 19
antho-cyanosides, 201
antibiotics, 148, 179
anticonvulsants, 185
antidepressants, 151, 213
antihistamines, 213
anti-oxidants, 171, **176**, 185, 197, 199, 201,
    202
antipsychotics, 151
anxiety, 184, 211, 212, **215–16**, 223
Apidra, 75, 154, 155
appetiser/ snack recipes, **252–5**
appetite increase, 17
appetite loss, 148, 184
appetite suppression, 239
apples, 91, 98
apricots, 97, 98
arm nerve damage, 184
arthritis, 38, 112, 114
artificial pancreas, **244**
artificial sweeteners *see* non-nutritive
    sweeteners
Asian diet, 94
Asian ginseng, 198
asparagus, 91
Aspartame, 90, 104

aspirin, 151, 171, **173–4**, 182, 185, 193,
    202
Assessing Fitness to Drive, 225, 226
atherosclerosis, **170, 172**
attitude, 26, **106**, 220–1
Australasian Podiatry Council, **274**
Australian Diabetes Educators Association,
    24, 274
Australian Diabetes Obesity and Life
    Study, 44
Australian Driving Guidelines, **225–6**
Australian Indigenous HealthInfoNet, 275
Australian Islet Transplantation Program,
    243
Australian Register of Therapeutic Goods
    Association, 203
autoimmune diseases, 13, 38, 39, 238
autoimmune responses, 38, 238
autonomic neuropathy, **183–4**
Avandamet, 153
avocados, 84, 92, 96, 175, 176, 185

B

B cells, 60, 238
baby lift (exercise), **124**
back pain, 118
balance, 185
balance and mobility exercises, **125–33**
balsam pear *see* bitter melon
bananas, 97, 98, 99, 101, 185
Banting, Frederick, 38
bariatric surgery, 163, 164
barley, 91, 92
basal-bolus regime, 156
basal insulin, 153, 156, 157, 160
batteries, 69, 71
B cells, 60, 238
BCMA, 238
BD safe clip, 160
beans, 91, **92**, 265
bed-wetting, 165
beef, 103, 201, 203
Beef waldorf (recipe), **260**
beer, 101
Bell's palsy, 183
bent-arm row (exercise), **121**
Best, Charles, 38
beta-blockers, 151
beta cells, 35, 36, 37, 38, 39, 40, 147, 153,
    236, 237, 242–3
Beyond Blue, 275

biceps curl (exercise), **133**
bicycling, 22, 113
bilberries/ blueberries, **198**, **201**, 251
binge eating, 88
biofeedback, **205**
biological skin substitutes, **242**
birth defects, 222
biscuits, 100, 105
bitter melon, **197**
black beans, 91
blackberries, 201, 273
bladder function, 184
blindness, 25, 34, 179, 240
bloating, 148, 150, 152, 184
blood clots, 170, 171, 173, 175, 176, 182, 202, 229
blood filtering, 176–7
blood glucose
  advances &, 232, **233–4**, 235–6
  alcohol &, 60, **74**, 101
  aloe vera &, 198
  alternative sweeteners &, 104
  artificial pancreas &, 244
  attitude &, 220
  bilberries &, 198, 201
  biofeedback &, 205
  bitter melon &, 197
  carbohydrates &, 89, **90**, 95
  children &, 60
  chromium &, 204
  cinnamon &, 197
  circulation problems &, 169, 170, 171
  complementary therapies &, **195–9**, 204, 205
  complications &, 11, 32, 59, 60, **169–70**, 171, 175, 176, 178, 179, 180, 183, 184, 189, 240, 241
  control of, 19, **58–81**
  coriander &, 199
  dental disease &, 189
  diabetes burnout &, 218
  diabetes symptoms &, **34**, 36
  driving &, 63, **225–6**, **227**
  emergencies &, **52–3**
  emotions &, 212, 216, 218
  energy source, 31, 32
  excess of, **32**
  exercise &, 58, 61, **74–5**, **76**, 86, 110, 111, 112, 113, **114**, **115**, 116, 119, 144, 145, 146, 212
  eye problems &, 11, 19, 32, 34, 59, 169, **179–80**, 181, 240, 241
  fats &, 92
  fenugreek &, 196
  fibre &, 92
  finding the balance &, **13–14**
  five steps to success, **63**

food &, 13, 31, 55, 58, 61–2, **72–4**, 75, 84, **85–6**, 89, 90, 92, 94, 144, 145, 146, 175, 222
gestational diabetes &, 45
ginseng &, 198
goals, **60–3**, 85
gymnema &, 196
hormones &, **33**
illness &, 32, 60, 63, 74, **75–6**, 212, **224**
importance of, **31–2**
insulin &, 20, **33–4**, 58, 150, 153, **156**, **157**, 160, 212, 232, **235–6**
keeping tabs on, 20
kidney disease &, 176, **178**
lifestyle &, 11
management of, 11, 13, 14, **19–22**
meal times &, **61–2**, 79
medications &, 11, **144–57**
medications that may interact with, 144, 145, 146
monitoring and screening, **47–51**, 58–81, **224**, 233–4
mornings &, **76**
muscles &, 110, 111
myths about, 54
nerve damage &, 11, 19, 32, 59, 169, 171, 183, 184, 226
numbers to know, **79**
over-the-counter remedies &, 225
pancreas transplants &, 162
pre-diabetes &, 18, 169
pregnancy &, 62, **222**
prickly pear &, 199
protein &, 95
Pterocarpus marsupium &, 199
quality of life &, 210
record keeping &, 65, 68, **70**, 115
self-monitoring of, 58, **59–62**, 63, **64–76**, 77–8, 86
sex &, **221–2**
stress &, 63, 74, 75, 216
swings and spikes in, 11, **14**, **16**, 20, 33, **37**, 41, 58, 60, **72–5**, 77, 86, 153, 212, 221–2, 224, 226, 236
testing, 11, **13**, 14, **17**, 18, 22, **47–51**, **58–81**, **85–6**, 114, 115, 145
travel &, 227, 228
type 1 diabetes &, **37**, 169, 196, 222, 224
type 2 diabetes &, 17, **18**, 40, **41**, **145–6**, 169, 196, 197, 198, 199
uncontrolled diabetes &, **32**
water intake &, 76
weight loss &, 87
weight-loss surgery &, 163
what it is, **19**
see also glycaemic index
blood glucose, fasting, 18, 145, 197, 198

blood glucose meter calibration, 67, **70**
blood glucose meter cost, 69
blood glucose meters, 13, 19, 20, 50, 58, 64, 65, **66**, **67–9**, 70, **71**, **72**, 226
blood glucose tests, 11, **13**, 14, 15, **17**, 18, 19, **20**, 22, 145
blood pressure
  alcohol &, 101
  brain aneurysms &, 172
  cardiovascular risk &, 11, 42, 44, 87, 157
  complementary therapies &, 202, 205
  complications &, 11, 42, 44, 40, 157, **172**, **178**, 182
  deep breathing &, 219
  depression &, 212
  diet &, **22**, 97, 171
  exercise &, 112, **115**, 118, 171, 172
  high, 11, 19, 21, **22**, 42, 44, 80, 86, 97, 101, 112, 118, 171, **172**, 173, 174, **178**, 182, 202, 219
  low, **115**, 183
  management of, 14
  monitoring of, **80**
  overweight &, 21, 22
  salt intake &, 97
  target levels for, 80, 172
  type 2 diabetes &, 172
blood pressure medications, 151, **174**, **178**, 213, 223
blood thinners, 196, 197, 198, 202
blood vessels, 170, **171**, **172**, 173, 176, 178, 179, 180, 186, 202, 216, 240, 241
blueberries/ bilberries, 198, 201, 251
blurred vision, 17, 20, **34**, 174, 180, 181, 225
body clock, 76
body fat *see* fat (body)
body mass, 238
body mass index (BMI), 43
body temperature regulation, 184
borderline diabetes *see* pre-diabetes
Bowman's capsule, 177
boxing, 113
brain
  blood glucose &, 31, 34, 183
  obesity &, **239–40**
brain aneurysms, 172, **174**
brain chemicals, 213, 239
bran cereal, 91
bran muffins, 103
Brazil nuts, 97
bread, 73, 90, 98, 99, **100**, 105
breakfast, 76, 88
breakfast recipes, **248–51**
breastfeeding, 39, 104, 149, 150, 151, 196, 197, 204, 237
breathing problems, 36, 78, 113, 114
broccoli, 91, 97

buoyancy belts, 141
burnout, 218–21
butter, 94, 103
buttock toner (exercise), **128**
Byetta, 150–1

C

C75, 239
caffeine, 222
calcium, 97
calcium channel blockers, 151
calf-raise (exercise), **126**
cancer, 162, 197
canola oil, 92, 93
capillary action tests strips, 64, 66, 72
capsaicin, 185
capsicums, 97
car exercises, **129**
car travel, 228, 229
    see also driving
carbohydrates
    alcohol and mixers &, 101–2
    counting, **90–1**
    energy &, 31, 89–90
    food exchanges &, 99–100
    food labels &, 105
    gestational diabetes &, 45
    GI &, 98, 173
    healthy eating plan &, **89–90**, 91, **95–6**,
        173
    hypoglycaemia &, 53, **73**, 114, 145, 227
    insulin finetuning &, 75, 156, 160
    low-carbohydrate controversy, 95–6
    medications &, 149, 150, 152, 156, 160
    myths about, **88**
    oral glucose tolerance test (OGTT) &, 49
    pancreas &, 35, 45
    physical activity &, 86, 114
    travel &, 227
    type 1 diabetes &, 13, 21, 90, 156
cardiovascular emergencies, 174
cardiovascular problem prevention, **172–6**
cardiovascular problems, 11, 19, 21, 22, 59,
    79, 87, 92, 94, 101, 183, 202, 241, 242
cardiovascular risk, **170**
carpal tunnel syndrome, 183
Carrot, apricot and pecan muffins (recipe),
    248
carrots, 91, 98, 100
casual plasma glucose tests see random
    plasma glucose tests
cat pose (exercise), **140**
Caucasian people, 16, 36, 38, 41
Caverject, 223
central nervous system, 183
cereals, 76, 99, **100**

cerebrovascular disease, 170
Charcot's foot, 186
check-ups, **78**
cheese, 94, 99, 100
Cheese and onion rarebit (recipe), **249**
chewing gum, 189
chicken, 93, 100, 103, 185
chicken recipes, **256**, **264**
children
    artificial pancreases &, 244
    blood glucose targets for, 60
    blood glucose tests &, 15
    cow's milk &, **39**
    future &, 234, 236, 244
    insulin &, 15, 46
    obesity in, **46**
    pre-teen and adolescent, **15**
    primary school, **15**
    toddler and pre-schooler, **15**
    type 1 diabetes &, **15**, 16, 36, 37, **39**, 161,
        236, 237
    type 2 diabetes &, 10, 15, 16, 36, 41, **46**
Chinese medicine, 197, 199, 206
Chinese people, 16, 41
chocolate, 98, 104
cholesterol, 87, 92, 94, 101, 157, 170, 171,
    173, 175, 176, 198, 201–2 see also high
    cholesterol
cholesterol/ triglyceride blood tests, 16, 17,
    22, **78–9**
chromium, **204**
Cialis, 223
cibenzoline, 151
cinnamon, **197**
circulation problems, 169, **170**, 171, **172**, **173**
Citrus and spinach salad (recipe), **258**
claudication, 170
clinical depression, 213
coeliac disease, 13, 38
colds and flu, 36
colour perception, 181
combined training, **113**
commitment, **54–5**, **118**
complementary therapies
    acupuncture, **206**
    biofeedback, **205**
    blood glucose control &, **195–9**, 204, 205
    definition of, **193–4**
    diabetes complications &, **201–4**
    eye problems &, **201**, 204
    heart and kidneys &, 196, **201–4**
    history of, 192, 194, 197
    judging, **193–4**
    magnets &, **206–7**
    medications interacting with, 193, 196,
        197, 198, 202
    mind–body approach &, **204–7**

neuropathy &, **199–200**, 201, 206, 207
placebo affect &, 194, 195, 200, 204
quality control &, 203
regulation of, 203
research on, **194–5**, **196**, 200
safety risks &, 193, 195, 197, 198
types of, **195–204**
see also pregnancy
complications of diabetes
    anti-oxidants &, **176**
    blood glucose &, 11, 32, 59, 60, **169–70**,
        171, 175, 176, 178, 179, 180, 183, 184,
        189, 240, 241
    complementary therapies &, **201–4**
    driving &, 53, 225, 226
    exercise &, 116
    food &, 84, **175–6**
    non-diagnosis &, 16
    pre-diabetes &, 169
    pregnancy &, 222
    prevention of, **167–89**
    research and advances, 234, 237, **240–2**
    type 1 diabetes &, **169**, 178, 181
    type 2 diabetes &, 168, **169**, 172, 178, 181
    types of, 168, 169, **170**, **172–6**
    weight-loss medications &, **172**
    see also blood vessels; cardiovascular
        problems; eye problems; kidney
        disease; nerve damage
concentration, 110
confectionary, 90
    see also jelly beans
confusion, 14
constipation, 36, 184, 185
contacts directory, **274–5**
continuous glucose monitors, 72, **233–4**,
    244
core body exercises, **123–4**
coriander, **199**
corn, 90, 98, 99, 100
corn chips, 93
cornflakes, 98
coronary artery disease, 42
corticosteroids, 151, 162
cortisol, 33, 216
cost
    blood glucose meters, **69**
    CGMS, 233
    test strip, 69–70
counsellors/ counselling, 13, 214
counterregulatory hormones, 33
cow's milk, **39**, 237
    see also milk
coxsackievirus, 39
crab filo parcels, Gingered (recipe), **254**
cramps, 183, 184
cranberry juice, 179

cream cheese, 103
creatinine, 178
Credentialled Diabetes Educator, 24
cryotherapy, 182
cultural groups
   type 1 diabetes &, 36, 38
   type 2 diabetes &, **16**, 41, 44, 50
cycling, 22, 113
cyclosporine, 162
cytokines, 238

D

dairy products, 84, 94, 95, 97, 100, 103, 185,
   201, 203
DAISY study, 237
damage control, **19**
dancing, 113
deep breathing, **219**
dehydration, 76, 224, 225
dementia, 112
denial, 214, **220**
dentists and dental care, 16, **25**, **189**
depression, 12, 112, 211, **212–14**, 223
desk exercises, **129–31**
dessert recipes, **268–73**
desserts, 88, 90
Determir, 232
Dexcom G4® Platinum, 234
'diabesity' dangers, **44**
diabetes at a glance, **37**
diabetes burnout, **218–21**
diabetes by numbers, **49**
Diabetes Control and Complications Trial,
   59, 169, 179
Diabetes Counselling Online, 220, 275
diabetes defined, **30**, 31
diabetes educators, 13, 14, 19, 20, **23–4**, 27
diabetes epidemic, 10–11
Diabetes Exercise and Sport Association
   of New Zealand, 275
Diabetes New Zealand, 24, 160, 192, 274
diabetes organisations and associations,
   24, 67, 192, 220, **274**
Diabetes Prevention Program, 51–2, 87, 148
Diabetes Prevention Trial, 236
Diabetes Services Scheme, 27
diabetes specialists, 14, **23**, 226
diabetes support groups, 12, 220, **274–5**
diabetes tablets, 73, 75, 144, 146, **147–50**
diabetes team, 13, 17, 19, 20, **26**, 27, 60, 71
Diabetes Youth New Zealand, 24, 274
diabetic ketoacidosis, **52**, 77, 160, 224, 225
diabetic retinopathy, 16, 162, **180–1**, 182,
   201, 237, 241, 242
diagnosis
   dealing with, **12–13**

depression after, **213**
diabetes, **12–14**, 216
emotions and feelings &, **12**, 13, 26,
   211–12
type 1 diabetes, **13–14**, **16**
what you can expect, **13**
dialysis, 176, 178
diaries and journals, 70, **85**, 217
diarrhoea, 36, 148, 150, 151, 152, 184, 185
diastolic pressure, 80
diet
   deconstructing your, **21**
   exercise &, 111
   heart health &, **175**
   low-carbohydrate, **95–6**
   tips on, **21**, 22
   type 1 diabetes &, 21, 39
   type 2 diabetes &, 42, 44, 46
   see also food
'diet' products, 104, 189
dietary myths, **88**
dietitians, 14, 19, 23, **24–5**, **85**, 86, 90, 91,
   107
Dietitians Association of Australia, 274
Dietitians NZ, 274
digestive problems, 148, 149, 150, 151, 152,
   184, 185
dinner recipes, **260–7**
dipeptidyl peptidase-4 inhibitors, **150**
distal symmetric neuropathy, 183
dizziness, 185
DO IT study, 111, **119**
doctors
   activity plans &, 113, 118
   anxiety &, **216**
   blood glucose meters &, 66, 67, 68
   check-ups with, **78**
   complementary medicines &, 193, 194
   diabetes management &, 14, 19, **23**
   full assessment by, 17
   goal setting &, 63
   medications &, **145–6**, 147, 151, 153
   nerve damage &, 184, **188**
   reporting to, 65, 66, 67
   self-monitoring &, 60, 65
   support from, 23
   travel &, 228
dopamine, 239–40
double-blind tests, 195, 200, 201
double vision, 181
doughnuts, 98, 103
download capability (meter), 66, 67, 68
doxepin, 151
driver responsibility checklist, **226**
driving, 53, 63, **225–7**
drugs *see* medication(s)
dry swimming (exercise), **123**

E

Eastern therapies, 193, 197, 199, 204, 206
eating/ meal plans, 21
   attitude &, **106**
   blood glucose &, 55, 63, **72–3**, **85–6**, 89
   building blocks of, 89
   complications risk &, 84, 86, 173, 185
   dietitians &, **85**, **86**, 99
   food diary &, **85**
   food exchanges &, **99–100**
   foods on the menu, **89–99**
   GI &, **97–8**
   medications &, 84, 86
   putting together, **86**
   special considerations, 55, 84, 86
   weight control &, 55, 87, 89, 93, 95, 96,
   102
Edgar National Centre for Diabetes and
   Obesity Research, 274
Edmonton Protocol, 243
Egg and anchovy pan bagna (recipe), **257**
eggs, 94, 100, 185
emergencies
   cardiovascular, **174**
   diabetes, **52–3**
emotions and feelings
   attitude &, **220–1**
   blood glucose, 212, 216, 218
   calming your, 214, 215
   coping with, **212–16**
   diabetes burnout &, **218–21**
   diagnosis &, **12**, 13, 26, **211–12**
   exercise &, 112
   negative, 211, 212, **214–16**
   positive, 211
   relationships &, **217**
   self-talk &, **216**
   stress &, **216–17**
   talking about, **213–14**, 218
   triggers &, 215
endocrinologists *see* diabetes specialists
endothelium, 241
energy management, 87, 88, 89
energy needs, 21
energy sources, 31, 101, 111, 216, 224
environmental triggers, 235, **237**
epicatechin, 199
epinephrine, 216
erectile dysfunction *see* sexual dysfunction
evaporated non-fat milk, 100
evening primrose oil, **200**, 204
Exenatide, **150–1**
exercise
   action stations, **114–15**
   activity schedule, **117**
   aerobic, 22, **112–13**, 118, 141
   beginning, **116–18**, 141

blood glucose &, 58, 61, **74–5**, **76**, 86, 110, 111, 112, 113, **114**, **115**, 116, 119, 144, 145, 146, 212
blood pressure &, 112, **115**, 118, 171, 172
body fat &, **111**, 112
combined training, **113**
commitment and motivation, **118**
dementia &, 112
energy &, 111
eye problems &, 182
general health &, 110, **112**
hypoglycaemia &, **114**, **115**
illness &, **76**
medications &, **74**, 110, 114, **115**
metabolism &, **110–11**, 112
mood and memory &, 112
muscle &, 111, 112
myths about, 88
pain conditions &, 113, 115, 116, 118
resistance, 112, **113**, **114–15**, 117, 118
safety precautions, **113**
short- and long-term effects of, **111**
travel &, **229**
types of, **112–15**
waist girth &, **111–12**
weight loss &, 22, **106**, **111–12**, 113
see also physical activity
Exercise and Sports Science Australia, 275
exercise specialists, 19, 23, **26**, 114, 115, 118, 182
exercises
    balance and mobility, **125–33**
    strengthening and toning, **120–4**
    stretching, **134–40**
eye organisations and associations, 274
eye problems
    aspirin &, 182
    blood glucose &, 11, 19, 32, 34, 59, 169, **179–80**, 181, 240, 241
    breakthroughs of the future, **240–1**
    complementary therapies &, **201**, 204
    focal neuropathy &, 183
    high blood pressure &, 22, 80, 171, 180, **182**, 201
    kidney disease &, 178
    physical activity &, **182**
    prevention of, 168, **171**, **179–82**
    surgery for, **182**
eye specialists, 14, 19, 23, **25**
eye tests, 14, 16, 20, 22, **25**, 78, 171, **181–2**

F
faintness, 185
family history, 14, **16**, 37, **38**, 48, 51, 110, 235, 236, 237 see also genetics
fast food, 21, 22, 46, **88**

fasting blood glucose, 18, 145, 197, 198
fasting plasma glucose test, **47**, 49
fat (body), 110, **111**, 112, 113
    see also abdominal fat; obesity and overweight
fat (dietary), 21, 31, 84, 86, 87, 89, 90, 91, **92–4**, 95, 96, 99, 102, 173, **175**, 228
    see also monounsaturated fats; polyunsaturated fats; saturated fats
fat-soluble vitamins, 92, **96–7**
fatigue, 17, 19, 32, **34**, 36, 37, 48, 58, 212, 218
fatty acids, 31, 42, 200
feelings see emotions and feelings
feet
    caring for, **188**
    checks of, 16, **25**, **186–7**
    nerve damage to, 118, 168, 169, 172, 183, 184, **185**, **186–8**, 207, 225
    numbness in, 183, 184, 186, 188
    organisations and associations, **274**
    pain in, 116
    preventing problems in, **171**, 173, **186–8**
    swelling of, 178
    tingling in, 17, **36**, 37, 183, 184, 188
    see also podiatrists
fenugreek, **196**
fever, 78
fibre (dietary), 21, 90, **91–2**, 96, 105, 173, **175**, 228
finger prick tests, **50–1**, 64, 66, 68, **69**, 160
Finnish Diabetes Prevention Study, 52
fish and seafood, 95, 97, 175, 185
fish and seafood recipes, **254**, **257**, **262**
flatulence, 92, 148, 150, 152
flavonoids, 176, 201, 202
flexible insulin therapy, 156
fluid intake, **224**
fluid retention, 149
focal neuropathy, **183**
food
    blood glucose levels &, 13, 31, 55, 58, 59, 61–2, **72–4**, 76, 79, 84, 85, 222
    cardiovascular disease &, **173**, **175–6**
    children &, 15
    consistency &, 72–3, **86**
    cooking of, 93
    cultural diversity &, 94
    diabetes burnout &, 219
    diabetes cause &, 39
    dieting myths &, **88**
    exercise &, **74–5**, 86, 114
    gestational diabetes &, 45
    illness &, **224**
    insulin &, 86, 156
    kidney problems &, **178–9**
    lipids &, 86
    management of, **84–107**

nerve damage &, 185
nine strategies &, 21
nutrients in, 85, 86, 90, **97**, 99, 100, 201
pre-diabetes &, 18
premenstrual syndrome &, 222
salt-free, 97
staggering your, **94**
sugar-free, **90**
travel &, **228**
trimming fat from, **93**
type 1 diabetes &, 13, 84
type 2 diabetes &, 18, 62, 86, **87**, 92
vitamins and minerals in, **96–7**
what's on the menu, **89–99**
    see also breakfast; carbohydrates; eating/ meal plans; glycaemic index; kilojoules; product labels; recipes
food and nutrition organisations and associations, **274–5**
food diaries, 85
food exchanges, **99–100**, 102, 156
food portions, 46, 85, 88, 99, 102, **105**
Food Standards Australia and New Zealand, 104, 274
food substitutes, **103**
foot ulcers, 173, 186, 188, 242
foreign policy, 64
fortified wines, 101
free radicals, **39–40**, 199
friends, 114, 115, 116, 214, 217, 220
frozen yogurt, 103
fructosamine tests, **77**
fruit, 21, 22, 73, 76, 84, 90, 91, 92, 97, 98, 99, 100, 171, 173, 175, 176
fruit cocktail, 100
fruit juice, 224
fruit peel, 91
frustration, 214, 215, 218
fungal infections, 188
future, **232–44**

G
Galvus, **150**
gamma-linolenic acid, **200**, **204**
gancyclovir, 151
gangrene, 170, 186
garlic, **202**
gastric banding, 163, **164**
gastric bypass surgery, 163, **164**
gastric sleeve, 163, **164**
gastrointestinal problems, 168
gastroparesis, 184, 185
gelatine, 100
genetic therapies, 38
genetics, 38, **41**, **44**, **237**, **238–9**
    see also family history

gestational diabetes, **37**, **45**, 62
gingivitis, 25, 189
ginkgo, 202
ginseng, **197–8**
Glargine, 232
Glaucoma Australia, 274
glibenclamide, 153
glitazones *see* thiazolidinediones
glomerular filtration rate, 176
glucagon, 33, 228, 236
Glucobay, **149–50**
glucolipotoxic environment, 111
Glucophage, 87
glucose intolerance/ tolerance, 46, 47,
     51–2, 148, 169
glucose meters *see* blood glucose meters
glucose tablets/ powder/ gel, 73, 114, 149,
     227
Glucovance, 153
glycaemic control targets, **60**, **61**
glycaemic index, 73–4, 94, 95, 96, **97–9**, 173
Glycaemic Index Foundation, 275
glycated haemoglobin, **49–50**
glycogen, 35
glycosylated haemoglobin test *see*
     HbA1c tests
glycosylation, 77
goals
     blood glucose, **60–3**, 85
     weight, 86, 87
Goat's cheese toasts (recipe), **252**
grains, 95, **105**
grapes, 100, 201
grapeseed extract, 202
Grave's disease, 38
green beans, 100
growth hormones, 33, **241–2**
Guardian-REAL-Time continuous glucose-
     monitoring system, 234
gum disease, 36, **189**
gymnema, **195–6**

H

haemoglobin, 77
hands
     nerve damage in, 17, 36, 37, 183, 184
     swelling of, 178
HbA1c tests, 14, 17, 18, 22, **47**, **49–50**, 58,
     77, 78, 79, 81, 145, 146, 169, 198, 217,
     225–6, 234
HDL cholesterol, **78**, 79, 95, 96, 101, 148
headaches, 148, 149, 150, 174
healing impairment, 19, 22, 37
health funds, 67, 69, 72, 85, 161, 233, 245
health insurance, 67, 72, 85
Health Navigator New Zealand, 275

healthcare professionals, 14
A Healthy and Active Australia, 275
heart attacks, 19, 21, 22, 78, 110, 168, 169,
     170, 171, 173, **174**, 175, 176, 183, 196,
     202, 203, 216
heart disease
     blood glucose &, 44, 198, 225, 226, 234
     blood lipids &, 78
     complementary therapies &, 198, 201,
          202–3, 204, 206
     diet &, **175**
     emotions and feelings &, 211, 212, 215, 217
     exercise &, 112, 114, 118
     fats &, 92
     medications &, 146
     obesity &, 44
     proinsulin levels &, 241
     reducing risk of, 170, **172–6**
     see also cardiovascular problems
heart failure, 148, 149
Heart Foundation (Australia), 275
heart organisations and associations, **275**
heart rate, 216, 219
heartbeat irregularities, 175, 183
herbal supplements *see* complementary
     therapies
herbs, 105, 225
high blood pressure *see* blood pressure
high cholesterol, 11, 14, 17, 21, 22, 42, 44,
     86, 94
HIV medications, 151
hives, 148
home testing, 50, 58, **59–62**, **64–76**
honey, 73
'honeymoon' period, **36–7**
hormones, 33, 75, 94, 150–1, 164, 174, 216,
     217, 224, 236, 238, 239, **241–2**
HRT, 223
Humalog, 75, 154, 155
Humalog Mix, 154
human insulin, 155
human leukocyte antigens, 236
Humulin, 154, 155
hunger, 37, 89, 164
hyperglycaemia, 15, 75, 160
hyperosmolar hyperglycaemic state, **224**
hyperosmolar syndrome, **52**
hypoglycaemia, 212
     alcohol &, 74, 101, 145
     artificial pancreas &, 244
     carbohydrate snacks &, 53, **73**, 114, 145,
          227
     children &, 15
     complementary therapies &, 195
     driving &, 27, 53, 225, 226, **227**, 228
     exercise &, 74, **114**, **115**
     explanation of, 33, **52–3**

food portions &, 88, 145
insulin &, 33, 74, 155
insulin pumps &, 160, 245
medications &, 59, 73, 74, 115, 145, 147,
     148, 149, 150, 151, 152, 153, 236
sex &, 221
symptoms of, 53, 73, 114, 216
testing for, 27, 59, 61, 64, 72, 73, 79, 114,
     226
travel &, 227, 228
treating, **73**
type 1 diabetes &, 52, 61
type 2 diabetes &, 53, 61
hypoglycaemic unawareness, 163, 184, 244
hypotension *see* blood pressure
Hypurin Isophane, 154, 155

I

ibuprofen, 179
ice cream, 103
identical twins, 16, 38, 41
identification, 114, 226, 228
illness
     blood glucose &, 32, 60, 63, 74, **75–6**,
          212, **224**
     planning for, **224–5**
immune system, 32, 36, 37, **38**, **39**, 94, 162,
     204, 205, 211, 238, 242
immunosuppressant medications, 162, 163,
     242, **243–4**
impaired fasting glucose, 18, 47, **51**
impaired glucose intolerance/ tolerance,
     18, 44, **51–2**, 148
impotence *see* sexual dysfunction
inactivity, **42**
incretin mimetics, **150–1**
Indian people, 16, 41
indigenous health, **275**
indigestion, 185
infection-fighting medications, 151
infections, 17, 19, 36, 37, 162, 168, **179**, 188
information sources, **24**
     see also diabetes educators; diabetes
          support groups
inhaled insulin, **234–5**
injection alternatives, **159–61**
injection sites, **158**, 159
injections, 147, 151, **158**, 159
     see also insulin injections
insoluble fibre, 92
insulin
     advances in, **232**
     artificial pancreas &, 244
     balance &, 13
     blood glucose &, 20, **33–4**, 58, 153, **156**,
          157, 160, 212, 232, **235–6**

children &, 15, 46
choice of, **154–5**
complementary medicines &, 195, 196
diabetes burnout &, 218
discovery of, **38**, 144
DKA &, 52
doses of, 154, **156**
driving &, **226**
eating plans &, 84, 86, 156
exercise &, 74, 75, 110, 111, 114, 156
finetuning, **75–6**, 233
future &, **234–5**, 243
gestational diabetes &, 45
glycaemic control &, 61, 73
hypoglycaemia &, 59, 73
illness &, 76, 225
improvements in, 154–5
ins and outs of, **155–8**
inside job of, **33–4**
mornings &, 76
overweight &, 21
pancreas &, 33, 35, 145, 150, 151, 152, 153
pregnancy &, 62, 222
research on, **235–6**, 243
self-monitoring of, 60, 61, 63, 233
side-effects of, 73, **157**
timing of, **75**, 76, 86
transplant surgery &, 162, 163, 243
travel &, 227, 228, **229**
treatment changes &, 63
type 1 diabetes &, **11**, 13, 30, **36**, 37, 60, 61, 62, 86, 90, 144, 153, 154, **156–7**, 161, 236, 242
type 2 diabetes &, 11, **17–18**, 21, 36, 37, **40**, 41, 42, 46, 62, 86, 88, 90, 144, **146**, 149, 153, 154, **157**, 222, 236, 242
types of, 11, **154**, **155**, **156**
insulin antagonists, 33
Insulin Aspart, 154, 155, 232
insulin boluses, 153
insulin-dependent diabetes *see* type 1 diabetes
Insulin Determir, 154, 155
Insulin Glargine, 154, 155
Insulin Glulisine, 154, 155
insulin injections, 13, 15, 30, **36**, 37, 45, 59, 60, **75**, 86, 88, 144–5, 146, 156–7, **159–61**, 234, 243
insulin patches, 235
insulin pens, **159**, 229
insulin pumps, 60, 114, 156, 157, **160–1**, **165**, **222**, 233, 234, 244, **245**
insulin receptors, 40
insulin resistance, 21, **33–4**, **40**, **42**, 44, 45, 47, 51, 72, 86, 87, 88, **94**, 111, 148, 153, 212, 217, 222, 224, 235, 237, 239
insulin response, 48

insulin sensitivity, 110, 113, 148, **149**, 152, 175, 239, 241
intensive therapy, 59
intermediate-acting insulin, **154**, **155**, 156, 157
Internet chat groups, 220
Intranasal Insulin Trial, **14**, **236**
iron, 97
irritable bowel syndrome, 150
islet cell transplants, **162–3**, **242–4**
islets of Langerhans, 35, 162–3
isoniazid, 151

J

Janumet, 153
Januvia, **150**, 153
JDRF Type 1 Diabetes Pump Program, 161
jelly beans, 73, 114, 227
jet injectors, needle-free, **159–60**
jogging, **141**
joint problems, 110, 112, 113, 115, 141
Joslin Diabetes Center, 237
journals and diaries, 70, **85**, 217
Juvenile Diabetes Research Foundation, 24, 274
juvenile-onset diabetes *see* type 1 diabetes

K

karella *see* bitter melon
ketoacidosis, **52**, 77, 160, **224**, 225
ketones, 52, **77–8**, 79, 224, 225
kidney beans, 92, 98
kidney care, **176–9**
kidney disease, 168
    blood glucose &, 11, 19, 32, 34, 59, 162, 169, 176, **178**
    blood pressure &, 22, 80, 172, **178**
    complementary therapies &, **201–2**
    diet &, 56, 95, 96, **178–9**
    exercise &, 112
    genes &, 237
    medications &, 146, 148, 150, 151, **179**, 241
    smoking &, 22
    symptoms of, 178, 179
    type 1 diabetes &, 169
    type 2 diabetes &, 178
kidney disease prevention, **171**, 174, **176–9**
kidney failure, 162, 176, **178**
kidney function, **176**, 241
Kidney Health Australia, 275
Kidney Health New Zealand, 275

kidney tests, 16, 22, **178**
kidney transplants, 162
kilojoules, 86, **87**, **89–90**, 92, 96, 99, **102–3**, 106, 112, 238
knee raise (exercise), **132**
kumara, 90

L

L-carnitine, **201**, **202–3**
lactic acidosis, 146, 148
lamb with burghul, Spiced, **261**
lancets, 20, 27, 64, **65–7**, 68, 69, 227, 228, 229
lancing devices, 66
Lantus, 154, 155, 232
lapbanding surgery, 163, **164**
laser eye surgery, 182
L-carnitine, **201**, **202–3**
LDL cholesterol, **78**, 79, 94, 98, 148, 175
legs
    atherosclerosis &, **170**, 172
    cramps in, 183, 184
    nerve damage &, 184
legumes, 90, 91, 92, 95, 173, 175, 196
lentils, 100
leptin, **239**
Levemir, 154, 155, 232
Levitra, 223
Lifeline (Australia), 275
Lifeline (New Zealand), 275
lifestyle changes, 11, 30, 37, 41, 51, 110, **116–18**, 145
Lift for Life program, 115
linolenic acid, 204
lipid tests, **78–9**, 86
liqueurs, 101
Liraglutide, **150–1**
Lispro, 154, 155, 232
lithium, 151, 179
liver and liver problems, 32, 35, 101, 148, 149, 150, 174, 178
liver tests, 22
'living bandages', 242
logbooks, 70, **85**
lollies, 90
long-acting insulin, 144, 154, **155**, 156, 157
low-carbohydrate diets, **95–6**
low-fat dairy products, 84, 93, 100
low glycaemic index, 21
lower body strengthening and toning exercises, **122**
Lucentis, 240
lunch recipes, **256–9**
lupus, 38, 238
lying twist (exercise), **137**

M

MacLeod, John, 38
macular oedema, 181, **240**
magnesium, 97, **204**
magnet therapies, **206–7**
Mango mousse (recipe), **270**
MAO inhibitors, 151
Maori people, 16, 36, 38, 41, 44
margarine, 103, 175
Marsala chicken with fennel (recipe), **264**
MDI, 156
meal planning, 24–5
meal skipping, 88
meat, 21, 22, 84, 91, 93, 94, 95, 97, 99, **100**, 179, 185, 199, 201, 203
Medic Alert Foundation (Australia), 274
Medic Alert Foundation (New Zealand), 274
medical history, 13
medical identification, 27
Medicare, 85
medication(s)
    advances in, **232–7**, **240–1**
    alcohol &, 101, 145, 148, 150
    allergies to, 148, 151, 154–5
    blood pressure, 151, **174**, **178**, 213, 223
    cardiovascular disease, **173–4**
    children &, 46
    choice of, **145–6**, 147, 151, 153
    cholesterol &, 148, 149
    combinations of oral, 146, 148, 149, 150, 151, **152–3**
    complementary medicine interactions with, 193, 196, 197, 198, 202
    depression &, 151, 213
    diabetes burnout &, 218
    diabetes complications &, 171, 173
    dosages of, 147, 151, 153
    double-duty, **241**
    driving &, 27, **226**
    eating plans &, 84, 86
    effectiveness of, 147
    emotions &, 216, 218
    exercise &, 74, 110, 114, **115**
    eye problems &, 182
    finetuning of, 60, **75–6**
    glycaemic control &, 60, 61, 62, 74
    hypoglycaemia &, 59, 73, 74, 115, 145, 147, 148, 149, 150, 151, 152, 153, 236
    illness &, **225**
    immunosuppressant, 162, 163, 242, **243–4**
    intensive therapy &, 59
    interactions, 25, **151**, 174
    kidney disease &, 146, 148, 150, 151, 178, **179**, 241
    multiple conditions &, 60, 63

    need for, **145–6**
    neuropathy &, **185**
    newer types of, 11, 153
    oral contraceptives &, 222
    oral glucose tolerance test (OGTT) &, 49
    overview of, **146–51**
    pancreatic function &, 35
    pharmacists &, **25–6**
    pre-existing conditions &, 150, **151**
    pregnancy &, 148, 149, 150, 151, 222
    sex-related problems &, 222, **223**
    side effects of, 145, 146, **147–8**, **149**, 150, **151**, 152, 153, **157**, 172, 174, 185, 213, 223, 244
    snacks &, 75
    taking advantage of, 55
    timing of, **75**, 76, 115
    tracking effect of, 60
    travel &, **227–8**, 229
    type 1 diabetes &, **36**, 37, 144
    type 2 diabetes &, 11, **17–18**, 37, 46, 51, 144, 145, **146**, 148
    weight-loss, 148, **172**
    see also blood thinners; insulin
Mediterranean diet, 94
Medtronic Minimed, 234
mefloquine, 151
megesterol acetate, 151
meglitinides, 150
Melon, fetta and orange salad (recipe), **259**
memory, 112
men
    abdominal circumference chart for, 43
    alcohol &, 101
    energy requirement of, 89
    kilojoules required by, 89
    sexual dysfunction &, 184, 185, **223**
    type 1 diabetes &, 38
    weight for height chart for, **43**
mental confusion, 73, 174
mental fatigue, 34
mental health organisations and associations, **275**
metabolic engine, **110–11**, 112
metabolic problems, 94, 238, 239
metabolic rate, 106
metabolic switch, 34
metabolic syndrome, 42, **44**, 217
metformin, 51, 146, **148**, 151, 157, 185, 193, 197, 226
metformin combinations, **152–3**
microalbumin, 86
microalbuminuria, 16, 177, 178
Middle Eastern people, 16, 41
milk, **39**, 73, 90, 91, 93, 99, 100, 103, 237
minerals, 90, 96, **97**, **204**

MiniMed Paradigm® REAL-Time System, 234
minoxidil, 151
miscarriages, 45
mixed insulin, **154**, 156
Mixtard, 154
mobility and balance exercises, **125–33**
molecular messages, 235
mononeuropathy, 183
monounsaturated fats, 94, 95, 175
mood, 112, 212, 213, 214, 222
morphine, 193
motivation, 63, 116, **118**, 215, 218, 220
Motrin, 179
mountain pose (exercise), **134**
muesli, 103
muffins, Carrot, apricot and pecan (recipe), **248**
multiple health problems, 60, 63
multiple sclerosis, 38
mumps, 39
muscle mass, 106
muscle strength, 111, 115
muscle wastage, 185
muscles
    exercise &, 110, 111, 112, 113, 118
    insulin sensitivity &, 110, 113
myelin sheath, 183
myths, 54, 88

N

nanoshells, 235
naproxen, 179
National Amputee Associations and Support Groups (Australia), 275
National Diabetes Services Scheme, 24, 69–70, 161, 274
National Health and Medical Research Council, 101
National Stroke Foundation (Australia), 275
natural therapies *see* complementary therapies
nausea, 36, 37, 78, 148, 149, 150, 151, 152, 174, 184, 185, 206
needle-free jet injectors, **159–60**
needles, 158, 159, 160, 227
negative emotions, 211, 212, **214–16**
nephrons, 177
nephropathy *see* kidney disease
nephrotic syndrome, 178
nerve damage, 168, 242
    alcohol &, 186
    B vitamins &, **185**
    blood glucose &, 11, 19, 32, 59, 169, **171**, 183, 184, 226

complementary therapies &, **199–200**, 201, 206, 207
driving &, 225, 226
exercise &, 118, 171
healthy eating plan &, 185
high blood pressure &, 22, 80
major types of, **183–4**
medications &, **185**
pain relief for, **185**
prevention of, 171, **184–6**
sexual dysfunction &, 184, 185
smoking &, 22, 171, 186
tests of, **184**
type 1 diabetes &, 59, 169
UTIs &, 179, 184
see also feet
nervousness, 216, 228
neurologists, 184
New Zealand Nutrition Foundation, 275
New Zealand Society for the Study of Diabetes, 274
no-added sugar, 105
no-prick meters, **72**
non-fat products, 100, 103
non-nutritive sweeteners, **104**
non-proliferative retinopathy, 180
non-stick pans, 93
noodles, 90, 94
nopal *see* prickly pear
Novomix, 154
Novonorm, **150**
Novorapid, 75, 154, 155
numbness, 170, 174, 183, 184, 186, 188
nutrients, 31, 85, 86, 89, 90, 96, **97**, 99, 100
Nutrition Australia, 275
nutritive sweeteners, **104**
nuts and seeds, 84, 95, 96, 97, 175, 176

O

oats, 91, 92
obesity and overweight
blood vessels &, 170
brain &, **239–40**
children &, 46
carbohydrates &, 95
genes &, **238–9**
type 2 diabetes &, 16, **21**, 37, 40, **42–4**, 45, **46**, 51, 55, 235, 238, **239–40**
weight-loss medications &, **172**
weight-loss surgery &, **163–4**
obesity rates, 42
Obesity Surgery Society of Australia and New Zealand, 164
obsession, 220
OEA (oleyleth-anolamide), 239
oestrogen, 222, 223

oils, 92, 175
oligomeric proanthocyanidin complexes, **202**
olive oil, 84, 92, 93, 94, 96, 175
Omega-3 fats, 175
onion tartlets, Caramelised (recipe), 252
OPC supplements, **202**
ophthalmologists, 14, 25, 181, 182
optometrists, 14, 25, 181
Optometrists Association Australia, 274
oral contraceptives, 222
oral glucose tolerance tests (OGTT), **18**, 47, **48–9**, 145
oral insulin, **235**
organisations and associations, 24, 67, 192, 220, **274**
orlistat, 172
orthostatic hypotension, 183
over-the-counter remedies, **225**
overeating, 240
overhead press (exercise), **130**
overseas policy, **64**
overseas travel, **229**
overweight *see* obesity and overweight
oxidation, 176

P

Pacific Islander people, 16
pain relievers, 151, 173, 185
pain signals, 171
palm clasp (exercise), **131**
pancreas, 33, **35**, 36, 37, 38, 40, 60, 147, 150, 151, 236
pancreas, artificial, **244**
pancreas transplants, **162–3**, **242**
Paradigm Veo System, 234
pasta, 90, 98, 100, 175
pastrami, 103
PCO supplements *see* OPC supplements
Peach and blackberry filo pizzas (recipe), **273**
peakless long-acting insulin, **155**
peanut oil, 92
peanuts, 92, 97, 98
pears, 100
peas, 90, 98, 99
pedometers, 141
peer reviewed studies, 195
pen injectors, **159**, 160
pentamidine, 151
peptides, **237–8**
periodontitis, 189
peripheral neuropathy, 114, 183, 201, 207
peripheral vascular disease, 170, 173
Pharmac, 67
pharmacies, 67

pharmacists, **25–6**
phenothiazines, 151
photocoagulation, 182
physical activity
beginning, **116–18**, 141
blood glucose &, 18, 22, 55, 58, 59, 60, 62, 63, **74–5**, **76**, 86, 110, 212
children &, 46
dementia &, 112
depression &, 214
illness &, **76**
increasing your, 110, **116**
insulin &, **42**, 74, 75
medications &, **42**, 74, 110
organisations and associations, **275**
travel &, **229**
type 2 diabetes &, **42**, 43, 62
weight &, 22, 55, **106**, 240
see also exercise
physical fatigue, 34
physiotherapists, 14, 118
Pikelets with berries and yogurt (recipe), **251**
pioglitazone, 149, 152
placebo effect, 194, 195, 200, 204
plasma glucose concentration, 67
plasma glucose tests, **47–8**, 49
platelets, 173
podiatrists, 14, 19, 23, **25**, 186, 187, 188
Podiatry New Zealand, 274
polycystic ovary syndrome, 45
polyneuropathy, **183**, 199
polyphenolics, 197
polyunsaturated fats, 94, 175
pork, Five-spice (recipe), **267**
porridge, 98
potassium-containing foods, 86, 97
potato chips, 85, 93
potatoes, 91, 98, 185
potbelly peril, **42**
poultry, 95, 97, 185
power, 59
pramlintide, 236
pre-diabetes, 18, 44, **51–2**, 87, **169**
pregnancy
blood glucose &, 62, 222
complementary therapies &, 196, 197, 204
diabetes complications &, 222
glucose targets &, 60
medications &, 148, 149, 150, 151, 222
planning for, **222**
sweeteners &, 104
see also gestational diabetes
premenstrual syndrome, 222
pre-schoolers and toddlers, **15**
prescriptions, 228
pressure sores, 188

pre-teens and adolescents, **15**
prickly pear, **199**
primary school children, **15**
processed foods, 173, 175
product labels, 90, 91, **105**, 194, **203**
progesterone, 222
progestin, 222
proinsulin, 241
proliferative retinopathy, 180–1, 182
prostaglandins, 200
protamine, 155
Protaphane, 154, 155
protease inhibitors, 151
protein, 31, 35, 77, 80, 86, 89, **94–5**, 99, 171, **178–9**, 201
protein PTPIB, 239
psychologists, 13, 14
Pterocarpus marsupium, **199**
public screening, 50–1

Q

quality of life, 210, 211, 215, 220
quinine, 151, 193
quinolones, 151
The Quit Group (New Zealand), 275
Quit Now (Australia), 275
Quitline, 173, 275

R

radishes, 100
raisins, 98, 100
ramipril, 175
random plasma glucose tests, 47, **48**, 49
ranibizumab, 240
rapid-acting insulin, **154**, **155**, 156, 157, 160, 232, 234–5
rapid-onset diabetes, **36**
recipes
    breakfast, **248–51**
    dessert, **268–73**
    dinner, **260–7**
    lunch, **256–9**
    snacks/ appetisers, **252–5**
Recommended Daily Intake (kilojoule), 89
record keeping, 65, 68, **70**, **85**, 217, 222
red blood cells, 77
Registered/ Accredited Practising Dietitians, 24–5
'regular' insulin, 153
    see also short-acting insulin
relationships, **217**, 219
relaxation pose (exercise), **139**
religious belief, **217**
renal insufficiency, 178
repaglinide, 150

research, 20, 194–5, 196, 200, 233, **235–42**, 243, **244**
resistance bands, 114
resistance exercise/ training, 112, **113**, 114–15, 117, 118
resources directory, **274–5**
respiratory problems, 36, 78, 113, 114
responsibility, **27**, 215, 220–1
retinal damage, **179–81**
retinal detachment, 181
retinal photography, 25
retinopathy, 16, 162, **180–1**, 182, 201, 237, 241, 242
rheumatoid arthritis, 38
Rhubarb and saffron crème brûlée (recipe), **268**
rice, 90, 94, 97, 98, 175
rifampin, 151
rights and responsibilities, **27**
rosiglitazone, 152, 153
rowing, 113
Royal Australian and New Zealand College of Ophthalmologists, 274
Royal New Zealand Foundation for the Blind, 274
rubella, 39
running, 22
rye bread, 98

S

safflower oil, 94
salad greens, 100
salad recipes, **258–60**
salami, 103
salmon and asparagus, Summer (recipe), **262**
salt intake, 21, 22, 86, 93, **97**, 173
sandwiches, Open-faced chicken (recipe), **256**
saturated fats, 21, 86, 91, 92, 93, 94, 96, 98, 104, 105, 173, 175, 228
seafood *see* fish and seafood
self-discipline, 214
self-esteem, 15
self-knowledge, 221
self-monitoring, 58, **59–62**, **64–76**, 77, 86
self-monitoring testing tools, **65–70**
    see also under tool eg lancets
serenity, 220–1
sex
    blood glucose &, **221–2**
    men &, 184, 185, **223**
    women &, 184, 185, **221–3**
sex drive, 184
sex hormones, 222
sexual dysfunction, 17, 19, 168, 184, 185, **223**

shaking, 114, 184
sharps disposal, **160**
shift workers, 150
shoes, 141, 171, **186**, **187**, **188**, 229
shopping, **103**, **105–6**
shopping lists, 103, 105
short-acting insulin, **154**, **155**, 156, 157, 160
Siberian ginseng, 198
sildenafil, 185, 223
siphon-style tests strips *see* capillary action tests strips
sitagliptin, **150**, 153
Sjogren's Syndrome, 238
skim milk, 93, 98, 100
skin problems, 148, 150
skin substitutes, biological, **242**
sleep, 112, 216
sleeve gastrectomy *see* gastric sleeve
smoking, 14, **22**, 171, **173**, 178, 186, 189, **275**
snack/ appetiser recipes, **252–5**
snack attacks, **34**
snacks, 75, 76, 86, 89, 93, 94, 102, 114, 145, 147, 189, 221, **227**, 228
social eating, 85
social support, 217
socialising, 214
socks, 171, **188**
soft drinks, 73, 90, 102, 103, 114, 189, 224
soluble fibre, 92, 175
sorbitol, 90, 199, 241
soy products, 95, 98, 175
spaghetti, 98
Special K™, 98, 103
specialists, 14, **23**, 226
speech difficulties, 170, 171
spices, 105
spinach, 97, 199
spirits, 101, 102
SSRIs, 213
standing abdominal squeeze (exercise), **127**
standing side stretch (exercise), **135**
starches, 90, 91
statins, 175
stationary bike riding, 114
statistics, 10, 41
stomach pain, 78, 150
stomach ulcers, 174
steering wheel press (exercise), **129**
strawberries, 97
strength training, 106
strengthening and toning exercises, **120–4**
stress, 63, 74, 75, 112, 204, 205, 216–17, **219**, 224
stress hormones, 33, 216, 217, 224
stress-management programs, 217
stretching exercises, **134–40**

Stroke Foundation of New Zealand, 275
strokes, 19, 21, 22, 78, 110, 112, 168, 169, 170, 171, 173, 174, 217
sugar-free foods, **90**, 104
sugar intake, 21, 54, 84, **90**
sulfa medication allergies, 148
sulfonamides, 151
sulfonylurea combinations, **152–3**
sulfonylureas, 144, **147–8**, 149, 151
sunburn, 74
support
  diagnosis &, 12, 13
  enlisting, 219–20
  exercise &, 114, 115, 116, 220
  family and friends &, 27, 116, **217**, 220
  hypoglycaemia &, 114, 115
  professional, **22–6**, 274–5
support groups, 12, 220, 274–5
surgery
  eye, **182**
  islet cell transplant, **162–3**, **242–4**
  pancreas transplant, **162–3**, 242
  pros and cons of, **163**
  type 1 diabetes &, **162–3**
  type 2 diabetes &, **163–4**
  weight-loss, 163–4
  see also biological skin substitutes
sweet corn *see* corn
sweet potatoes, 98, 99, 100
sweeteners, **90**, 104
swimming, 45, 229
symptoms, 54, 58
  aneurysm, **174**
  common diabetes, **16–17**, 32, **34**, **36**, **37**, 48, 165
  depression, **213**
  exercise &, 110, 111, 112, 114
  heart attack, **174**
  hypoglycaemia, 53, 73, 114, 115
  ketoacidosis, 225
  nerve damage, 183, 184
  stroke, **174**
  type 1 diabetes &, **34**, **36**, **37**
  type 2 diabetes &, **16–17**, **34**, **36**, **37**, **40–1**, **42**, 224
syndrome X *see* metabolic syndrome
syringes, 160, **161**, 227, 229
systolic pressure, 80

T

T-cells, 39, 238
tadalafil, 223
take-charge tips, **20**
take-charge tool kit, **10–11**
talking, 213–14
taro, 90

tartar, 189
T-cells, 39, 238
tea, **175–6**
Team Care Arrangements, 85
technological testing advances, **71–2**
TEDDY, 39, 237
test strips, 19, 20, 64, 65, **69–70**, **71**, 72, 227
testimonials, 194
testing schedules, 62
testing tools, **65–70**
tests
  additional, **177–80**
  blood flow &, 68
  blood-glucose, 11, **13**, **14**, **17**, 18, 19, **20**, 22, **47–51**, **58–81**, **85–6**, 114, 115, 145
  blood pressure, 17
  cholesterol/ triglyceride, 16, 17, 22, **78–9**
  eye, 14, 16, 20, 22, **25**, 78, 171, **181–2**
  frequency of, **60–2**
  home, 50, 58, **59–62**, **64–76**
  importance of, **14**, **16**
  kidney, 16, 22, **178**
  liver, 22
  nerve damage, **184**
  oral glucose tolerance, 18, 47, **48–9**, 145
  overview of, **47–51**, **58–81**
  taking charge of, **68**, **69**
  thyroid, 22
  types of, **14**, **16**
  urine, 22, 50, **77–8**, 178, 224
  see also under test eg fasting plasma glucose test
tetracyclines, 151
thiazide diuretics, 151
thiazolidinedione combinations, **152–3**
thiazolidinediones, **149**, 237, 241
thigh toner (exercise), **131**
thirst, 17, 32, **34**, **36**, **37**, 48, 58, 165
thyroid disease, 13
thyroid function tests, 22
time zones, 229
tingling, 17, 36, 37, 183, 184, 188
tissue stiffening, **242**
tobacco smoke, 40
toddlers and pre-schoolers, **15**
toenails, 188
tomatoes, 97, 100
tooth decay, 189
  see also dentists and dental care
total carbohydrates, 90
total cholesterol, 78, 79
touch sensitivity, 184
touchdown tilt (exercise), **136**
trace minerals, **204**
trans fats, 175
transplant surgery, **162–3**, **242–4**
travel, **227–9**

travel insurance, 228
tree pose (exercise), **125**
tricyclics, 151, 185
triglycerides, 22, 44, **79**, 95, 96, 98, 148, 149, 157, 170, 198, 202, 217
TRIGR study, 237
tuberculosis medications, 151
tuna, 100, 103
type 1 diabetes
  age at onset, **36**, **37**
  attitude &, 221
  autoimmune co-conditions &, 13
  balance &, **13–14**
  BCMA &, 238
  blood glucose &, **37**, **169**, 196, 222, 224
  blood glucose meters &, 72
  carbohydrate intake &, 13, 21, 90, 156
  causes of, **37**, **38–40**
  CGM system &, 234
  children &, **15**, 16, 36, 37, 39, 161, 236, 237
  complementary therapies &, 196
  cow's milk &, 39
  diabetes specialists &, 23
  diagnosis of, **13–14**, **16**
  diet &, 21, 39
  emergencies, **52**, 53
  food &, 13, 84
  free radicals &, **39–40**
  frequency of tests, **60–2**
  genetics &, **38**
  glycaemic control targets &, **61**
  health complications &, **169**, 178, 181
  highs and lows &, **14**, **16**
  HLAs &, 236
  'honeymoon' period, **36–7**
  hypoglycaemic risk &, 52, 61
  INIT II &, **14**
  insulin &, **11**, 13, 30, **36**, **37**, 60, 61, 62, 86, 90, 144, 153, 154, **156–7**, 161, 236, 242
  islet-cell transplants &, **162–3**, 243
  ketoacidosis &, 23, 78, 224
  medications &, **36**, **37**, 144
  overview of, **36–40**
  pancreas transplants &, **162–3**, 242
  peptides &, **237–8**
  pregnancy &, 222
  prevention of, **236**, **238**
  rapid onset of, **36**
  research &, 235, 236, **237–8**
  rising incidence of, 41
  self-monitoring of, 59, **60–2**
  sex-related functions &, 221
  surgery &, **162–3**, 242, 243
  symptoms, **34**, **36**, **37**
  transplant surgery &, **162–3**, 242, 243
  treatment for, **36**, **37**
  triggers, 235, **237**

urine microalbumin tests &, 80
vaccine trial &, **14**, 236
viruses &, **39**
Type 1 Diabetes Genetics Consortium, 237
type 2 diabetes
  abdominal fat &, 110, 112
  age of onset, 37, **41**, 42, 46
  blood glucose &, 11, 17, **18**, 40, **41**, **145–6**, 169, 196, 197, 198, 199
  blood glucose meters &, 68
  carbohydrate intake &, 90
  causes of, 16, **21** 41–2
  CGM systems &, 234
  children &, 10, 15, 16, 36, 37, 41, **46**
  complementary therapies &, 196, 197, 198, 199, 200, 204, 206
  complications &, 168, **169**, 172, 178, 181
  cures for, **53**
  dementia &, 112
  diagnosis of, 13
  diet &, 42, 44, 46
  eating plans &, 86–7
  emergencies, **52**
  emotions and feelings &, 13
  exercise &, 62, 110–11, 112, 113, 114, 115
  food &, 18, 62, 86, **87**, 92
  frequency of tests, **62**
  genetics &, 16, 41, **44**
  glycaemic control targets &, **61**
  HHS &, 224
  hypoglycaemia risk &, 53, 61
  inactivity &, **42**, 110
  insulin &, 11, **17–18**, 21, 36, 37, **40**, 41, 42, 46, 62, 86, 88, 90, 144, **146**, 149, 153, 154, **157**, 222, 236, 242
  insulin resistance &, 33, 34
  medications &, 11, **17–18**, 51, 86, 144, 145, 146, **147–51**
  obesity &, 16, **21**, 37, 40, **42–4**, 45, 46, 51, 55, 235, 238, **239–40**
  onset of, 37, **40–1**, 42, 46
  overview of, **40–4**
  pramlintide &, 236
  pregnancy &, 222
  research &, 235, 236, 237
  rising incidence of, **46**
  risk factors for, **16**
  self-monitoring of, 59, 68
  specialists &, 23
  stress &, 217
  surgery pros and cons, **163–4**
  symptoms of, **16–17**, **34**, **36**, **37**, **40–1**, **42**, 224
  undiagnosed, 16, 20, 47
  urine microalbumin tests &, 80
  weight loss &, **21**, 87, 88, 113, 165, 238
  weight-loss surgery &, **163–4**

U
ulcerative colitis, 150
ulcers, 173, 174, 186, 188, 242
United Kingdom Prospective Diabetes Study, 59, 169
United States of America measurements, 64
upper back push-down (exercise), **129**
upper body strengthening and toning exercises, **120–1**
upward raised legs (exercise), **138**
urea, 179
urinary tract infections, 36, 179, 184
urination problems, 17, 32, **34**, 36, 37, 48, 179, 185
urine, 176, 177, 179
urine ketones, **77–8**, 224
urine microalbumin test, 78, 80
urine tests, 22, **50**, **77–8**, **80**, 178, 224

V
vaginal dryness, **223**
vaginal yeast infections, 36, 223
vaginitis, 223
vardenafil, 223
vegetable and bean stew, Roast (recipe), **265**
vegetables, 21, 22, 84, 90, 91, 92, 93, 95, 97, 98, 99, 100, 171, 173, 204
Viagra, 185, 223
Victoza, **150–1**
Vildagliptin, **150**
viruses, **39**
visceral adipose tissue, 42
Vision Australia, 274
vision problems, 11, 19, 25, **34**, 171, 174, 179, **180–1**, 226, **240–1** see also blurred vision
vitamin B, 200
vitamin B6, 185
vitamin B12, 97, 185
vitamin C, 97, 176
vitamin E, 97, 176, 202
vitamin supplements, 97
vitamins, 90, 92, **96–7**, 204
vitrectomy, 182
vomiting, 37, 52, 78, 149, 151, 184, 185

W
waist measurement, 42, **111–12**, 115
walking, 22, 45, 55, 76, 81, 113, 114, **116**, 117, **141**, 220, 229
wall push (exercise), **120**
wallslide with raised arms (exercise), **122**
warfarin, 197, 198, 202

waste disposal, 27, 66, **160**
water-aerobics, 141
water intake, 76, 92, 179, 189
water running, **141**
water-soluble vitamins, 96, 97
watermelon, 98
weight gain, 17, 37, **157**
weight goal, 86, 87
weight lifting/ training, 75, 112, **113**, 114
weight loss
  alternative sweeteners &, **104**
  attitude &, **106**
  eating plans &, 55, **87**, 89, 93, 95, 96, 102
  exercise &, 22, **106**, 111–12, 113
  importance of, **21**, 22, 55
  kilojoules &, **102–3**
  making it work, **102–7**
  medications &, 148, **172**
  myths about, **88**
  pre-diabetes &, 18
  research on, **238–40**
  smart shopping &, 103, **105–6**
  substitutions &, **103**
  type 2 diabetes &, **21**, 87, 88, 113, 165, 238
  working on, **238–40**
  see also obesity and overweight
weight-loss surgery, **163–4**
wheatgerm, 91
whole blood glucose, 67
whole grains, 21, 22, 84, 90, 91, 97, 105, 173, **175**, 204
Willis, Thomas, 211
willpower, 106
wine, 101
women
  abdominal circumference chart for, 43
  alcohol &, 101
  blood glucose control &, 62
  energy requirement of, 89
  gestational diabetes &, 37, **45**
  kilojoule requirement of, 89
  menstrual cycle irregularities &, **45**
  sex-related functions &, 184, 185, **221–3**
  type 1 diabetes &, 38
  UTIs in, 179
  vaginal dryness &, **223**
  vaginitis &, 223
  weight for height chart for, **43**
  yeast infections &, 36, 223
  see also pregnancy

X–Y
Xenical, 172
X-ray crystallography, 39
xylitol, 90
yogurt, 73, 90, 91, 100, 251

Taking Charge of Diabetes

**CONSULTANTS FOR AUSTRALIA
AND NEW ZEALAND**

Carole Webster, National Publications Manager, State and Territory Diabetes Organisations

Dr Alan Barclay, BSc, Grad Dip, PhD, Accredited Practising Dietitian & Nutritionist

Dr. Shelley Kay, Accredited Exercise Physiologist, PhD (USyd), M.Sp.Sc (Hons); B.Sp.Sc; BA; ISAK Level 3 anthropometrist

Dr Kate Marsh, Advanced Accredited Practising Dietitian and Credentialled Diabetes Educator

Alison Pask, New Zealand Registered Dietitian

Writer Richard Laliberte
Senior Editor Samantha Kent
Designer Susanne Geppert
Cover Designer Joanne Buckley
Proofreader Susan McCreery
Nutritional Analyses Toni Gumley
Indexer Diane Harriman
Senior Production Controller Monique Tesoriero

READER'S DIGEST GENERAL BOOKS
Editorial Director Lynn Lewis
Art Director Carole Orbell
Managing Editor Rosemary McDonald

Taking Charge of Diabetes
Published by Reader's Digest (Australia) Pty Limited
80 Bay Street, Ultimo, NSW 2007
www.readersdigest.com.au
www.readersdigest.co.nz
www.readersdigest.co.za

First Australian and New Zealand edition 2004
Reprinted 2005 (twice), 2005 (paperback),
2006 (paperback), 2008 (hardcover), 2009 (hardcover).
Revised edition 2011. Revised edition 2013

National Library of Australia Cataloguing-in-Publication data:

Author: Laliberte, Richard, author.
Title: Taking charge of diabetes : a practical guide to managing your health and wellbeing / Richard Laliberte.
Edition: Revised edition.
ISBN: 978-1-922085-08-5 (paperback)
Notes: Includes index.
Subjects: Diabetes–Popular works.
Other Authors/Contributors: Reader's Digest (Australia), issuing body.
Dewey Number: 616.462

Prepress by Colourpedia, Sydney
Printed and bound in China by Leo Paper Products

We are interested in receiving your comments on the content of this book. Write to:
The Editor, General Books Editorial, Reader's Digest (Australia) Pty Limited, GPO Box 4353, Sydney, NSW 2001 or email us at bookeditors.au@readersdigest.com

To order additional copies of *Taking Charge of Diabetes* call 1300 300 030 (Australia)
or 0800 400 060 (New Zealand)
or email us at customerservice@au.readersdigest.com

NOTE TO READERS
The information in this book should not be substituted for, or used to alter, medical therapy without your doctor's advice. For a specific health problem, consult your doctor for guidance.

Book code 041-5255
Concept code US 4359 H